DAVID VINE, D.D.S.

(DOCTOR OF DENTAL SURGERY)

UNDERSTANDING

FIRST CLASS

DENTAL CARE

— A HUMAN INTEREST STORY —

Understanding First Class Dental Care — A Human Interest Story

All restorative, endodontic and surgical procedures within this book, with the exception of implant surgery, were performed by the author.

Publisher: David Vine, DDS

Sheridan Center

400 Arthur Godfrey Road

Suite 403

Miami Beach, Florida 33140

Ph. 305-538-1115

Fax 305-538-1129

email dvine@davidvinedentist.com

ISBN 0-9703471-0-3

Library of Congress Control Number LCCN-00-092856

First Edition 9 8 7 6 5 4 3 2 1

Printed in the United States of America.

Limits of Liability & Disclaimer of Warranty

Trademarks

This book is dedicated to **Michele Beth Applebaum** — for her help, her patience and understanding, and for her significant contribution as an elementary school counselor to the welfare of the children.

I thank the following dentists for allowing me to observe their procedures and taking time to answer my many questions. They are in no way responsible for any inaccuracies that may exist in this book.

Dr. Fredric J. Witkin, *Periodontics, Miami, Florida.*

Dr. Marvin M. Rosenberg, *Periodontics, West Palm Beach/Boca Raton, Florida. Co-Director, Post Graduate Periodontics Nova Southeastern College of Dental Medicine, Ft. Lauderdale, Florida. Co-author of "Periodontal and Prosthetic Management for Advanced Cases".*

Dr. Bernard W. Segall, *Maxillofacial Prosthodontics, Coconut Grove, Florida.*

Dr. Issaac Garazi, *Periodontics, North Miami Beach, Florida.*

Dr. Jack Mishkin, *Periodontics, Miami Beach, Florida.*

Dr. Jon L. Rauch, *Endodontics, Naples, Florida. Associate Clinical Professor, Nova Southeastern College of Dental Medicine, Ft. Lauderdale, Florida.*

Dr. Steven N. Green, *General Dentistry, Miami, Florida. President of the Holistic Dental Association, and author of "Eclectic Dentistry — Demystifying Medicine".*

Dr. Aquiles Mas, *General Dentistry, Miami, Florida. Co-director, Endodontics, Dade County Dental Research Clinic, Miami, Florida*

Also thanks to:

The Educational Staff at the Dade County Dental Research Clinic.
Dr. Frank J. Slavichak, *Director.*
Glenda Algaze, *CDA (Certified Dental Assistant), Instructor.*
Debra Morales, *R.D.H. (Registered Dental Hygienist), CDA, Instructor.*
Angel Diaz, *Dental Technician Instructor.*
Hilda Leyva, *CDA, Instructor.*
Emy Delgado, Wanda Morales, Maria Cox, Marcelina Shur, Lucy Peñate, Alex Solis.

To all my teachers throughout the educational system, I say <u>thank you</u>.
To all my patients — Thank you for your confidence.

Dr. Jerome Krivanick, in memory, University of South Florida, Tampa, Florida
The dental office of Dr. Robert Hill, Dorchester, Massachusetts, 1970–1973
    Joanne Boyle, dental assistant
    Judy Sherman, dental hygienist
    Robert Law, dental technician
    Wherever you are, thank you for helping me with my first real world dental experience.

Frederic G. Kirsch, D.D.S. Pediatric Dentistry, Coral Springs, Fla. *Thank you Rick for loaning me your car in college, for your sense of humor and your valuable contribution to this book.*

Dr. Donald N. Applebaum, Internal Medicine and Cardiology, Miami Beach, Fla.

Dr. Clark C. Mitchell, Ear, Nose & Throat Surgery, General Medicine & General Dentistry, Miami Beach, Fla.

Dr. Jimie A. Vance, General Dentistry, Melbourne, Fla.

Dr. Jeffrey D. Blum, Oral and Maxillofacial Surgery, Miami Beach, Florida

Dr. Jay J. Kopfe, Endodontics, Miami Beach, Florida

Dr. Lili Estrin, Internal Medicine and Geriatrics, Miami Beach, Florida

Dr. Howard Estrin, Gastroenterology, Miami Beach, Florida

Dental Depot, Inc. Jim and Peggy Ainslie. Joe Carlucci, Doug Gomez. *The best team for building and maintaining a dental office.*

Dr. Ramsey Saffouri

Mr. Sam Konell

Ms. Rita Paul

Dr. Kathryn Ann Bufkin. University of Miami, Coral Gables, Florida. *Thank you for your help in editing the manuscript.*

Dr. Edwin Flatto, Physician and Author, Miami, Fla.

Debra Brautman, R.D.H. (Registered Dental Hygienist)

Margaret Stringer, R.D.H.

Dr. Fred Kaytes, General Dentistry, Miami, Fla.

Dr. Barry Scholl, General Dentistry, Miami, Fla.

Dr. Stephen Chase, Periodontics, Miami, Fla.

Dr. Steven Kirsner, Rockledge, Fla. (honky-tonk music/general dentistry/real estate)

Howell A. Goldberg, D.D.S., F.A.G.D. (Fellow, Academy of General Dentistry), Plantation, Fla. — *The frat brother from Long Island.*

Stuart R. Mishkin, Esq., Miami, Fla. — *My Bar Mitzvah partner, fraternity brother and friend.*

Dr. Robert J. Cohen, Aventura, Fla. *(We prevailed under duress. Thank you, Bob)*

Dr. Paul Fletcher, Periodontics, New York City. *Thank you, Paul — The Baltimore Dental School years were quite an adventure.*

Dr. Richard Mautner, Endodontics Miami, Beach, Fla.

Dr. Steven Oppenheimer, Endodontics, Miami Beach, Fla.

Dr. Bernard E. Keough, Co-author of "Periodontal and Prosthetic Management for Advanced Cases". Private practice in Prosthodontics, West Palm Beach, Fla.

Dr. Melvin Kessler. Chairman, Orthodontics for General Practice, Dade County Dental Research Clinic.

Dr. Seymour Oliet, Dean, Nova Southeastern University, College of Dental Medicine.

Ann Page, Assistant to the Dean, Nova Southeastern University, College of Dental Medicine.

Dr. Robert Apfel, General Dentistry, Miami Beach, Fla.

Spectrum Dental Laboratory, Miami, Fla. Robert Goldberg, C.D.T. (Certified Dental Technician), Owner.

Angel Diaz, D.T. (Dental Technician), Yasmin Pietryak, Olga Moncaleano, Tatiana Saldarriaga, D.T., Pedro Astete Lara, D.T., Maria Fernanda Rojas, D.T., Jose Bravo, D.T.

Thank you Rob for your help in allowing me to provide First Class Dental Care.

Alberto and Josefa Valdez, Dental Lab., Miami, Fla.

Mejido Dental Lab., Miami, Fla. Rafael Mejido, President.

Uni-tech Dental Crafts, Margate, Fla., Allan Christian, D.T.

Miami Dental Arts, Dale Cornelison, C.D.T., President.

Glidewell Laboratories, Newport Beach, California.

Kimberly Katari, Esq. Boca Raton, Fla. — *For her superior legal talent.*
June and Danny Vargas (And David).
The Production Team, Sunrise, Fla. Stu Goldstein and Bob Peanka.
Marlin Fields, AT&T Media Services.
Charter Communications, Miami Beach, Fla.
Mr. Keith Richter — *For your friendship.*

Fred Gelfand, C.D.T. (Certified Laboratory Technician) — *Thank you Fred for your positive disposition during the early years (mid 1970's) in our downtown Miami walk up antique dental office.*

Dr. Richard Stein (and Janice), Wayne, New Jersey and Dr. Joseph Shapiro (co-author of the book "Out of Sight — Into Vision", New York City. *They left teaching positions in New York City and moved to Boston, Massachusetts to obtain optometry degrees in the early 1970's. Thank you Richie and Joseph for sharing life, "interesting" times and growing pains.*

Janet Osseroff — T. K. Productions Publicity Dept. (late 70's — early 80's). *Thank you, Janet.*
Jay Luber (wherever you are). *You heated up Baltimore and shared your enthusiasm for life. 1970 — 1972 Thanks, Jay.*
Mary Ellen Verdon and Glen & Linda Shuman — *Thank you for taking me in during the wild Coconut Grove years.*
Diane Breteau, publisher/editor Day & Night Publications Inc., Coconut Grove, Florida (early 1980's) — *Thank you Diane for publishing my music reviews and for treating me so kindly.*
Alan Maisel, Esq.
Aberbach's Photo, Miami Beach, Florida — Joel and Beverly Aberbach.
Arnie and Richie's Delicatessen, Miami Beach, Fla. *Arnie and Richie London, Wilbert Whilby, Thank you for delivering my delicious breakfasts.*
Irene Williams, Secretarial Services, Miami Beach, Fla. *Thank you Irene for your level headed advice and service.*
The Sheridan Center - Michael Diaz, Gilbert Carreno.
Natural Sound Recording Studio, Miami, Fla. Thomas and Linda Gamino, Scott Taylor. *Our time will come.*
Joseph's Hair Styling, Miami Beach, Fla. Joseph Laplaca
Stage Barber Shop, Miami Beach, Fla. — David Roberti.
Myrna Mogell — *Thank you Myrna, for your enthusiasm and your good humor.*
Louis Munez, Social worker, Dept. of Youth and Family Development, Metro Dade County, Fla.
Daye W. Sommers — *Thank you Daye, for helping me when I really needed help.*

State of Florida, Office of the Attorney General.
Victim Compensation Program, Tallahassee, Fla.
Thank you for allowing me to help injured crime victims.
    Jacquelyn Dupree, Bureau chief.
    Gwen Roache, operations and management consultant II
    and the following analysts: Bob Haas, Michele Mabry, Troy Nelson, Joe Miller, Frank Miller, Teresa McCloud, Ed Fangman, Angie Buchanan, Angela Jackson, Sharon Huttenstine, Susan Parmalee, David Sawh, Joanne Amos, Fay Basiri, Jennifer Walker, Susan Wheeler.

To the South Florida Hotel Guest Services — *I thank you.*
    Arsenio Jorge, Eduardo Roselli, John Lenis, Daphnee Abraham, Miguel Pena, Gregory Edge, Carlos Mejia, Miguel Peralta, Bernardo Gutierrez, Mary Jane Parry, John Nilbrink, Raquel Alvero, Stuart Hawkins, Gloria Kennedy, Natalia Paz, Andrew Wallin, Efrain Colindres, Angela Smith, Paula Arboleda, Gustavo Ortiz, Kleiber Topiol, Fred Ritter, Daniel Faillace, Jose Castellanos, Patricio Rosas, Mauricio Botero, Ariel Fonte, Eddie Brittingham, Sally Mitrani, Brian Hightower, Richard Rosen, Eduardo Rodriguez, Rick Garcia, Amparo Valbuena.

Midtown Pharmacy, Miami Beach, Fla. Jose Abut, Owner; Henry Abut, Pharmacy Technician; Wendi Thompson, Manager, Jose L. Pineda; Aida Mejia.

Tower 41 Condominium Residence — *Thank you for making this is a nice place to live.*
Mark Martel, General Manager; Oscar Martell, Chief Engineer; Samson Saintilmond, Sol Goldstein, George Armella, Jody Aguilar, Lazaro Navarrete, Sergio Diaz, Luis Hernandez.

Liliana Gonzalez Giraldo — *Thank you for keeping my dental office so clean. Gracias por mantener tan limpio mi consultorio.*

Special thanks to:

Nancy Morgan, President of Coral Gables Secretarial Service, Coral Gables, Florida, for her encouragement, wit and professionalism.
Marcia Brod, Amanda Barba, Vickie Sfalanga, Ellen Roden, Maria Ingelmo.

PrePress Consolidated Color, Inc., Miami, Florida. Leonardo M. Borsten, President, Gloria, Bernie and Dolly. *I thank you Leonardo for your talent, extreme patience and dedication to quality.*

Hallmark Press, Inc., Miami, Florida. Robin Hood — *Thank you for your professional handling of this project.*

Thank you, Ricky Di Pietro for your help with the original manuscript.

Nerida Di Pietro - Dental Assistant, office manager. *I thank you Nerida for your dedication, your intelligence and your hard work. To your Loyal and talented husband, Gino — Thanks.*

To my sister Jodie and her husband Jerry Levien — *Thank you.*

To Mom and Dad — *Thank you for your endless support, encouragement and love.*

C O N T E N T S

x — David Vine, D.D.S.

INTRODUCTION

I want to **earn** more money, which is why I'm writing this book.[1] However, I believe in a fair deal. My years of study and the labor expended in producing this book will provide you with information that could save your teeth, your money and your time.

So, why me—what is my background, my experience—what makes me qualified to write this book? And is there a need for a book like this? I believe there is and will show you why.

But let's start with my history, the background that led me to this point in life. I always like to know a little bit about an author besides his professional degrees.

Do you read the obituaries? I do, especially those in the New York Times. But it seems that whenever they describe someone's life, they always start off at the college and professional level—the beauty of childhood is passed by—how they played with friends, spent their summer vacations, who their best friends were—the important details that make up a total life!

I'm not going to tell you about bicycle trips with my best friend, Jay Plotkin, when I was 10 years old, or my summers at Camp Osceola in Horse Shoe, North Carolina, where I started as a camper in 1960, graduated to the position of C.I.T (counselor in training), then became a J.C. (junior counselor), and finally (!), a counselor.

Born April 26, 1947 in Brooklyn, New York, I moved with our family to Fairlawn, New Jersey, where I lived my early childhood years. My uncle owned a first-class nightclub on the cliffs of the Hudson River adjacent to the George Washington Bridge (Bill Miller's Riviera). With its retractable roof and window-lined circular design, it offered a most spectacular view of the Manhattan skyline. That, along with the top acts of the time, made it the premiere showcase attraction. My dad worked there for years until they tore it down to build a highway!

We moved to Miami Beach, Florida, in the mid-fifties. At that time, with vacant beachfront raw land, undeveloped suburbs and beautiful hotels and nightclubs, it was a great place to live.

But wait a second; this is a consumer's guide to dentistry—where do teeth enter the picture? Hold on, it's coming soon!

---

1. Three close friends advised me to eliminate this initial statement. After careful consideration, I decided that it is important to be honest regarding my motives—and honest regarding the entire content of this book.

When I attended Miami Beach Senior High School (1963-1965), choosing a lifetime career was not on my mind; playing music was. In junior high school, I had chosen tenor saxophone as my instrument when joining the school orchestra. I pursued music throughout my time at Beach High by joining the marching band, the orchestra, and the dance band. Besides that, I always performed and earned some money with small bands that I put together.

On the academic side, the usual high school curriculum didn't interest me too much. As a matter of fact, when a school counselor called my mom during my junior year to inform her of my poor performance and the good chance that I would not be accepted to a college, it was somewhat humiliating.

So I was forced to re-evaluate my position and make adjustments. Through diligent study and occasional help from a tutor, I reversed my academic ranking and ended my junior year with grades of A and a position on the coveted honor roll. I graduated in 1965 and headed for St. Petersburg, Florida, for my freshman year at the University of South Florida, Bay Campus (the main campus was in Tampa). I hadn't lost my love for music, but at this time I decided that a career in music was not necessarily where I wanted to go.

As a college freshman, I had to take the required basic courses if I wanted to earn a college degree. I also needed to choose a career and a corresponding curriculum, so I selected dentistry[2] and immediately began taking pre-dental courses, which included chemistry, zoology, physics, and a number of other science courses. It was tough going. Not only were these courses difficult, but in order to gain acceptance to a good dental school, it was necessary to achieve grades of A and B—anything below that level was not going to help.

One of my most challenging courses was advanced biology, taught by the infamous Dr. Jerome Krivanick. He was a feared instructor who occasionally passed around a microphone during his auditorium-filled lectures. If you were unprepared, your display of ignorance would be showcased. Anyway, when entering the auditorium on such a day, students would see the microphone and literally run from the auditorium as Dr. Krivanick vainly attempted to halt their retreat.

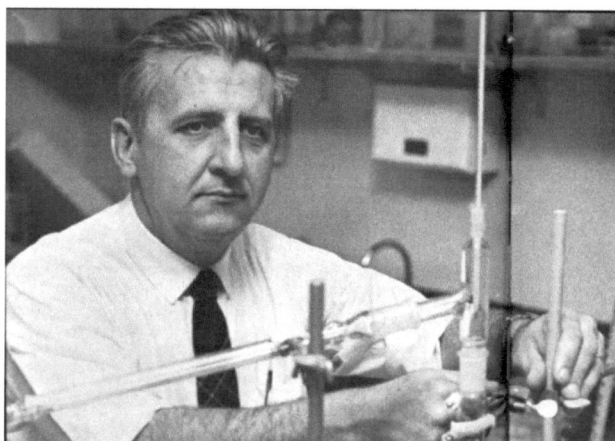

Dr. Jerome Krivanek — My most respected and influential college professor.

I excelled in Dr. Krivanick's class—rose to the challenge, got a grade of A, and earned his respect. But the thing that provoked my curiosity about the basic science of biology was the clinical relevancy he presented. Here we were learning about complex biochemical processes, the way human cells—the basic biological unit of the body—functioned. How this related to teeth I wasn't sure at the time, but these pre-dental/medical courses were stepping-stones to understanding more complex aspects of the human body. I was accumulating the tools necessary to help understand the puzzle of life!

Following a somewhat successful completion of my pre-dental curriculum (I had a tough time with physics due to difficulty in understanding mathematics, particularly calculus), I gained early acceptance to the Baltimore College of Dental Surgery, University of Maryland, on a scholarship program.[3]

2. My dental hygienist, questioned me about why I chose dentistry as a profession. Though I probably spent a lot of time subconsciously thinking about it, I guess an explanation about such a life altering choice is appropriate. Actually, this decision may have been a mistake. Recently, I read an autobiography about a man who questioned whether or not his whole life had been a mistake. Well, in life you may select a ***mountain*** to climb. If you question your selection as you climb, your doubts may interfere with your ability to navigate the difficult ascent. Dentistry has been a hell of a mountain for me. I thought it would provide a future that would allow me to pursue music under a more independent game plan.

3. Early acceptance means that due to taking extra courses during the summers (Miami-Dade Community College and the University of Miami) and attaining a good grade point average, I was able to skip my senior year of college.

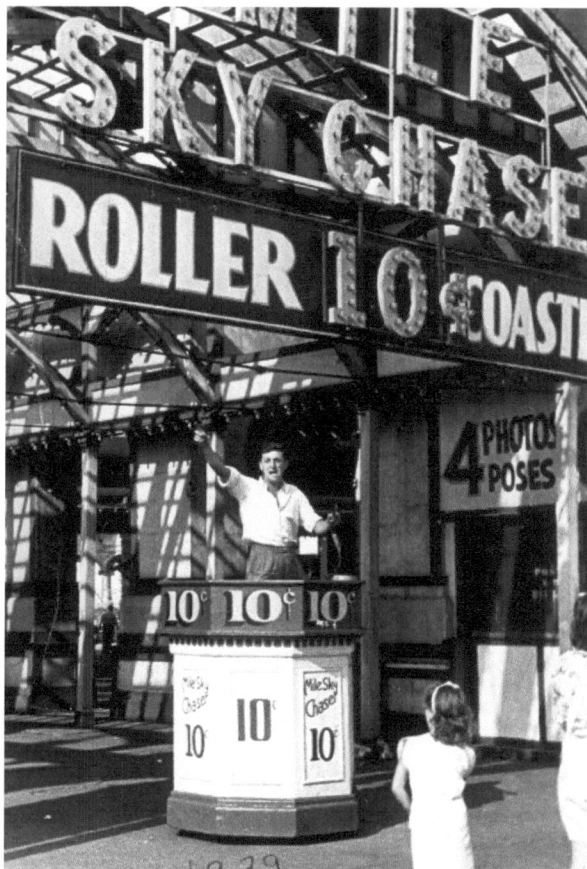

Dad at Luna Park, 1939 (Coney Island, N.Y.) where he met mom.

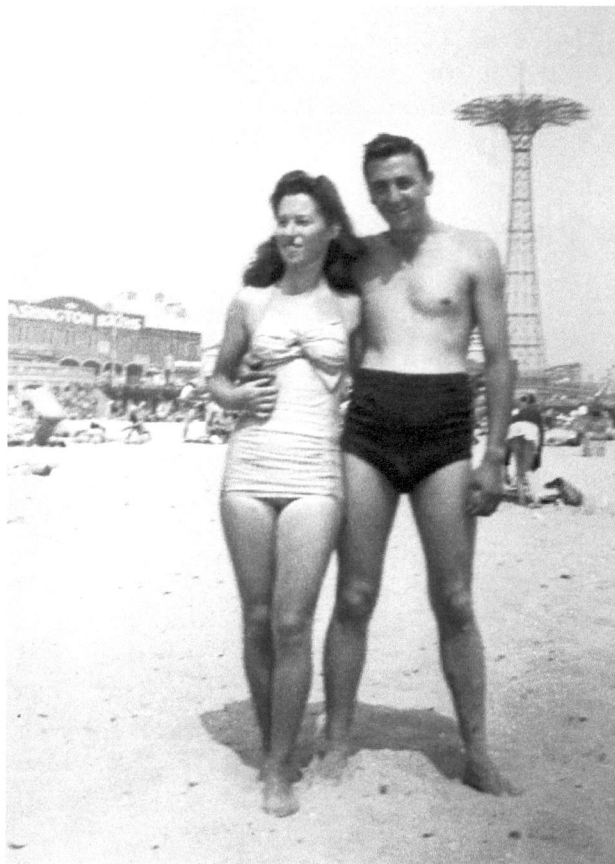

Mom and Dad, Coney Island, Parachute Jump. (1939)

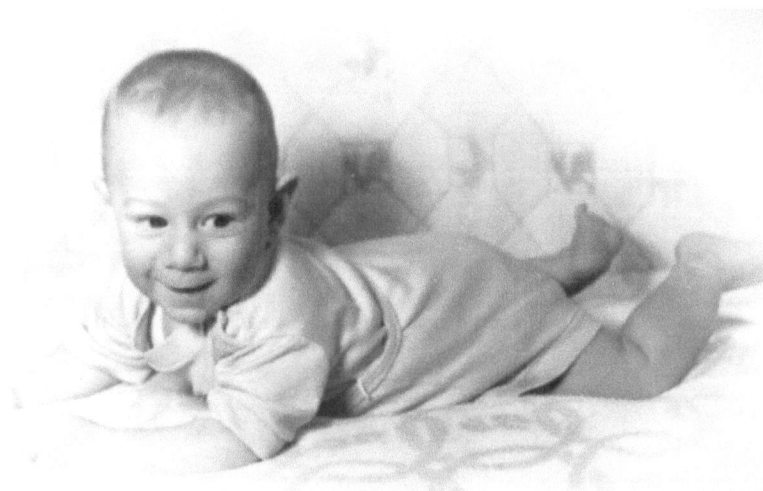

Me, 1947 – My most relaxing and enjoyable year

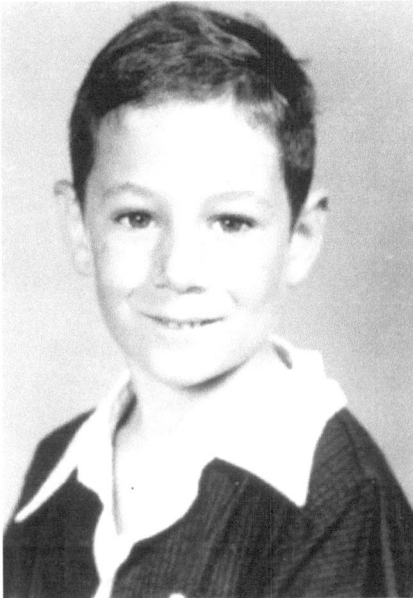

A young me – 1952

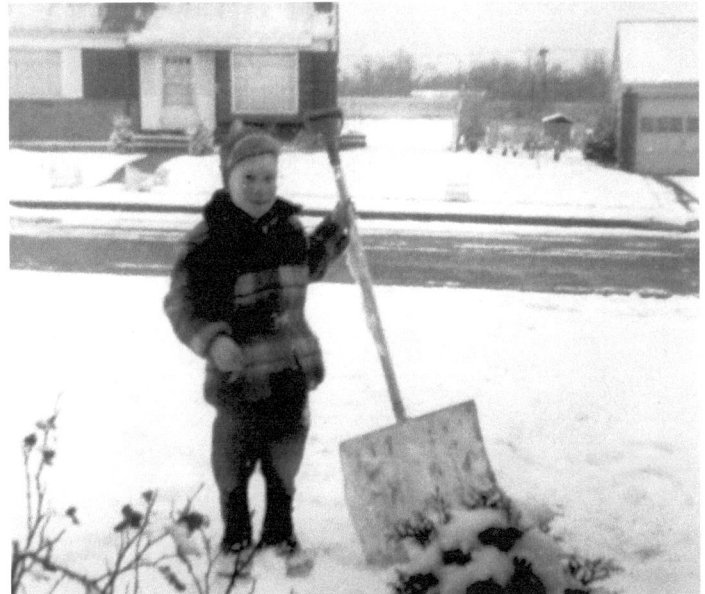

Having fun in Fairlawn, New Jersey winter. (early 1950's)

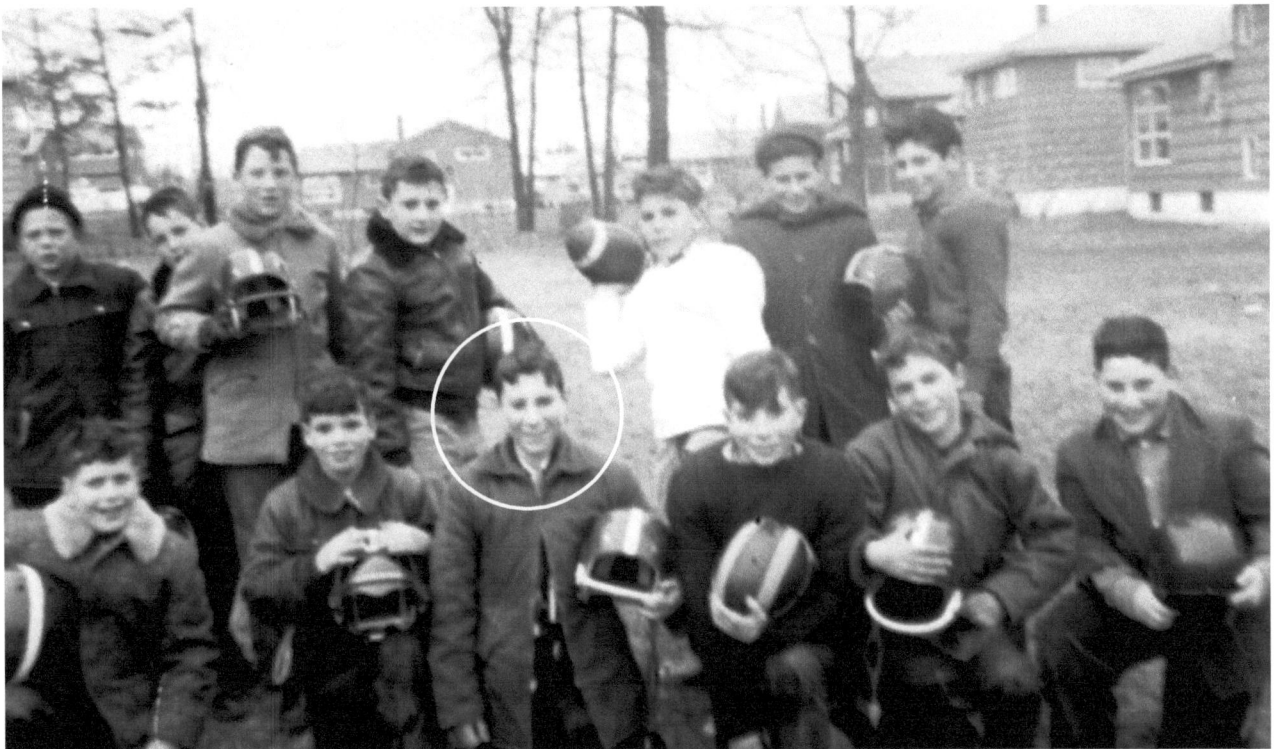

My limited football career with New Jersey friends

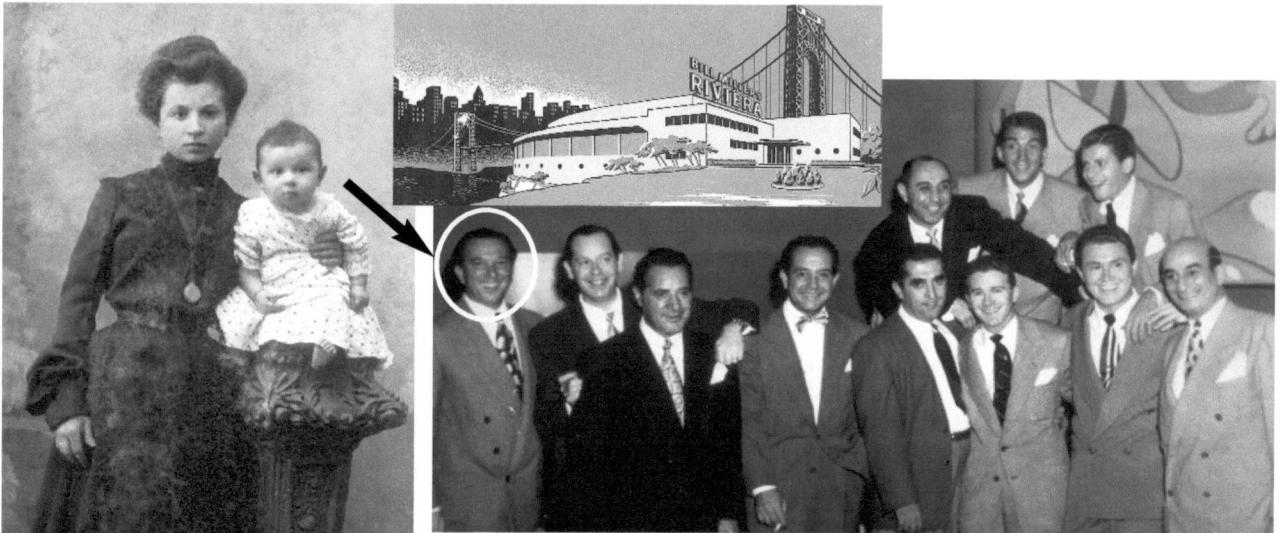

My uncle Bill Miller – far left. Milton Berle on his right. Myron Cohen – far right. Dean Martin and Jerry Lewis – top right, and entertainers at Bill Miller's Riviera, New Jersey nightclub – 1950's.

My grandmother with my uncle Bill Miller before he became a great vaudeville act and night club / hotel impresario, 1906.

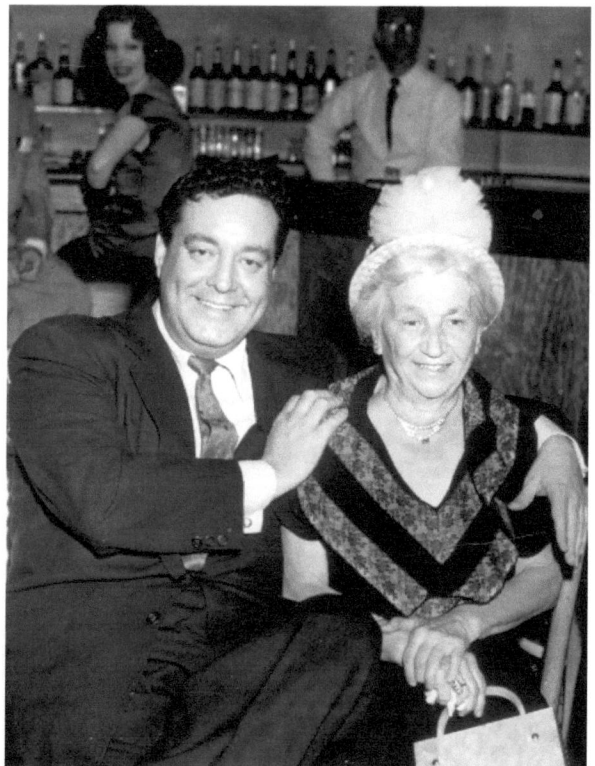

Lena Horne between Mom and Dad

Jackie Gleason and my grandmother at one of my uncle Bill Miller's night clubs. Upper left photo shows my grandmother in her youth.

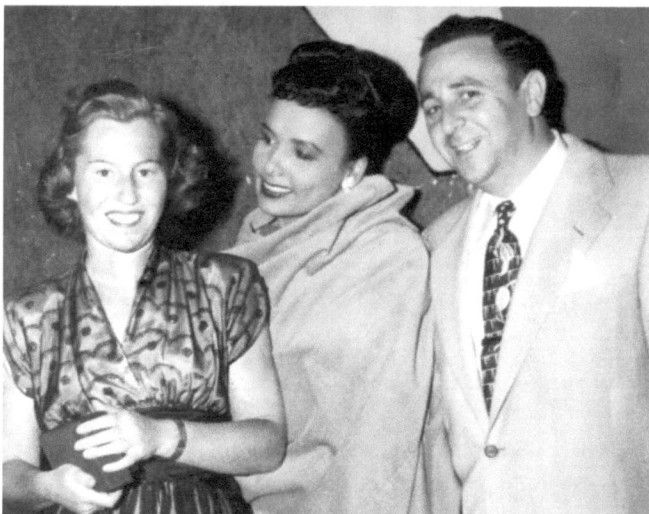

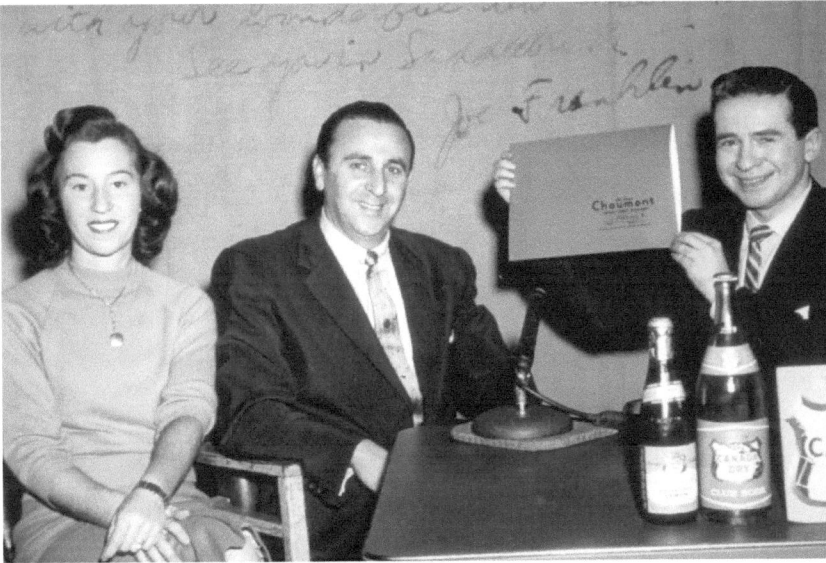

Mom and Dad promoting Dad's Chaumont Restaurant on Joe Franklin's classic television show. (early 1950's)

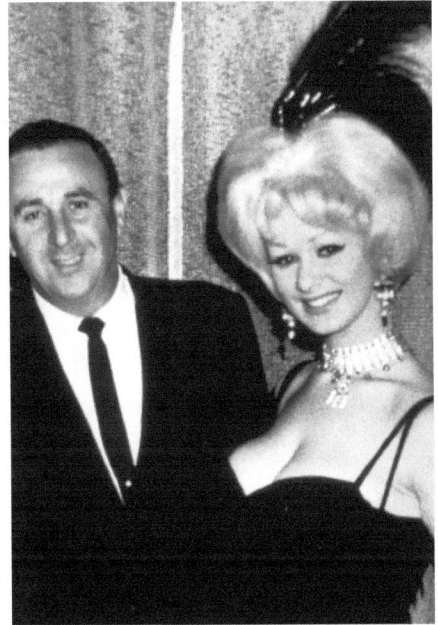

Mom and Dad – just kidding! – Dad with show girl from Le Crazy Horse Revue, at uncle Bill's Riverside Hotel, Reno, Nevada (1960)

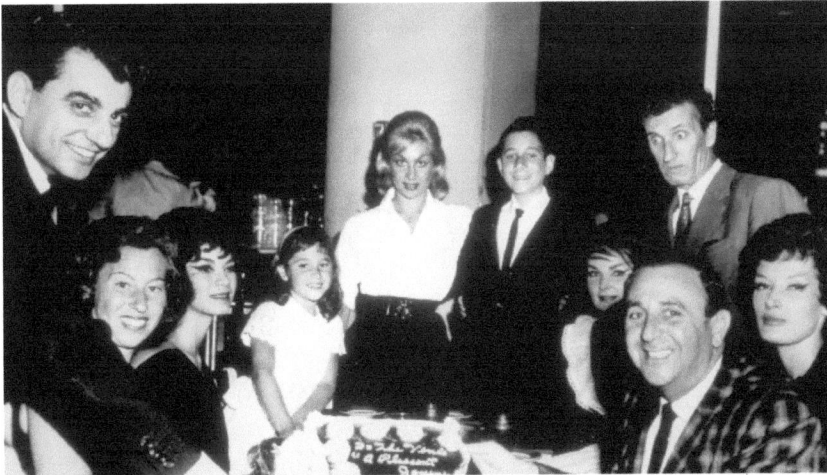

Me, standing in rear next to my favorite show girl – Diane, along with Mom and Dad, my sister Jodie and entertainers from Le Crazy Horse Revue. My great summer of 1960.

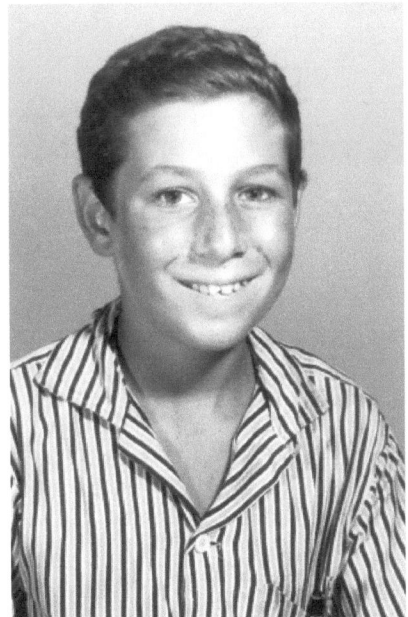

Me at Junior High age

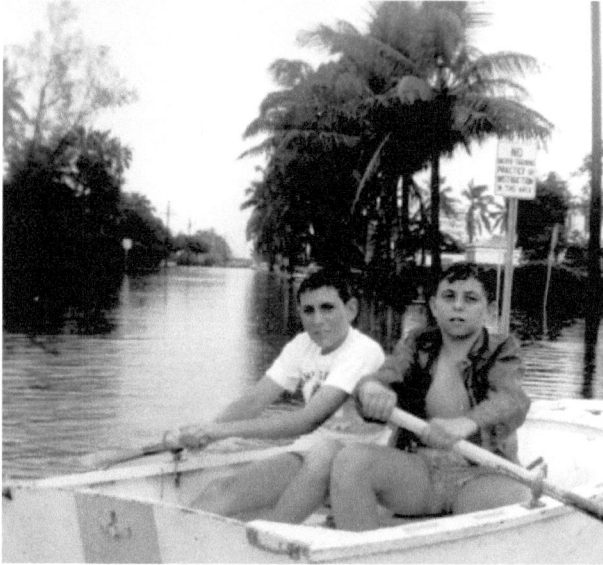

With my friend Jay Plotkin after a hurricane flooded our Miami Beach neighborhood.

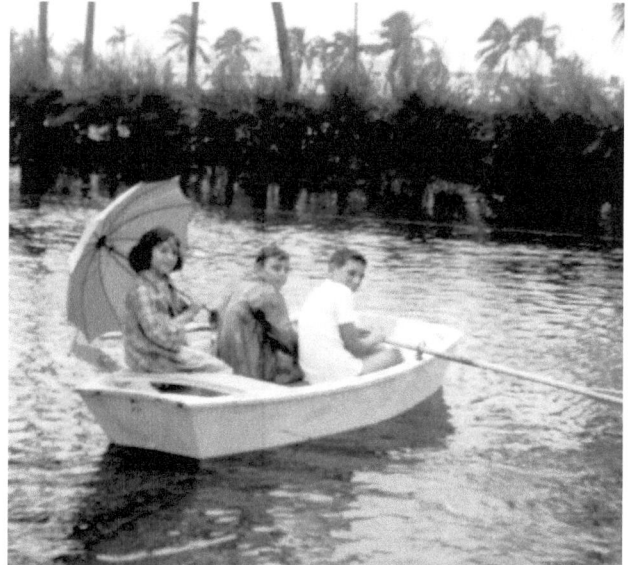

My sister Jodie joined us and The Miami Herald published this photo. (This is not a lake — it's our street!)

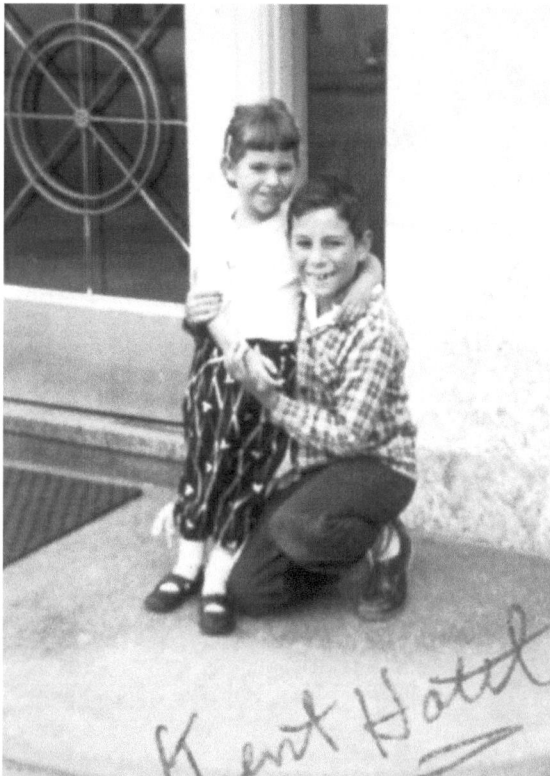

My sister Jodie and me in front of my dad's Kent Hotel, Miami Beach, 1955

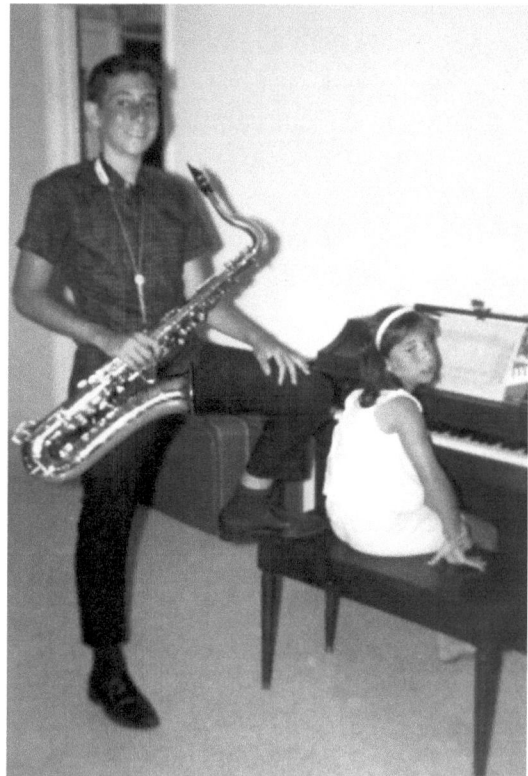

Hopeful sax superstar with my sister Jodie.

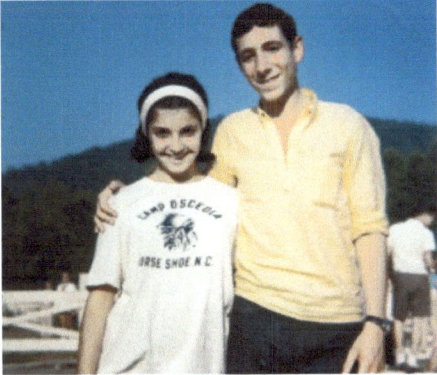

*With friend Joanne at Camp Osceola early
1960's. Horse Shoe, North Carolina.*

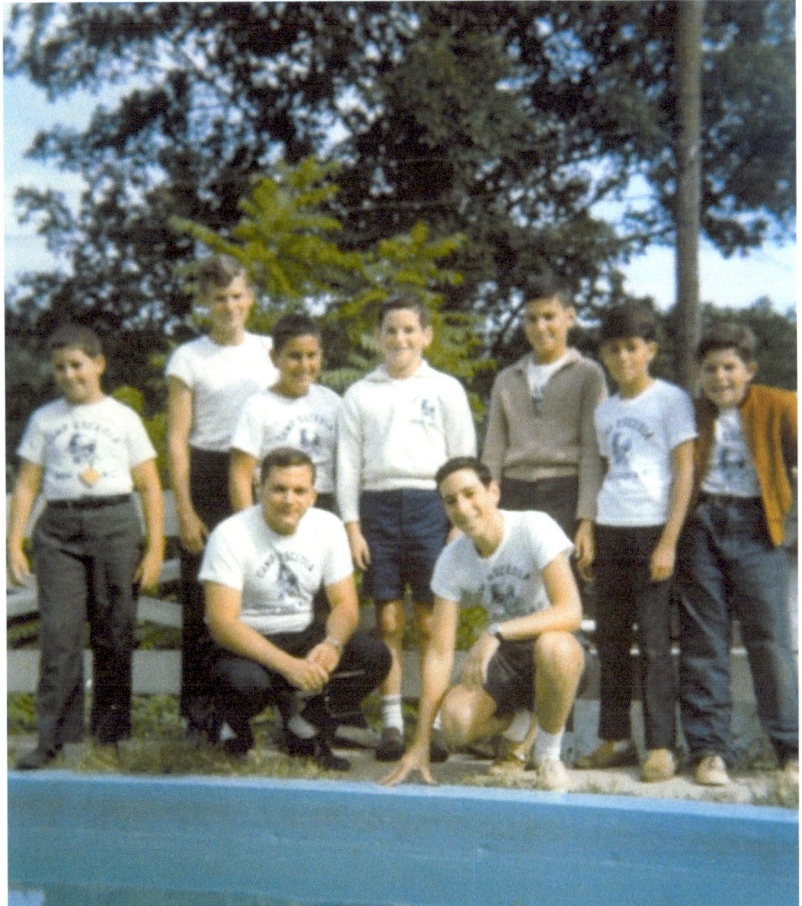

*Dennis Silver (kneeling left) Counselor, and me (to his right), Junior Counselor and
our campers.*

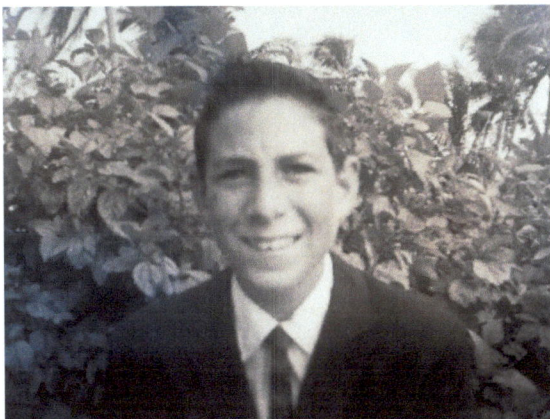

Me at age 13.

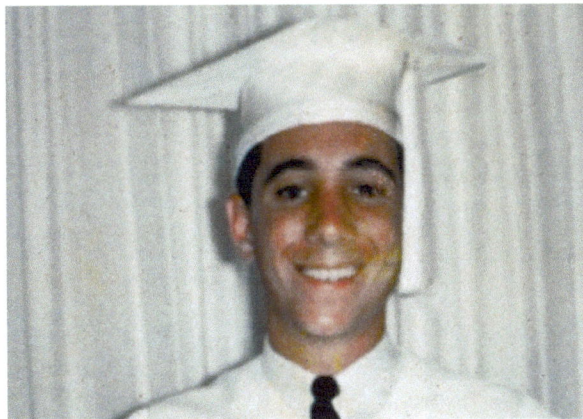

Miami Beach High School graduation, 1965.

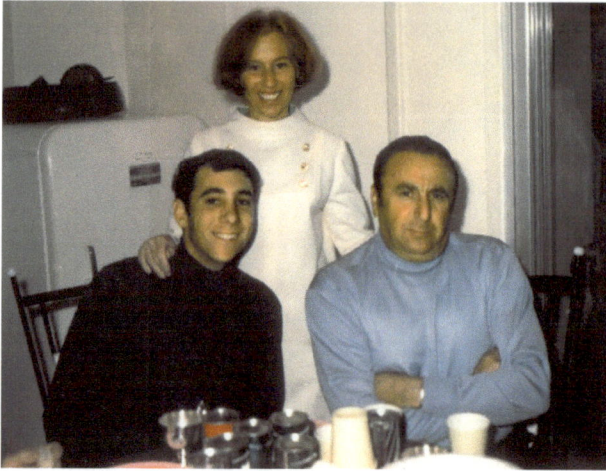

Mom, Dad and me – Late 1960's.

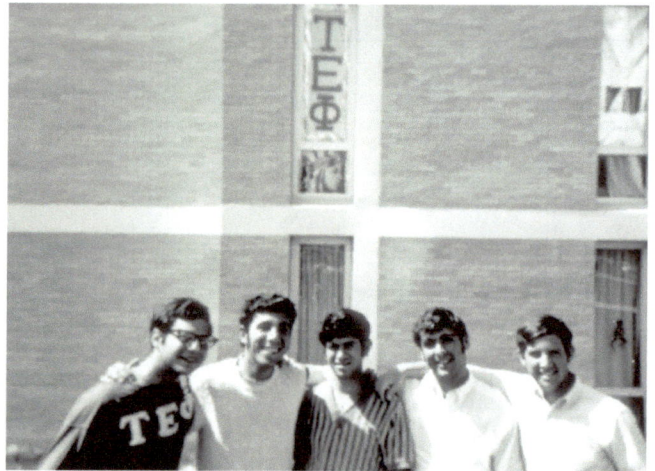

Friends/Fraternity Brothers – Tau Epsilon Phi, 1967. Some of my happiest times – We played hard yet maintained the highest academic level.

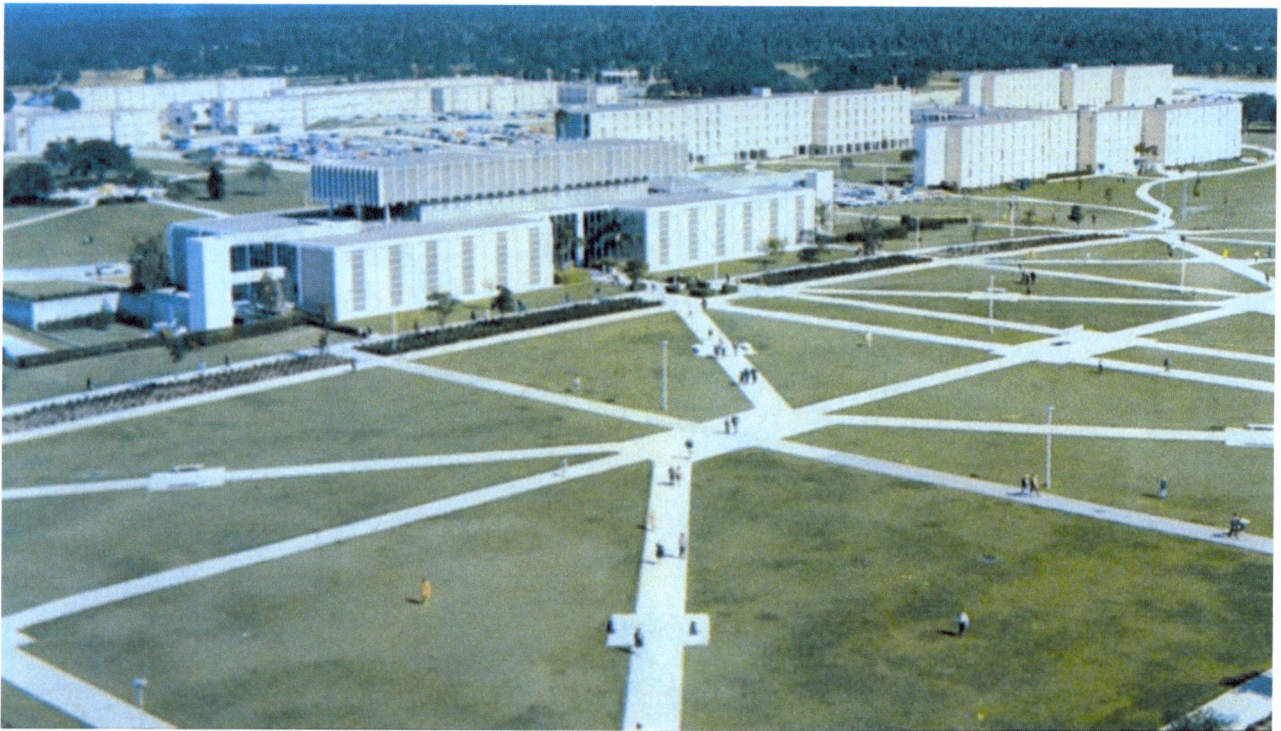

Main campus, University of South Florida, Tampa, 1966

THE DENTAL SCHOOL EXPERIENCE

The Baltimore College of Dental Surgery was the first dental school in the world. A grand and respected institution, it would be my home for the next four years. So in 1969 I drove north with my new found friend and fellow dental student, Barry Katzen, rented an old walk-up apartment in downtown Baltimore, and proceeded to learn how to be a dentist.

The Curriculum

The dental school curriculum was similar to the medical school curriculum—except the medical student's books were thicker! The first two years encompassed a complete study of the human body—its anatomy, physiology (how it functions) and pathology (how it deals with disease). The basic dental science courses involved developing a thorough familiarity with teeth and the oral cavity. We were taught how to "drill" cavity preparations, place "fillings," and become expert sculptural artists. We would spend hours carving wax into exact replicas of a tooth and then, as in the creation of fine jewelry, melt gold and cast this pattern into an artificial crown.

The third and fourth years continued with science courses, but students were taught dental procedures in clinics. Learning precise skills necessary to perform intricate dental procedures was the ultimate challenge.[4] Many students, who up to this point were capable of memorizing books and excelling in written tests, found this area of study quite stressful. To make things worse, many clinic instructors were extremely authoritarian and unsympathetic. If you didn't have "the hands," you were booted out of school. One friend, who succeeded beautifully in academics, was forced to repeat laboratory work during the summer in an old un-airconditioned basement classroom. Following this arduous and humiliating ordeal, he was subsequently thrown out of school (he went on to successfully complete medical school).

I managed to complete my courses and clinical requirements to the satisfaction of the faculty, and in 1972, graduated with a degree of Doctor of Dental Surgery — D.D.S. (Some schools award the D.M.D degree. The only difference between the two degrees is that the D.M.D. derives from Latin which stresses the medical basis for a dental specialty).

---

4. Challenge is not the term we young adults used at that time—more like nerve-racking, impossible and scary. Learning to use a high speed drill on an upper back tooth while looking through a small dental mirror is quite a feat. Add a little water spray (necessary so you don't overheat the tooth), and it is like driving in a rainstorm without windshield wipers! And remember, the mirror reverses your movements!

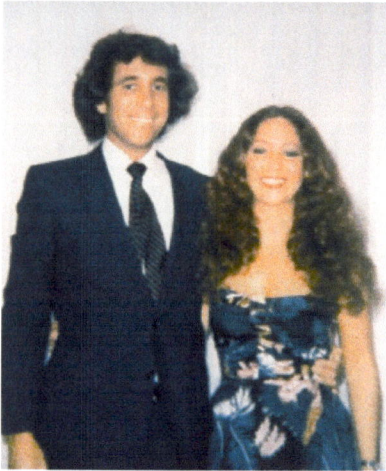

Me and my sister – Getting confused about life? (1970)

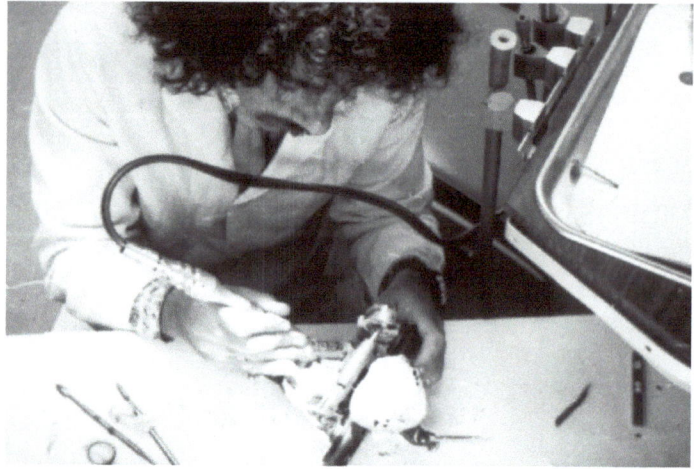

Me, learning to be a dentist. (1970)

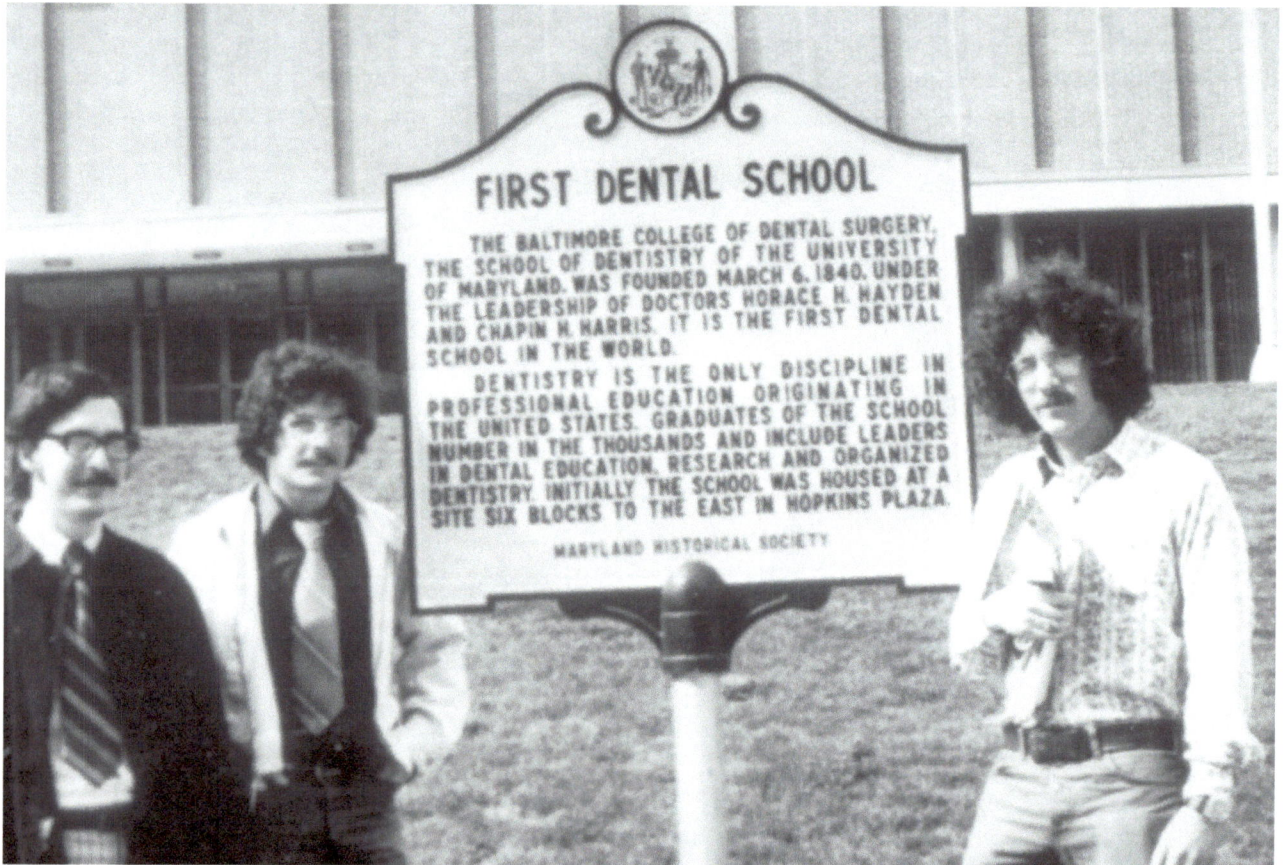

Brothers Steven and Mel Weinberg and me (on right). Today, we all have dental practices in South Florida.

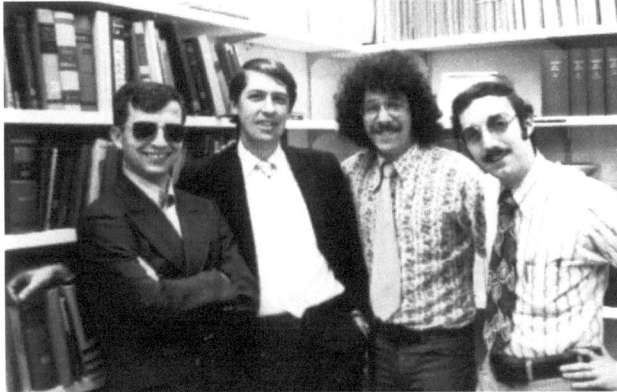

The Pathology department. The few professors that did not ridicule me about having long hair and wearing bell bottom pants. (1972)

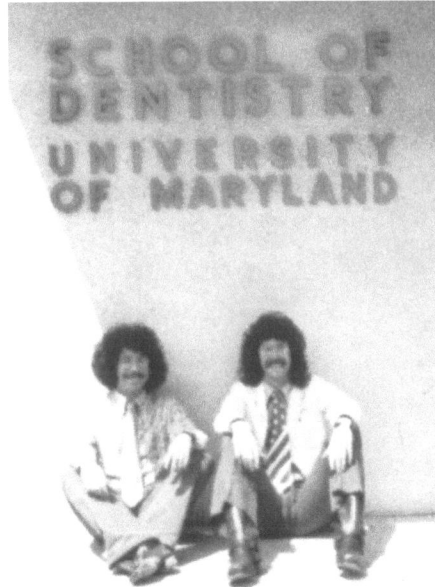

My roommate and friend Barry Katzen, on right. Barry now practices orthodontics in Ashland, Ore. (1972)

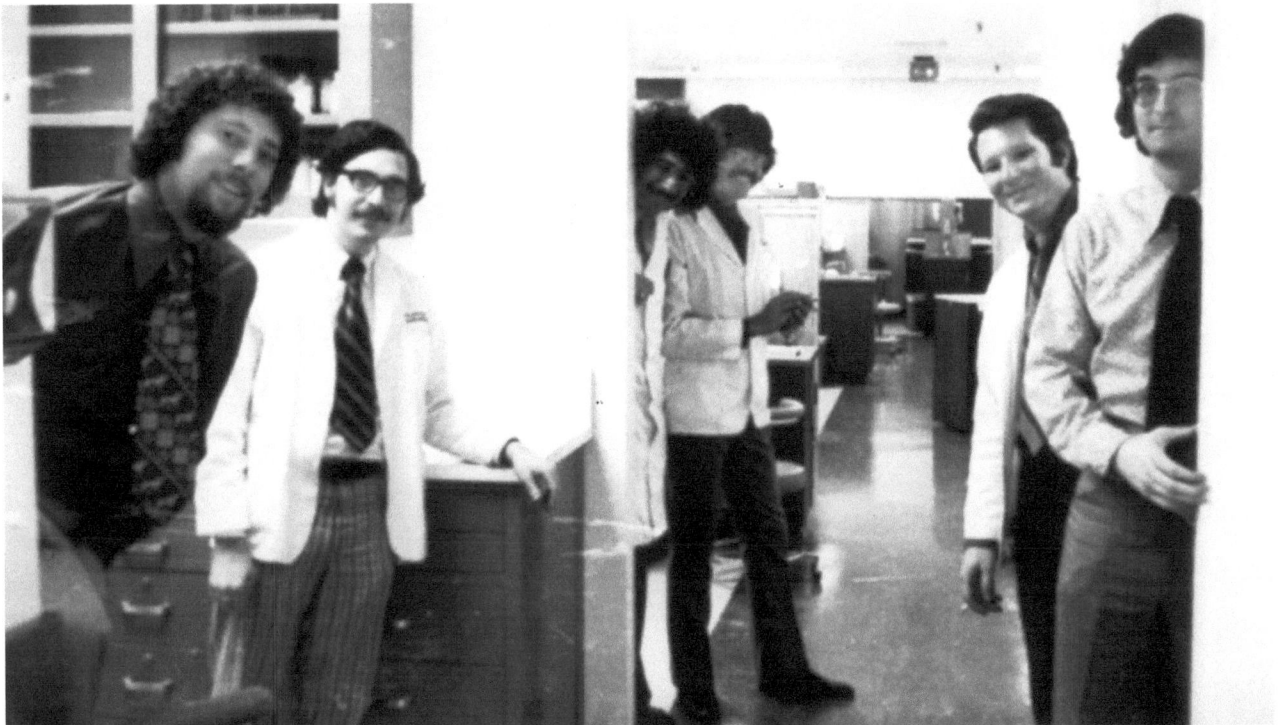

Fellow dental students in the clinic.

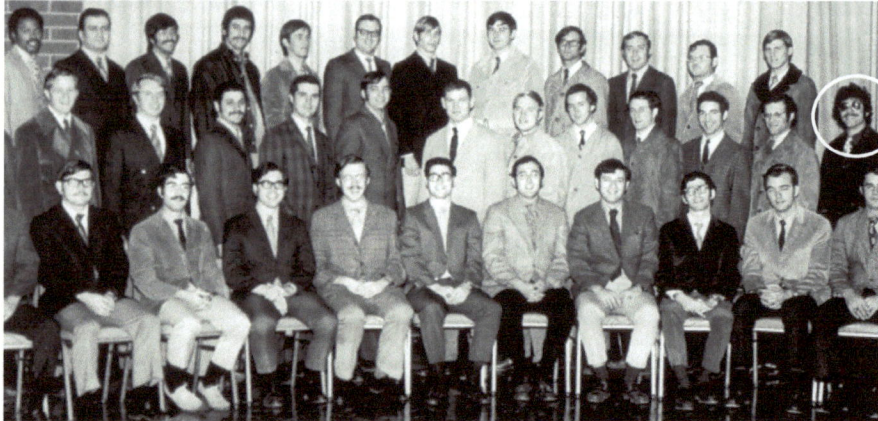

One half of our class (the second alphabetical section), early 1970's.

THAT YOU MAY KNOW US BETTER:

Four years ago, as lowly, short haired freshmen, we were the next to last class to enter the time worn halls of the Dental School on Lombard and Greene Streets. Now with our hair longer and at an average age of 25.5 years, we emerge as the second class to graduate from Hayden Harris Hall and the first class to be graduating with a class of Dental Hygienists.

Approaching graduation, our lines will average an even six feet and a comfortable 172 pounds. While it is true that 39% of us have gained an average of 9 pounds over the past 4 years, that really is not too neglectful considering the 3 years of happy marriage and home cooked meals that 79% of us have enjoyed. Our single members may not have enjoyed as many cooked meals but they did find time for slightly more than 2 dates per week during their senior year.

Our financial situation varied widely but on average 40% of our education was paid for by our parents. Upon graduation we still will be in debt by about $4,000.00 and we still have a few more payments to make on our 1968 car. Most of the $4,000.00 that we owe has come from educational loans that 79% of us have received. Scholarships have also aided some 74% of our class with an average of $1,200.00.

To help meet the payments on cars (27% of which are foreign made and 40% are Fords and Chevrolets), apartments and our many other expenses, 75% of us have held part time jobs during the school year and earned an average of $3.45 per hour for ten hours per week. While most of us worked as hospital laboratory technicians or blood bank technicians, some of us worked as ushers, pool room attendants or bartenders.

In our few hours of free time we either go to our favorite spot in Baltimore (which seems to be bed) or occasionally watch our favorite sports programs on T.V.

Our educational training is substantially greater than that of our parents; only 41% of our fathers and only 20% of our mothers are college graduates.

While in dental school, 6% of us considered our training superior and 69% of us considered it adequate. We feel that the strong points of our education have been in Pathology, Pharmacology and Pedodontics, while Physiology, Fixed Prosthodontics, Operative Dentistry and the coordination of the basic sciences and clinic left something to be desired.

Knowing four years ago what we know now, 70% of us would have pursued the same course of study.

As we approach graduation our future plans are still somewhat unsettled; 33% of us desire training in a dental specialty and many of us are waiting to hear from the Armed Forces. As for private practice, 60% of us plan to enter into group practices while only 10% plan to enter into a solo practice; the other 30% are still undecided.

This is the class of 1972.

From the Dental School Year Book profiling the graduating Class of 1972.

THE REAL WORLD

Most of my colleagues felt their dental education was adequate but that they needed more hands-on experience. Upon graduation, some entered the military, some pursued a two or three year post-graduate specialty (periodontics—gums, endodontics—root canals, pedodontics—children's dentistry, and so on), some dropped out of dentistry completely, and some, like me, got a job as an associate in a dental office. I had remained single during my years in Baltimore and, at age 25, equipped with a dental degree, a pent-up reserve of energy, and a quest for adventure, headed north to Boston, Massachusetts.

I had heard great things about Boston and the beauty of the New England area. I believed this was a good place to improve my dental skills and finally start living life (for the first time not as a formal student, although the learning experience is truly never ending).

When I arrived in Boston that summer of '72, I rented a beautiful apartment in the area known as Back Bay. Old brownstone houses throughout the neighborhood had been subdivided over the years to accommodate more residents. They were beautiful structures with spacious interiors, high ceilings and cozy fireplaces. The Charles River was around the corner and the adjacent park was a haven for sun worshippers. So I settled in, secured a job in a suburban dental practice and began commuting by train to Dorchester, Massachusetts.

29 Years Later

I feel confident in my abilities as a well-rounded dentist, but it took a long time to reach this point. Over the past 29 years, my attempts to learn as much as possible about dentistry have given me the knowledge necessary to perform with a more positive disposition. I have worked for many different dentists in varied settings—high-end offices, clinics, and middle-of-the-road suburban practices. I've kept up with dental advances, read professional journals and books, and visited with specialists on a continuing basis.[5] So, does all this make me qualified to write a consumer dentistry book? I believe so, and I hope that with the information you receive, you will be able to make more intelligent decisions and ultimately save your teeth and your money.

The Basic Science

Science likes to deal with proven facts. The problem is that very often there are too many facts and too many variables — things become difficult to prove. For instance, why is it that two people

---

5. When my patients needed a dental specialist, I accompanied them so I could learn the procedures correctly (and ease their anxiety).

of the same age living in the same town and having pretty much the same lifestyle develop radically different dental conditions? One has no cavities; the other develops many. Is it difference in diet, genetic makeup, unique stress patterns, or what? Probably all of these variables.

But if you wanted to set up an experiment to see exactly what causes cavities and wanted your results to be valid, you would need to follow certain specific conditions. Ideally, you would need two identical people (clones) in the same environment with the same diet and lifestyle. Then at a specific age, the diet of one clone would be changed to include heavy doses of some kind of refined sugar (lots of candy!). If this prolonged diet were maintained and all other variables remained unchanged and the clone developed cavities (as compared to no cavities in the other clone), then you could assume this sugar diet caused the cavities. But wait a second! Suppose the sugar clone didn't develop cavities? Would you then say the sugar diet doesn't cause cavities? Or do these particular clones possess an innate physiologic resistance to decay, perhaps due to the chemical composition of their saliva, the amount of saliva they produce, the unique physical makeup of their enamel, or any other unique variable?

Now let's do an in vitro experiment. As compared to in vivo, which refers to a living creature, in vitro means "not within the living organism." Because in vitro experiments occur outside the natural living organism, many important variables are lost—such as how the tooth would have been affected if it were still in a live body, protected by saliva, nourished by a good blood supply, and kept warm. We would take an extracted healthy tooth (removed from a patient to allow space for orthodontics treatment, or braces), set up some definite controls (to be accurate, scientific experiments have definitive rules of protocol that attempt to ensure the unbiased results of an experiment), and place this tooth in a sugar/acid solution for a prescribed period of time. We would evaluate the tooth structure afterward in a number of different ways. Normal visual evaluation would give us information concerning stains or texture of the tooth. A microscopic evaluation would show more details, or we could slice off sections of the tooth and prepare this specimen for histological interpretation (one of the ways that cancer is diagnosed, histology is the microscopic study of tissue specimens—it shows cellular structures, both normal and abnormal). If we really wanted to see smaller structures, we would use an electron microscope. Then we would need our knowledge of organic chemistry and physics to interpret the atomic "anatomy" of our specimen.

Once we obtained enough information from our experiment, we could finally reach a specific conclusion regarding the effect of the sugar/acid solution on tooth structure. Sometimes the conclusion drawn from an experiment is wrong. This reminds me of the researcher who was doing an experiment on a frog. He was very methodical with his notes. On day one, he cut off the front right leg of the frog and then yelled at the frog to jump. The frog jumped, and researcher wrote in his diary: Day 1- Cut off right front leg, frog jumped. On day two, he cut off the frog's left front leg and again told it to jump. He wrote in his diary: Day 2 - Cut off left front leg, frog jumped. On day 3, he cut off the frog's left back leg, yelled at it to jump, and again documented the result. On the final day, he cut off the frog's last leg and yelled at it to jump. The frog did not jump. He yelled louder, and the frog still didn't jump. After screaming at the frog to jump and getting no response, the researcher indicated in his diary that upon cutting off its last leg, the frog became deaf!

Properly done, scientific research is a great source of information that helps practitioners in all areas of medicine make intelligent decisions regarding their treatment of patients. Most practitioners, however, treat patients according to clinical judgment based on their experience. Published research can be—and many times is—biased and misleading. Dentists are required to study basic sciences (rather than how to simply "fix a tooth") so that they are equipped to evaluate the research and professional journals intelligently and make better decisions regarding the best treatment for their patients.

The Art and Science

A good example of how basic scientific principles are formulated, analyzed, and applied to clinical therapy is in the area of periodontology, the specialty that deals with the gums and the supporting bone surrounding the teeth. When these tissues become inflamed and infected—due mostly to accumulations of tartar, plaque and bacterial contamination—bone destruction can occur along with what are called pockets. A periodontal pocket is a separation between the gum and the tooth.

Therapy, which includes thoroughly cleaning out the tartar and plaque and eliminating bacterial toxins, normally results in eliminating the inflammation. However, the lost bone and altered anatomy leaves the patient in a compromised state.

The quest to re-grow this bone and restore normal anatomy has frustrated therapists in the past. Now, however, with the knowledge of basic cell biology, researchers have successfully devised a surgical technique that allows surgeons to partially restore the compromised normal anatomy. The development and use of a membrane placed into the surgical site is the key to this procedure. The membrane acts as a microscopic filter that prevents certain cells from repopulating an area so that slower moving cells can restore some of the damaged tissues.

When I first assisted a periodontist in this innovative surgery, I was amazed at the ingenious methodology. I was also quite impressed with the artistic skill of the surgeon. This periodontist (who allowed me over the years to assist and learn from him), was meticulous and had a precise surgical hand. He did not rush as he intricately placed the membrane, added a bone graft, and artistically sculptured and altered the bony architectural form to allow a healthier functional anatomy. This is the way good surgeons perform.

I have tried to emulate this method of thorough, accurate therapy within my general practice and have found that, not only does it provide me with satisfaction, but also my patients receive superior results. In today's fast-paced delivery of health therapy, it is important to understand the significance of a "thinking" practitioner who is in tune with preventive and conservative therapies. When intervention becomes necessary, precise and meticulous execution is paramount.

ANATOMY

The Mouth (Oral Cavity)

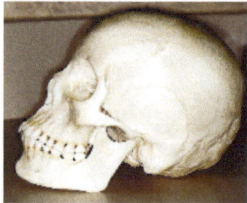

When I was in my first year of dental school 29 years ago, one of the most interesting courses was gross anatomy. Four of us were assigned a cadaver, and for the next six months meticulously dissected it from head to toe. Every nerve, artery, blood vessel and organ was isolated, studied, and re-studied. Of course, our ultimate concentration was on the head and oral cavity, but it was important to understand the relationship between the individual components and how they functioned successfully together.

A normal human being has two sets of teeth: the primary teeth (20 teeth) and the secondary dentition (32 teeth).

The primary, or baby, teeth function like permanent teeth: to chew food, to break down the substances placed in the mouth so salivary enzymes can begin the digestive process, and to support the facial architectural form. The primary teeth also maintain jaw space for the future eruption of permanent teeth. This is why it is so important that primary teeth be maintained and healthy until their natural exfoliation (when they fall out). When they do fall out over a period of years, they are replaced by the permanent or secondary teeth.

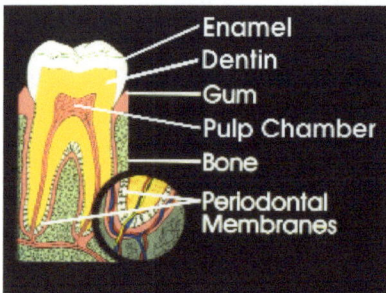

Though the teeth differ in size and shape, their physical makeup is the same: an outside layer of enamel covering a material called dentin. The pulp chamber occupies the next area of the tooth, and this harbors the blood supply and nerve tissue. Farther down the root (or roots, depending on which tooth you're talking about) is the termination in bone—the apex.

Electron microscopy allows further analysis of the tooth and has revealed, for example, microtubules penetrating through what at first seems to be solid dentin.

A typical molar tooth.

The Adult Dentition

The adult dentition has 32 teeth. There are deviations, of course. Some people have more; some have less.

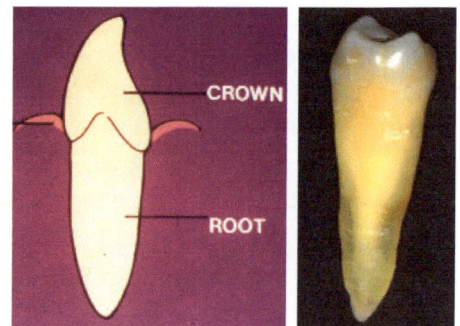

The real thing

Clinical Applications of Research

Researchers use their analyses to better understand how a tooth functions, and this information makes improvements in clinical dentistry possible, for instance, dental "bonding" procedures. This development was a result of researchers applying information gained by meticulous analysis of tooth micro structure and advances in the chemistry of plastics. Researchers determined that the application of certain non-harmful acids to tooth enamel could create a surface etching that allowed tooth-colored plastics to bond to the surface. This was a fantastic development, for if someone had a chipped front tooth, instead of cutting the remaining tooth down for fitting an artificial crown, a more conservative means of treatment was now available.

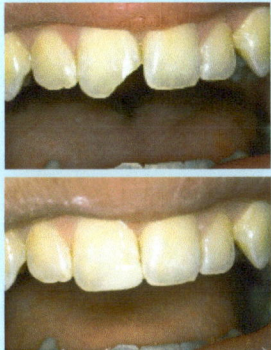

I remember when I was working in Dr. Robert Hill's office in Dorchester, Massachusetts, in 1972. He asked me to demonstrate this "revolutionary" procedure to a group of his colleagues. I was cautiously optimistic. Since then, through further advances in research, these procedures have proved to be quite successful. At first, they were only used on the front teeth where hard biting forces were less traumatizing. Today, state-of-the-art composites (made from reinforced durable plastics) are used in all areas of the mouth.

Teeth Are Not Just For Chewing

The ability to articulate sounds and speak legibly depends upon the interplay between the tongue, the teeth, and the adjacent soft tissues and muscles. Sounds are produced and manipulated by air flow patterns around a healthy dentition. Have you ever heard a whistling sound coming from someone who wears badly-constructed dentures? This and other speech problems develop when degenerative changes occur in the oral cavity. Romantics understand what may be the most important function of a healthy mouth. As an aesthetic and erogenous lure, a clean and healthy mouth is an obvious sexual attraction.

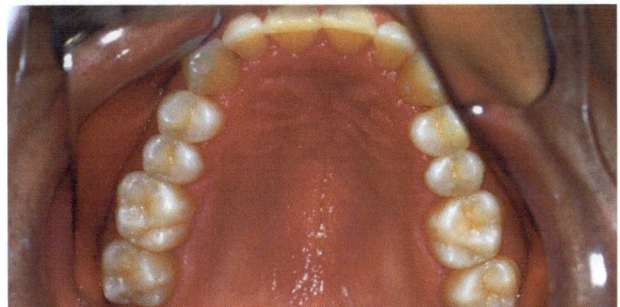

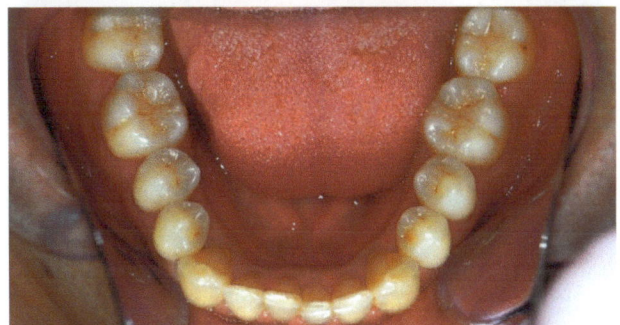

Typical upper and lower arches (wisdom teeth — 3rd molars not appearing). This is a relatively healthy adult dentition with no cavities and no fillings.

CHILDREN'S DENTISTRY

Children's teeth are called baby teeth, or as dentists refer to them, primary or deciduous. Generally, children have 20 teeth as compared with adults who have 32.

The teeth of children are important for several reasons. Like adult teeth, they are very important for proper food chewing, support of the facial muscles, and engaging smiles, but they are also needed to support jaw growth and provide adequate space for eruption of the permanent teeth. The premature loss of certain baby teeth may create crowding problems and malocclusions in the permanent dentition.[6]

When baby teeth first appear in a child's mouth, preventive hygiene measures become necessary to avoid decay. A child's first visit to the dentist is critical. Not only does the dentist need to evaluate the mouth, but also to expose the child to a friendly, non-traumatic experience. Though many dentists treat children, taking your child to a pediatric dentist initially may be a wise choice. Generally, the offices of pediatric dentists display a playground setting, and they are better equipped to handle the special needs of children.

Tooth Decay

Tooth decay is the primary cause of premature loss of baby teeth. A visit to the dentist will allow early detection and appropriate treatment. If decay is extensive and involves the nerve of the tooth, a procedure known as pulpotomy can be performed. In this procedure, a portion of the inflamed nerve tissue is removed. If successful, this procedure avoids premature loss of the space-

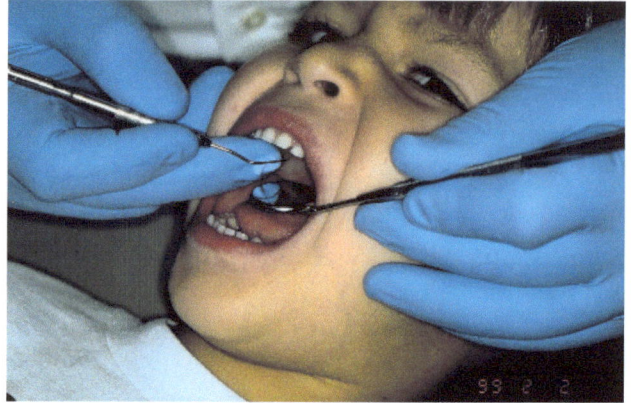

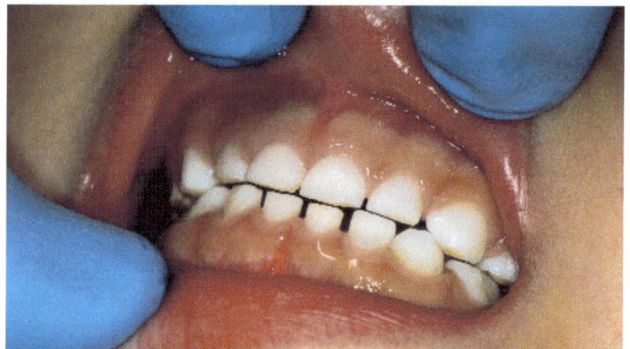

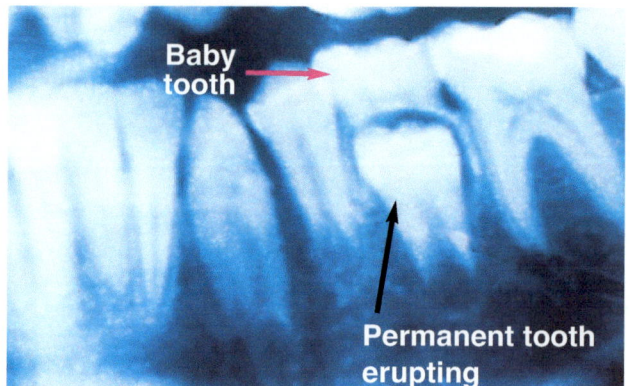

Baby tooth

Permanent tooth erupting

A mixed dentition. A radiograph showing eruption patterns of permanent teeth which will cause the exfoliation (loss) of deciduous teeth (baby teeth).

maintaining baby teeth.[7] Restoration of these badly damaged teeth may necessitate fabrication and cementation of artificial crowns.

Once decayed teeth are treated properly, a hygiene program can be established along with appropriate recall appointments to monitor the child's health and to provide preventive care.

Preventive Care

In addition to cleaning of the child's teeth and encouraging good oral hygiene, applying fluoride and sealers (bonded protective coverings over the cavity prone crevices of the teeth)[8] also affords protection from decay.

The dentist should discuss the child's eating habits and nutrition with the parent, as this is not only an important factor in avoiding decay, but also in maintaining an overall healthy state. It is worthwhile to note that one of the worst causes of decay in children is known as baby bottle syndrome. This syndrome occurs when a parent allows the baby to sleep while sucking the nipple of a milk bottle or any other sugar containing liquid.[9]

In addition to their child's nutritional habits, parents should also make the pediatric dentist aware of medications that either the mother had been taking during pregnancy[10] or that the child may be taking. One of the most serious dental cosmetic problems is tetracycline stain. This discoloration occurs as a result of taking the antibiotic tetracycline during periods of tooth formation, from the second trimester in utero to about eight years of age.

Finally, it is important not to underestimate the significance of a healthy and happy young dental patient. Proper, non-traumatic preventive care during these early years can have a tremendous positive influence on the psychological status of the patient for the rest of his or her life. Not fearing dental visits and receiving *conservative* care (less invasive therapies) will ultimately result in the preservation of a healthy mouth.

---

6. There are circumstances where for interceptive orthodontic reasons, premature loss may not be detrimental.

7. If baby teeth are lost prematurely, a device known as a space maintainer will prevent future crowding problems. It functions, as its name indicates, to maintain the space needed until the permanent teeth erupt.

8. Though not 100% effective, they do reduce susceptibility to decay.

9. Any food source that lies on the teeth exposes the enamel to the acids produced by specific oral bacteria.

10. Obviously the mother should have tried to avoid all types of medication (and unhealthy habits) during pregnancy.

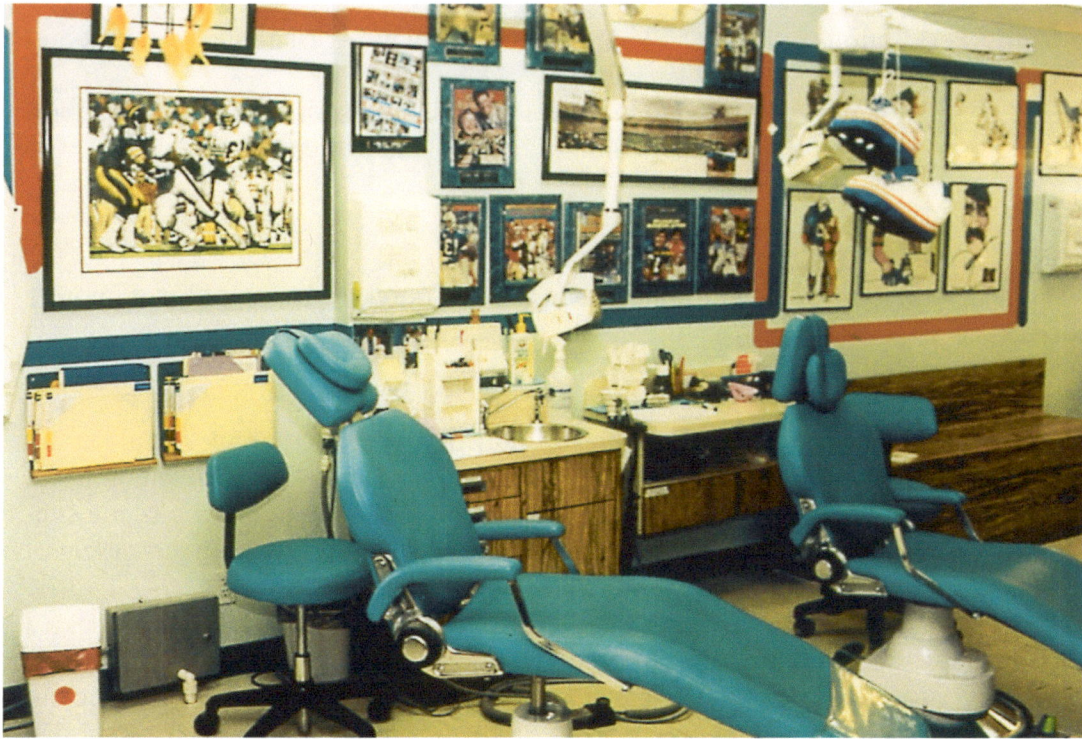

My college friend Rick Kirsch became a pediatric dentist. He is an avid Miami Dolphins football fan. He decorated his office with this upbeat, happy theme.

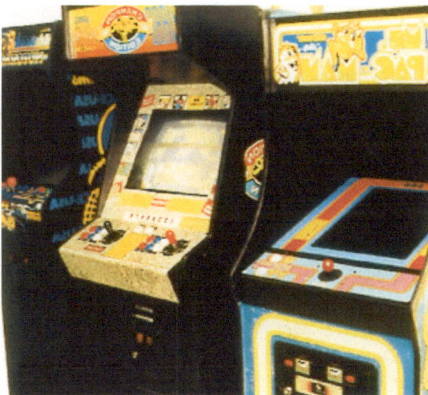

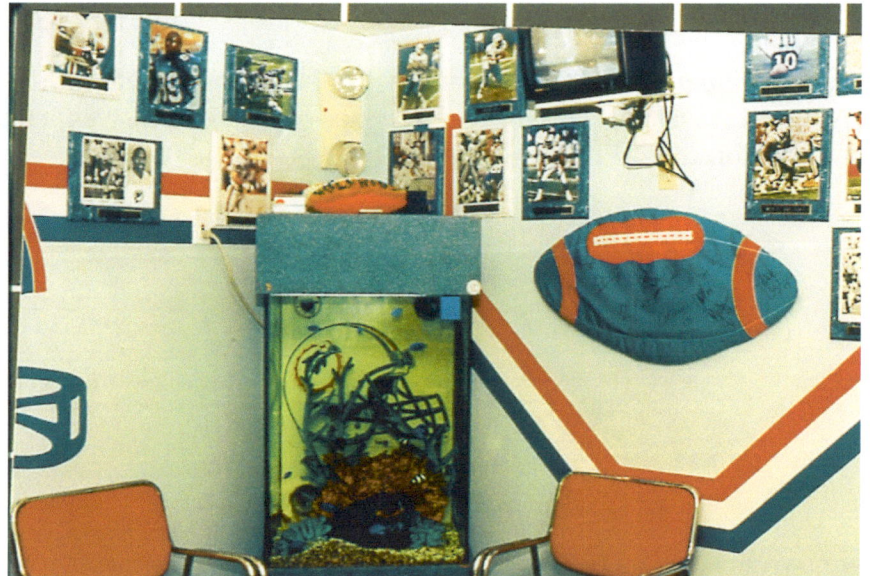

Frederic G. Kirsch, D.D.S., P.A.

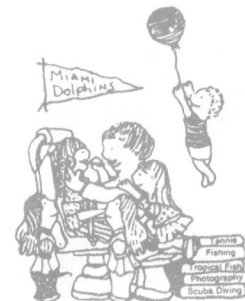

Pediatric Dentistry

Dear Parent,

As a Pedodontist, I Am Deeply Interested in the dental health, general health, and psychological well being of your child.

A child's first visit to the dentist is most important, and in many cases the most impressionable. Most children fear the dentist, either because of a previous unpleasant experience or because they naturally fear any new experience.

What will be done on the first visit?

During the first visit, the child is introduced to the dental environment. A thorough examination will be performed and x-rays will be taken. The results of the examination and x-rays will be discussed with you, a treatment plan established and financial arrangements made. Naturally, if this is an emergency visit, the immediate problem is cared for and the routine procedures are postponed.

What should I say to my child?

The feelings that parents show toward dental care may be crucial in determining how a child approaches his/her visit to the dentist. Generally speaking, it is best to avoid any unpleasant comments or thoughts. Tell your child the dentist is going to take pictures, and count his/her teeth. If the child asks, "will it hurt?" be honest and say, for example, "it won't be unpleasant if you help the doctor." Do not use fear-arousing words such as "needle, shot or drill." Above all, do not bribe your child and do tell the truth.

We ask you not to be upset if your child cries. Crying is a child's normal reaction to fear. We understand these fears and will work to erase them.

During treatment, we request that parents remain in the reception room. It has been our experience that children respond much better on their own. Many seem to acquire a pride in the knowledge that they are grown-up enough to undergo treatment by themselves.

Your aim as a parent, and mine as a dentist, are the same . . . to maintain your child's health and to make the process of doing so a pleasant one for the child, parent and doctor.

Looking forward to meeting you;

Sincerely,

Frederic G. Kirsch, D.D.S., P.A.

1881 North University Drive • Suite 201 • Coral Springs, Florida 33071 • 753-7770

Orthodontics

No one's anatomy is perfect, and only where there are deformities that either diminish a person's self esteem or interfere with proper functioning should corrective treatment be considered. But how is a parent to know if their child's development is normal?

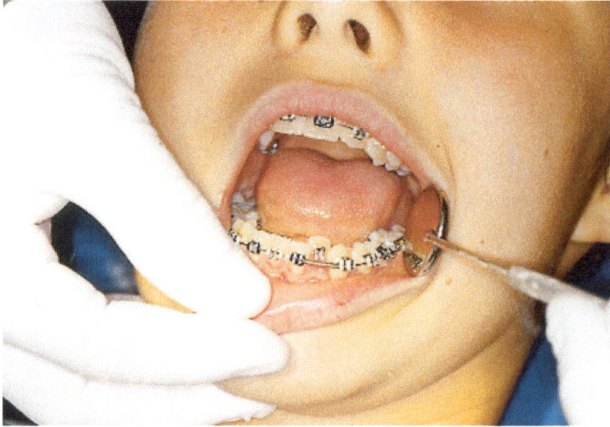

The child's dentist (pediatric or general) should be helpful in determining the need for an orthodontic consultation. Ask the dentist about his degree of experience and knowledge regarding the specialty of orthodontics. The level of orthodontic knowledge held by pediatric and general dentists varies widely. Some dentists have the training and background to diagnose orthodontic problems, and are also qualified to perform many of the orthodontic procedures. An honest practitioner will advice you appropriately.

Diagnostics

Jaw relations are analyzed.

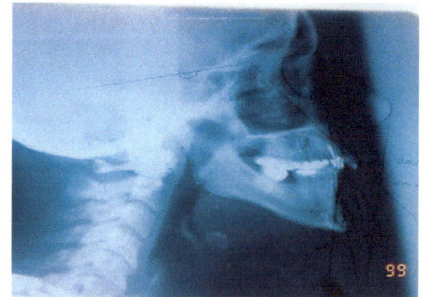

Special radiographs are utilized to analyze the relationships between anatomic structures.

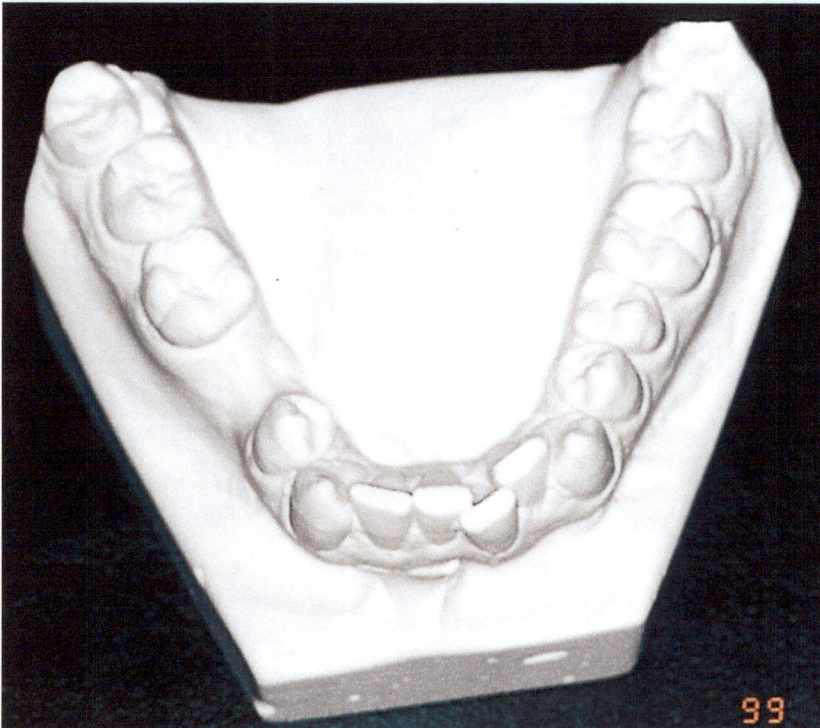

Study models allow careful evaluation of tooth position and potential problems.

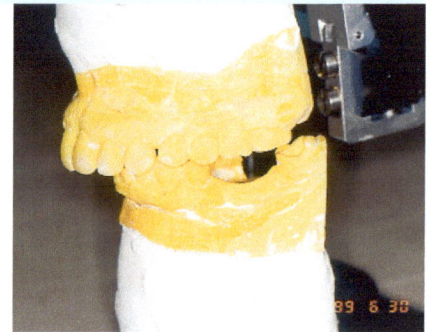

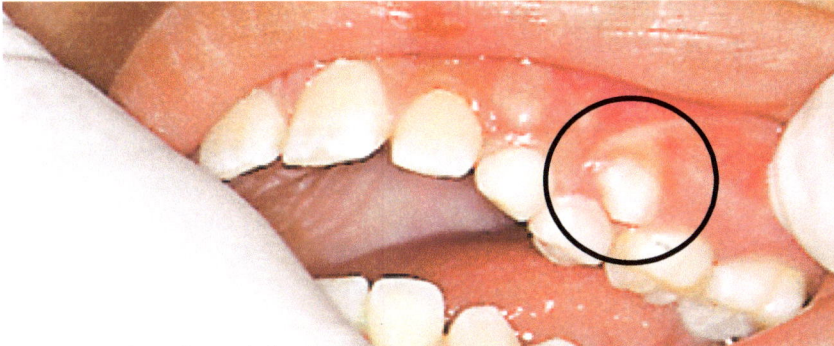

Ectopic eruption of a tooth (tooth erupting in an abnormal position)

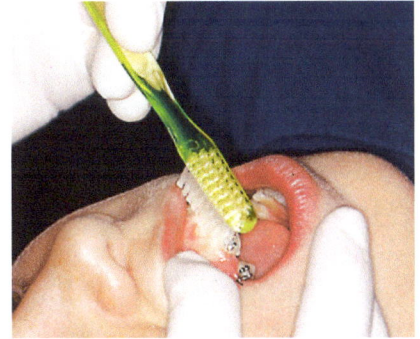

Proper oral hygiene is extremely important during orthodontic therapy.

Aesthetic braces are less visible

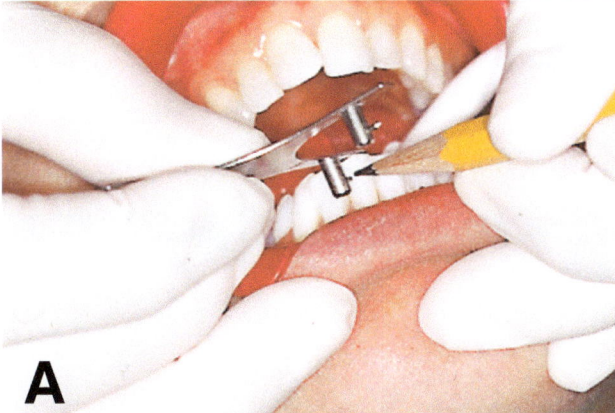

A

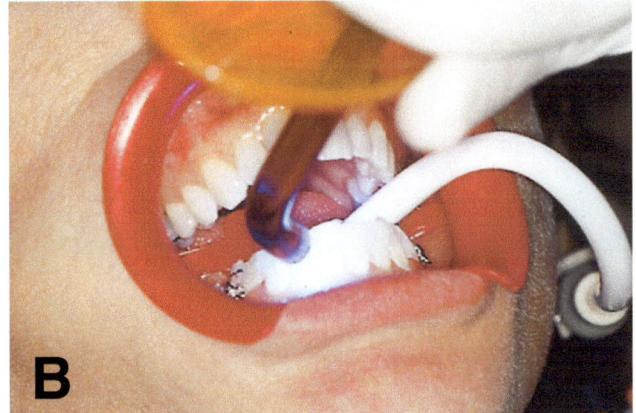

B

Clear brackets are bonded to the teeth

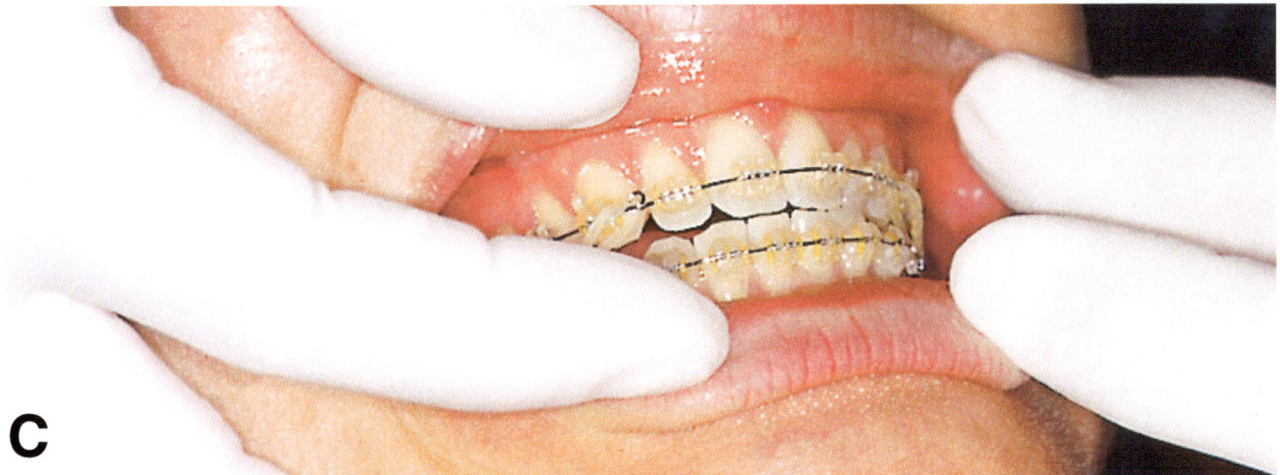

C

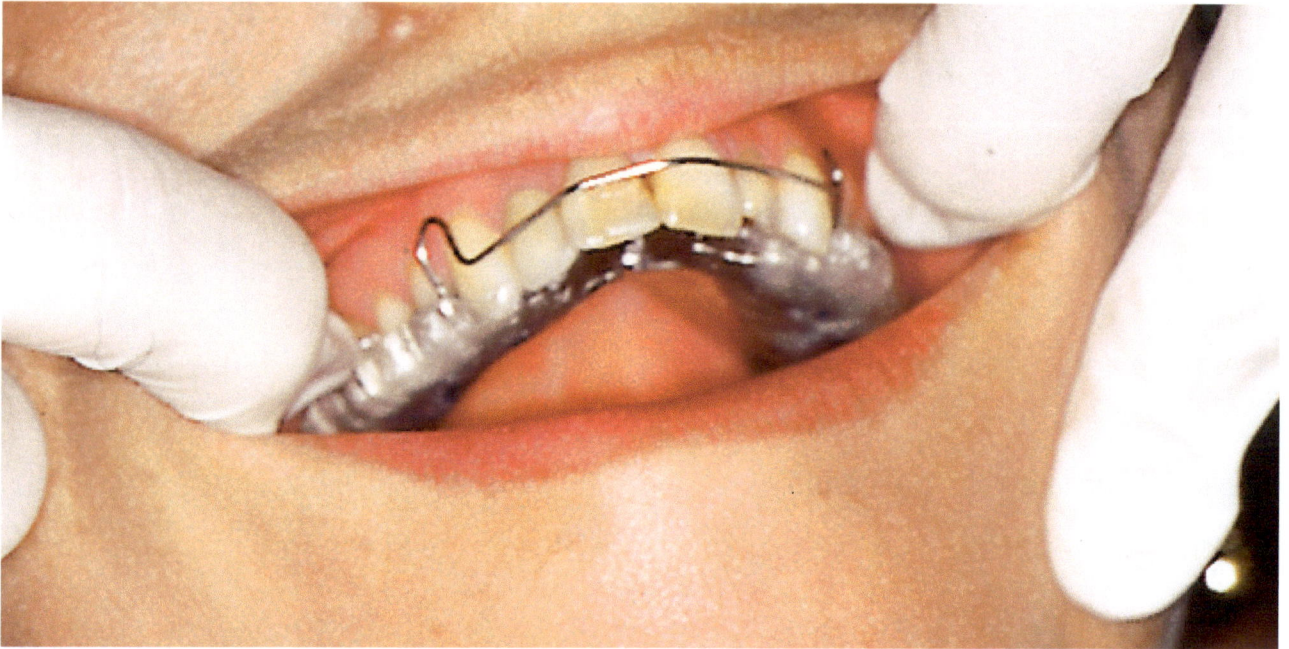

Different removable appliances are utilized to reposition the teeth and to retain the teeth in proper position following completion of orthodontic therapy.

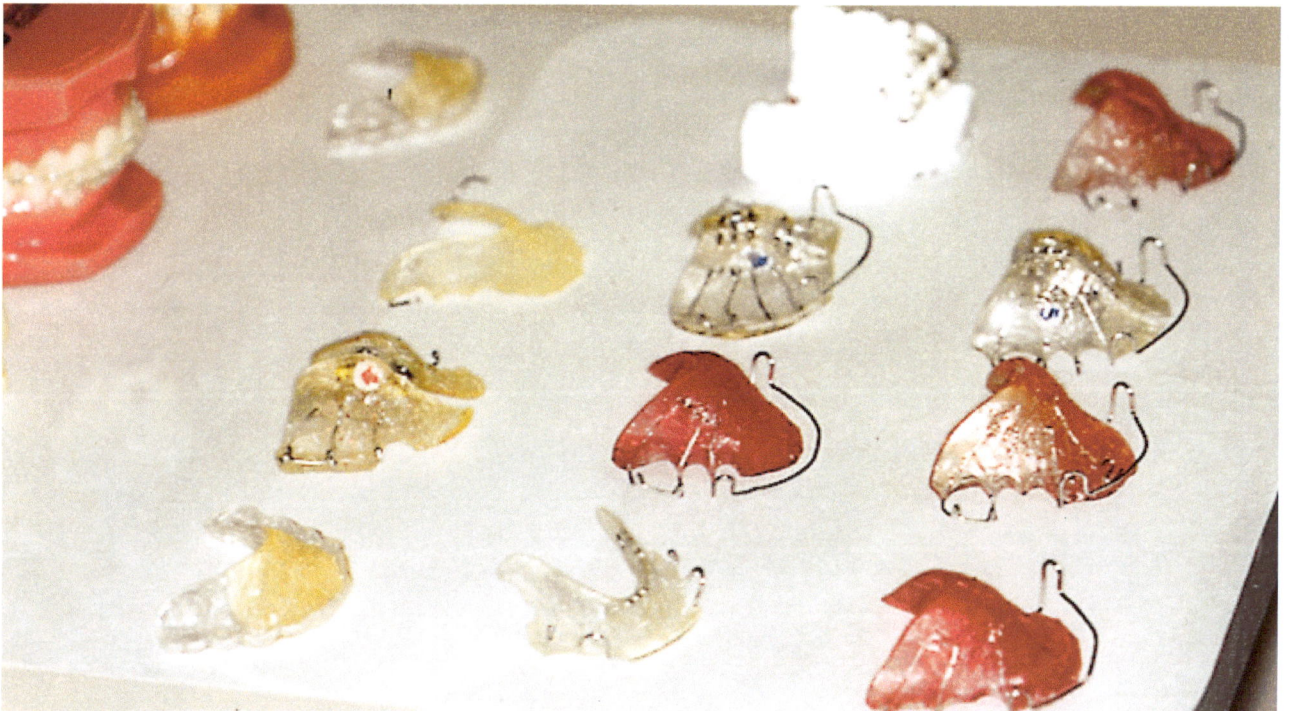

Adult Orthodontics

It is easier to move teeth when the patient is young, however, excellent results can be achieved with adult orthodontics. Specific treatment options can only be evaluated after a thorough examination is performed. This examination includes various types of radiographs and impressions made of the patient's mouth to produce study models.

In my practice, I find that when it comes to improving the appearance of front teeth, most patients prefer to avoid orthodontics when caps or veneers are an option.[11] It is up to the dentist to advise the patient concerning the advantages and disadvantages of alternative treatments.

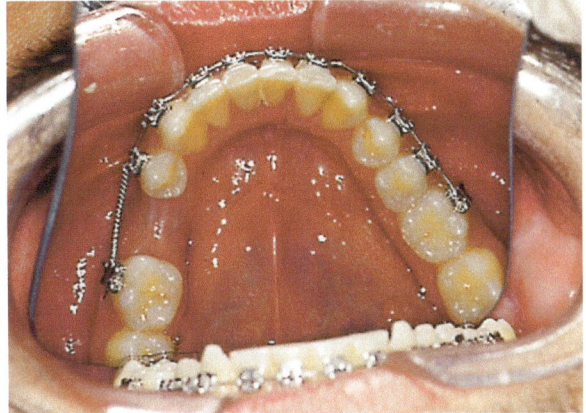

Orthodontic therapy is utilized to recreate proper arch form and elevate teeth that have collapsed into empty spaces.

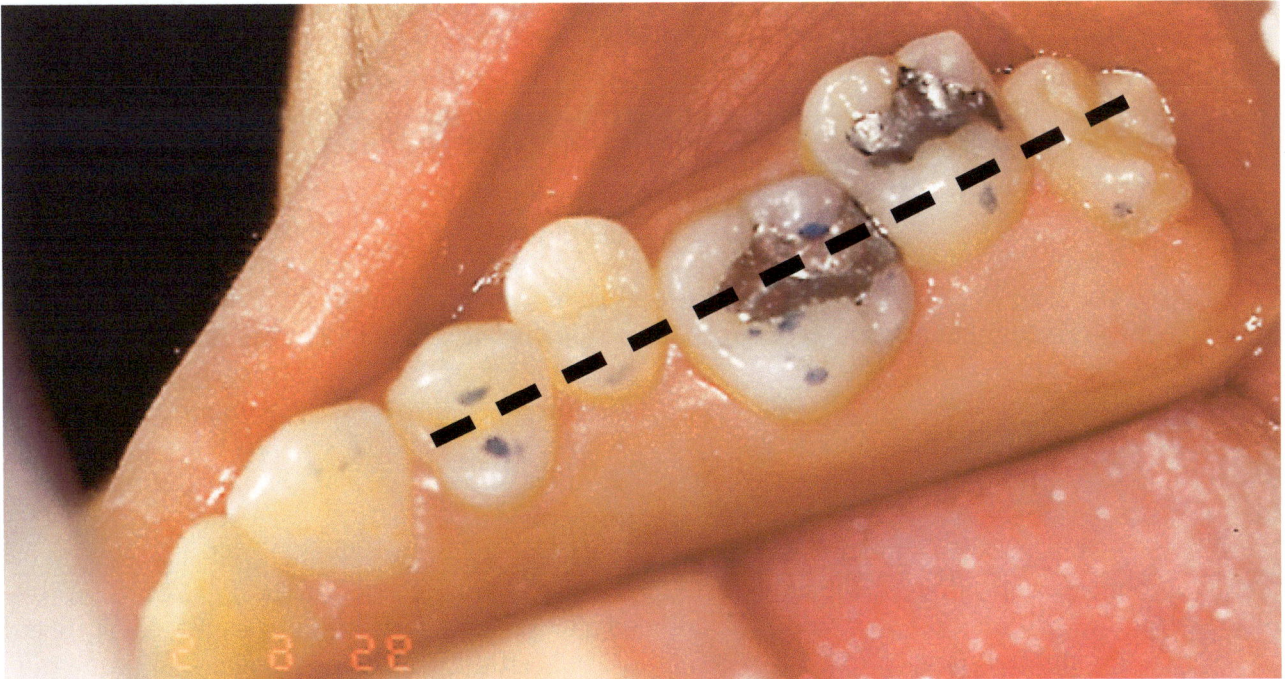

Crowding and misalignment of teeth can be corrected orthodontically. This may improve the biting relationship of the teeth thereby eliminating detrimental forces and reducing stress.

---

11. Caps or crowns are artificial coverings of natural prepared teeth. Chapter 8 on prosthetics provides a more comprehensive explanation. Veneers are thin porcelain shells bonded to natural teeth.

THE COMPLETE DENTAL EXAMINATION

Unless you want to wait until you experience discomfort, a checkup is the best preventive strategy. It is important that the dentist perform a thorough examination. In my office, I divide the exam into 10 segments:

1. Medical History
2. Dental History
3. Chief Complaint
4. Facial and Soft Tissue Exam
5. Tooth Mobility
6. Carious Lesions (cavities) and Existing Restorative and Prosthetic Status
7. Periodontal Screening
8. Occlusion and Diagnostic Study Models
9. Temporomandibular Joints
10. Radiographs

When I have completed this examination, the patient is scheduled for a consultation. Before the consultation appointment, I review all the information[12] and prepare a treatment plan or treatment options, depending on the complexity of the case.

Let's review the significance of each part of the examination.

---

12. Always with my dental assistant, Nerida. Her years of training, learning, and discussing treatment options with me have made her a significant contributor to sound dental analysis.

The Medical History

I have found very few medical conditions that preclude providing quality dental care and obtaining good results. Generally, very sick, aged, or disabled patients do not appear at a dental office because they are either bedridden and/or hospitalized, or they receive dental care at special facilities. Patients who come to my office complete a health questionnaire. I evaluate responses to see if health issues affect dental status or treatment needs. The complete medical history helps avoid unforeseen treatment complications. For instance, diabetic patients may be more prone to infections and heal more slowly. I must determine the severity of their disease and the medications they are taking. In treating most diabetic patients, I have not seen the dramatic detrimental conditions and treatment results textbooks suggested would occur. A history of liver dysfunction, may be significant in terms of a bleeding or healing problem in surgical procedures.

Allergies are significant, particularly, for instance, if my patient indicates an allergy to Penicillin. If my first choice for an antibiotic were Penicillin, I would administer Erythromycin instead. It is important to know what medications patients are currently taking in order to avoid interactions with drugs I may prescribe.

Occasionally, the dentist will discover undiagnosed medical conditions that show clinical signs of pathology in the oral cavity: i.e., cancer, AIDS, certain vitamin deficiencies, or numerous other conditions. If any of these conditions are apparent, the dentist should refer the patient to the appropriate physician.

Dental History

In taking a full account of patients' dental history, I look not only at the existing dental work, but at their past experience and how this will affect future care. If I see sloppy or sub-standard restorations (when they exist, they are usually obvious to a dentist), I wonder whether the patient is aware of the condition. I believe it's important to discuss this with them, look for reasons why this has occurred, and show them how quality care differs from their previous treatment. When their visit to my office is emergency based, patients are usually in pain. Then my primary objective is to deal only with their emergency needs in a gentle and compassionate manner. Once this is accomplished, I re-schedule them for a complete examination.

Fear of the dentist and financial constraints are two of the most common reasons for dental neglect. In order to provide proper therapy, the dentist must "discover" and deal with these factors individually.

Chief Complaint

Why did the patient come to my office? Though there may be many treatment requirements, prioritizing them is important. If a patient requests that I fix or do just "this one thing," it's up to me to evaluate the request as it relates to what may be best. For instance, if a patient's main concern is a chipped tooth, yet my examination reveals other areas of deterioration such as a deep cavity that left untreated will cause pain and require root canal therapy, I try to accommodate the original request while also educating the patient.

Facial and Soft Tissue Exam

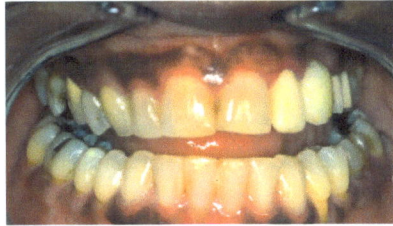

Natural gum pigmentation in an African American. This patient was concerned when she was told that these darkened areas on her gum were abnormal.

In this part of the examination, I look for anything abnormal—a swelling, facial lesions, and so on—that may require treatment or referral to a specialist.   Early detection of cancer can save a patient's life. Undiagnosed medical conditions are sometimes first observed during this part of the examination.

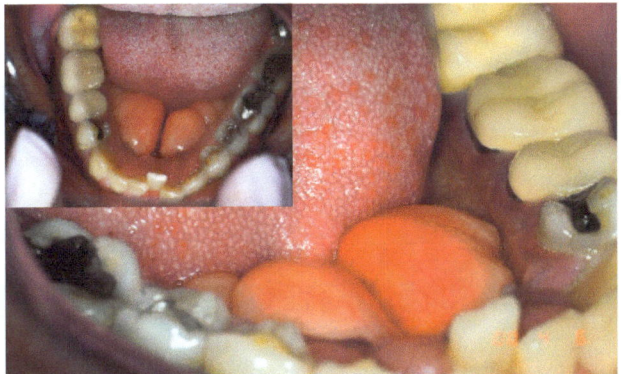

Mandibular tori – Excessive bone growth. This is benign and besides possibly interfering with this patient's ability to clean his lower teeth poses no major problems.

Tooth Mobility

Normally, teeth are not mobile. When I detect mobility, I immediately evaluate the biting relationship of the teeth. Is there traumatic occlusion? Have the teeth shifted due to loss of a tooth? Does the patient have periodontal disease with accompanying bone loss? Evaluation of the x-rays (radiographs) will help diagnose the problem.

Carious Lesions (Cavities) and Existing Restorative and Prosthetic Status

I use an explorer (a metal, pointed probe) to gently investigate the pits and fissures of the teeth to detect cavities. I check to see if present fillings (restorations) are sound with no recurrent decay or voids. I also evaluate bridges and other prosthetic appliances: Do they have proper anatomy? Is the fixed (cemented) bridge functioning properly? Can the patient perform required oral hygiene procedures under the bridge? Are the removable partial dentures irritating the soft tissues? Are the clasps designed properly, or are they traumatizing the teeth they contact?

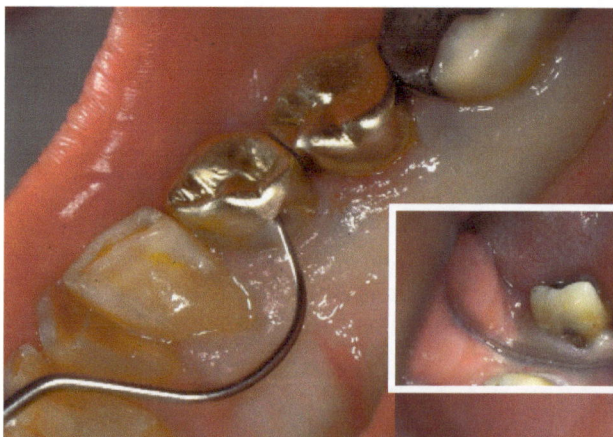

If the patient has no natural teeth (totally edentulous) and is wearing complete upper and lower dentures, how are these functioning? Bone and soft tissues tend to change over time, causing the dentures to shift from their original proper relationship. The bite may become traumatic, and tissues may become red and irritated. Preventive therapy may include everything from using soft relining materials to remaking the defective dentures. Ultimately, avoiding timely treatment in dealing with these problems exacerbates the condition. Neglect results in more complicated and expensive therapy with a diminished prognosis.

And what about dental implants? These restorative devices need periodic maintenance—for life!* This is one of the major disadvantages of any complex dental treatment. Keeping your own natural teeth healthy and avoiding any prosthetic replacement makes the most sense in relation to the time and expense of maintenance requirements.

* Advances in implant technology have eliminated many of the earlier problems that *were* occurring, including reducing many maintenance requirements. The I.T.I. implant system by Straumann seems to be in the forefront in this area. 1-800-448-8168. www.straumannusa.com

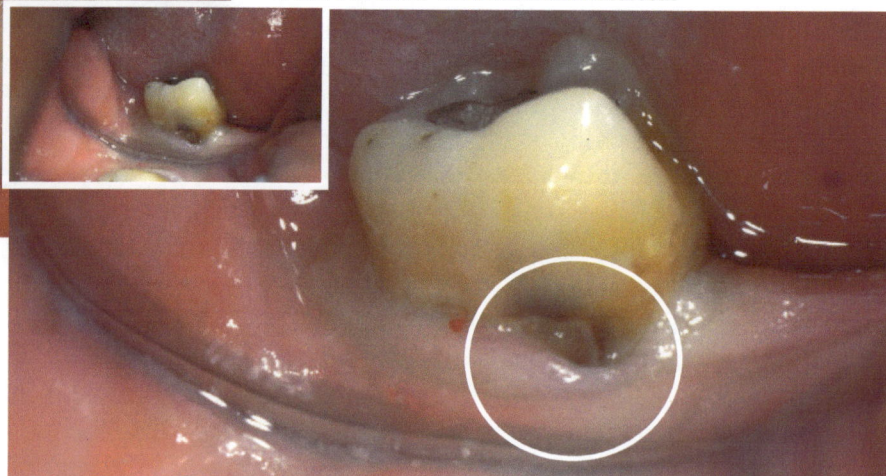

A probe is utilized to discover this defective margin under a gold onlay.

Hidden decay, not obvious on the first look. A dental mirror, properly placed, shows the true extent of the lesion.

Evaluation of existing restorative and prosthetic status

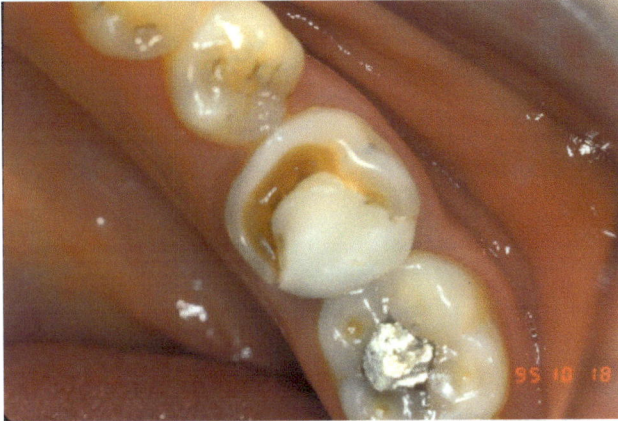

Erosion surrounding defective old "plastic" filling

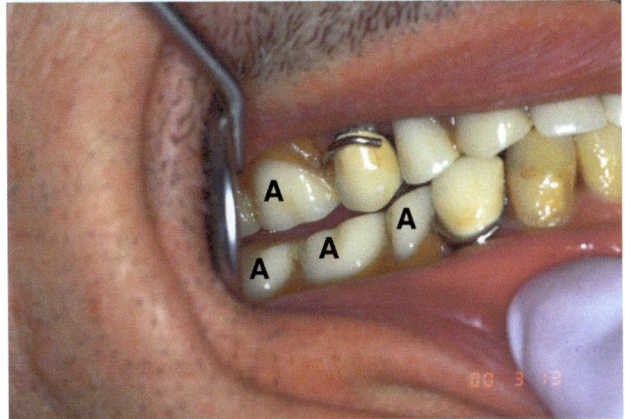

What's wrong with this picture? – Lack of occlusion, defective partial dentures. Artificial teeth (A) are not in proper contact.

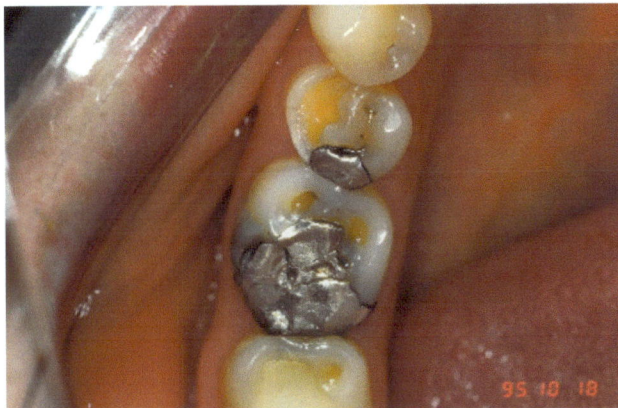

Old defective amalgam "fillings".

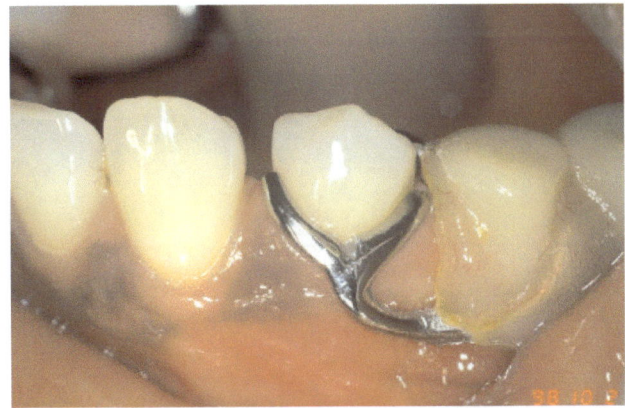

Defective partial denture clasp – Too bulky and too close to gum tissue.

Periodontal Screening

Screening involves a general appraisal as compared to a more complete and thorough examination. I evaluate the color, texture, and bleeding tendencies of the tissues adjacent to the teeth, noting the amount of plaque and tartar buildup. I use a measuring probe to detect periodontal pockets (pathologic separation between the gums and the teeth). The radiographic examination will reveal bone destruction, tartar beneath the gum line, and other pertinent information. If the periodontal status indicates a clinical deterioration, the patient will be scheduled for a more thorough periodontal examination where specific measurements and charting of pocket depths will be recorded.

Periodontal Evaluation

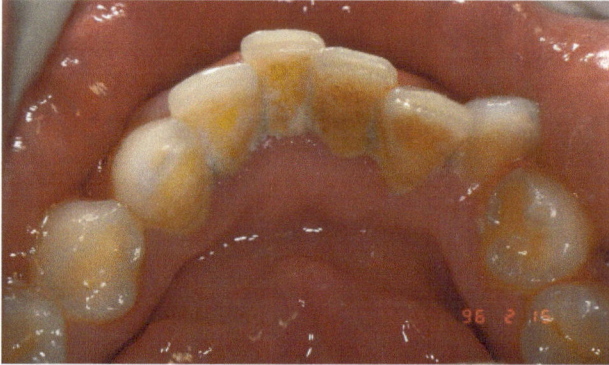

Extensive tartar accumulation...

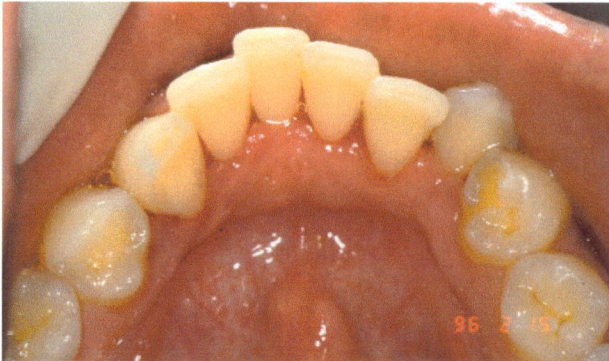

Following debridement (removal of all tartar and plaque).

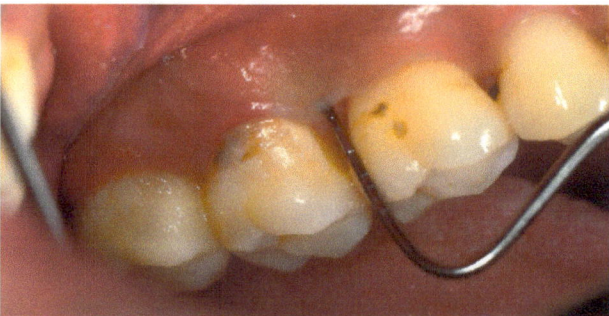

A periodontal probe measuring separation of the gum from the tooth (a periodontal pocket).

Occlusion and Diagnostic Study Models

Occlusion is the bite—the relationship between the upper and lower teeth. Though the teeth should occlude in a certain manner, deviations almost always exist; there is no absolutely normal biting relationship. When trauma is present with either tooth mobility or other clinically related factors, corrective treatment is indicated. When necessary, impressions are taken of the upper and lower teeth, poured in stone to make diagnostic casts, and mounted on a device that simulates the relationship of the jaws (an articulator). This makes it easier to evaluate the bite and demonstrate this information to the patient.

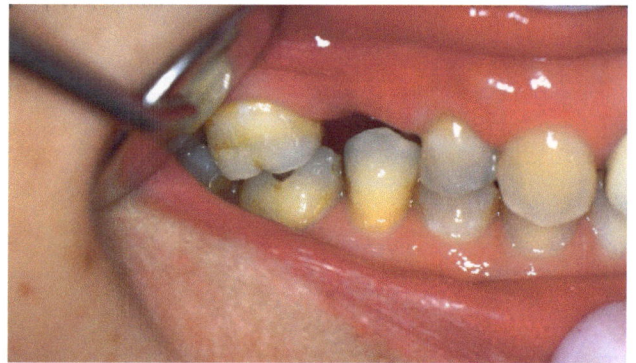

Clinical situation.

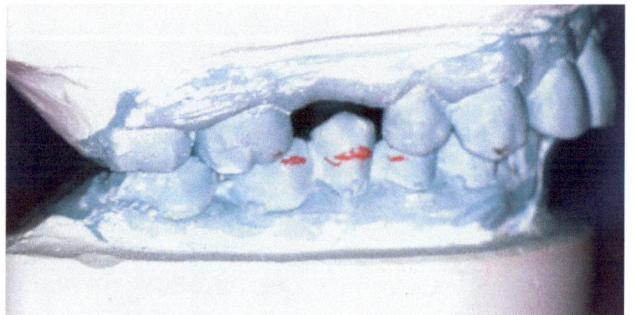

Diagnostic casts.

Temporomandibular Joint

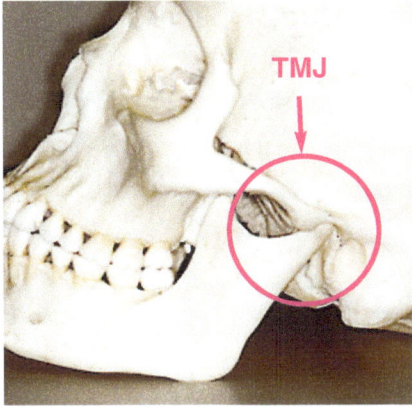

The temporomandibular joint (TMJ) is the ball-and-socket relationship that connects the movable lower jaw (the mandible) to the upper skull. Abnormalities in this joint may result in chronic symptoms such as headaches, clicking sounds, or muscle pain. The "inexact" nature of this problem has resulted in a cottage industry of TMJ therapists—some legitimate, others not. My exam evaluates the general status of this anatomic area. Rarely have I discovered subjective or clinical pathology.

Radiographs

A routine radiographic examination (peri-apical x-rays) usually involves about 16 radiographs, called a full series. Evaluation will generally show if cavities are present, the status of wisdom teeth (third molars), signs of periodontal disease or other areas of pathology. When a wider view is necessary, the dentist will request a panoramic radiograph.[13] Dental x-rays are very safe. Newer films requiring little radiation, along with the use of a lead apron, protect the patient. Moreover, digital radiography is rapidly replacing standard x-ray film. It requires even less radiation, and with computer enhancement, affords better diagnostic capabilities.

---

13. Though this radiograph shows a greater area, it doesn't show the fine details (called definition) as well as the smaller peri-apical x-rays.

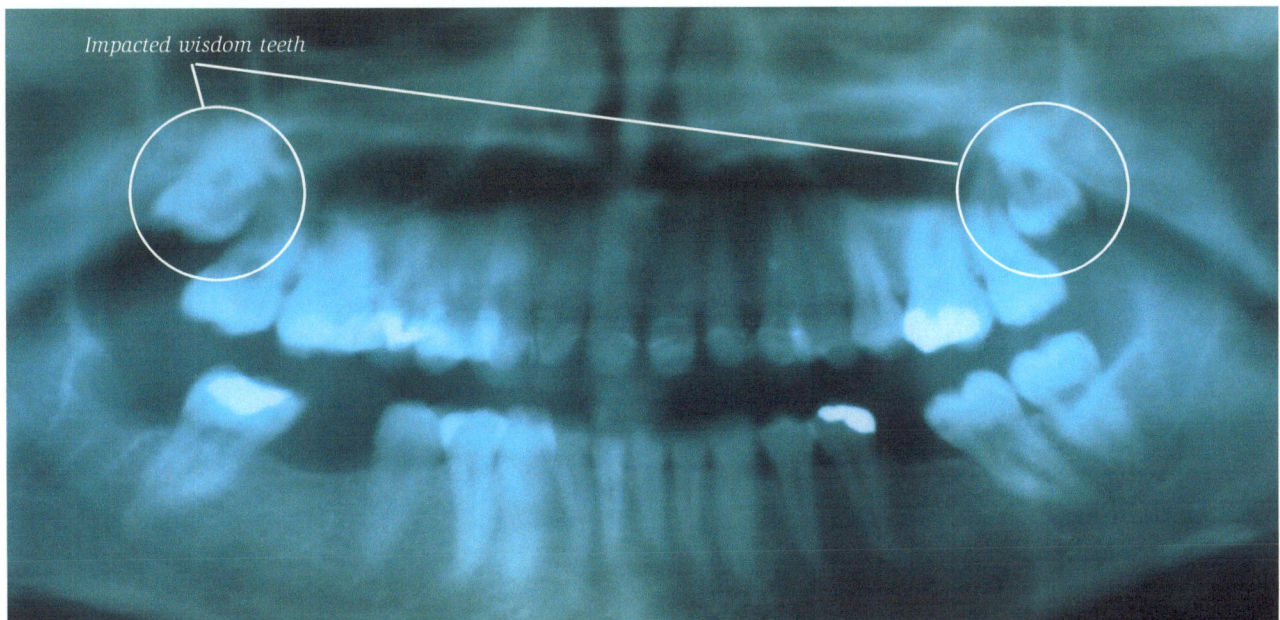

A panoramic radiograph.

What you don't see can be harmful

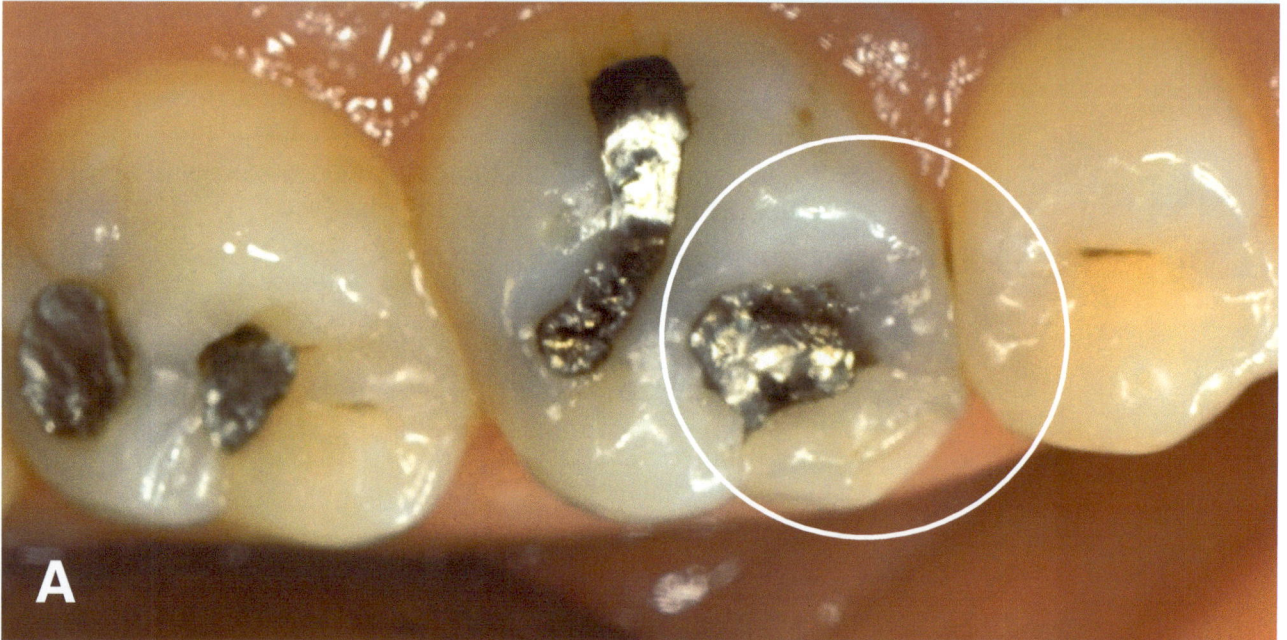

A

Visual exam of this old amalgam "filling" shows no obvious decay.

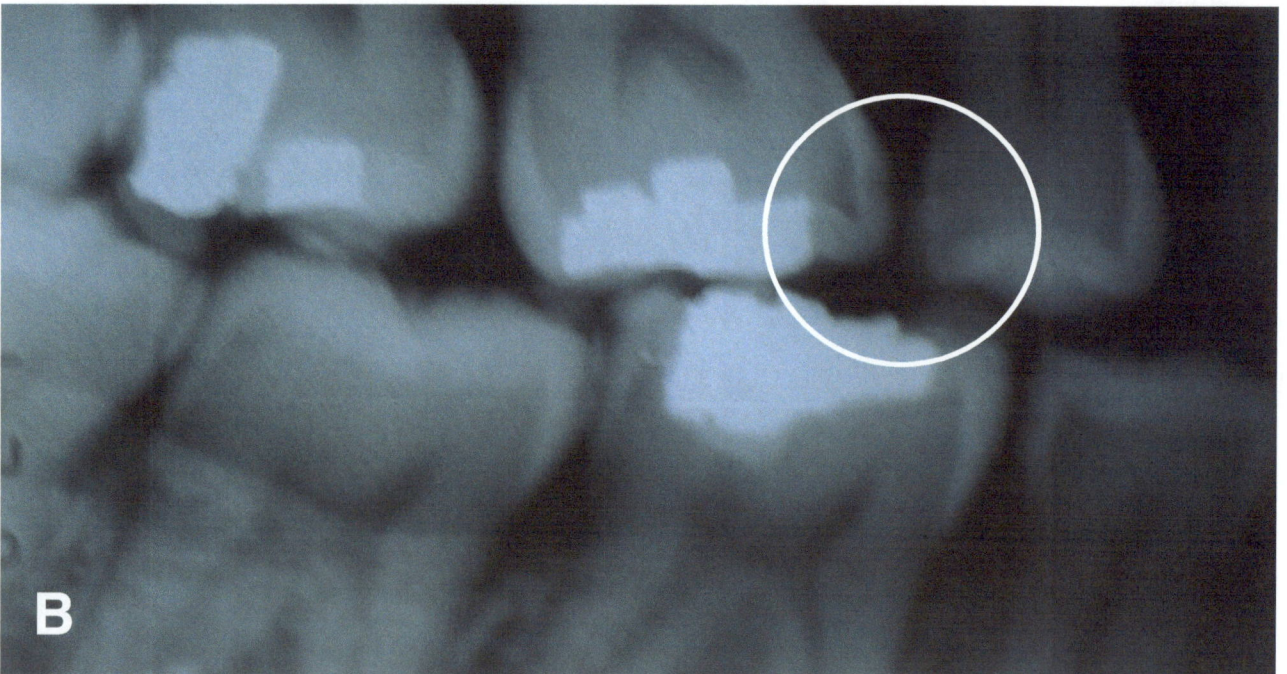

B

Radiograph reveals decay. If left untreated it will generally destroy more tooth structure and possibly result in a toothache.

What you don't see can be harmful   (Continued)

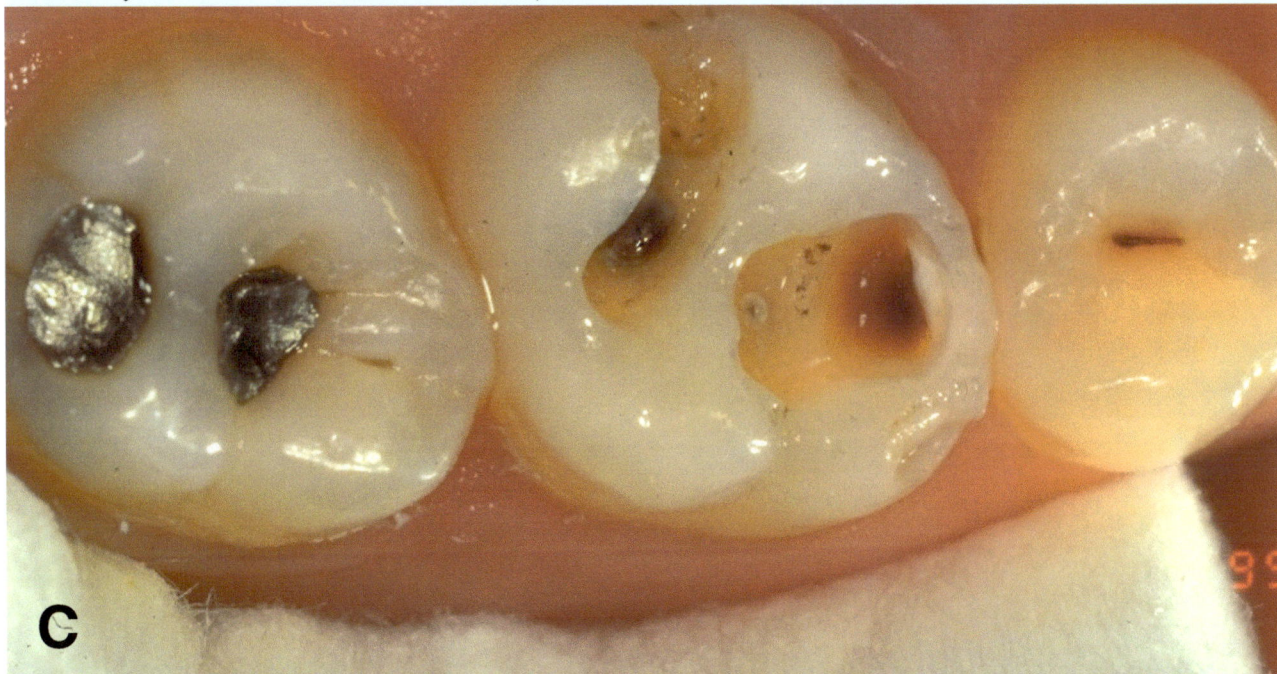

Removal of filling shows obvious decay.

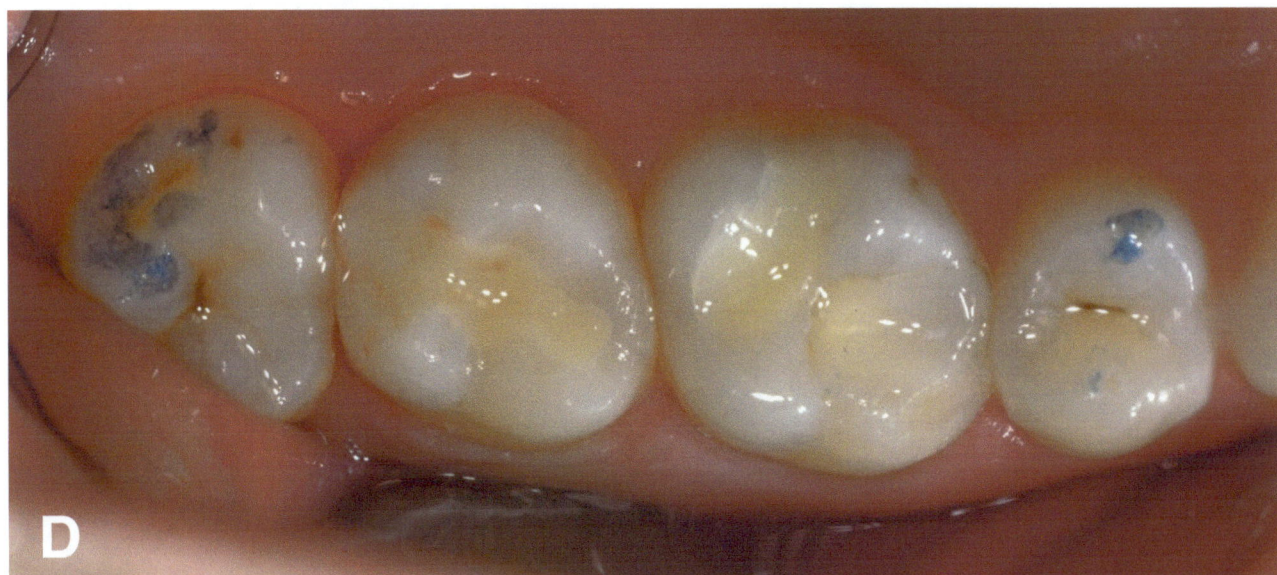

Following removal (excavation) of decay, a white composite filling is placed. Articulating paper registers blue spots on the teeth in order to evaluate and adjust the proper bite (occlusion).

What you don't see can be harmful   (Continued)

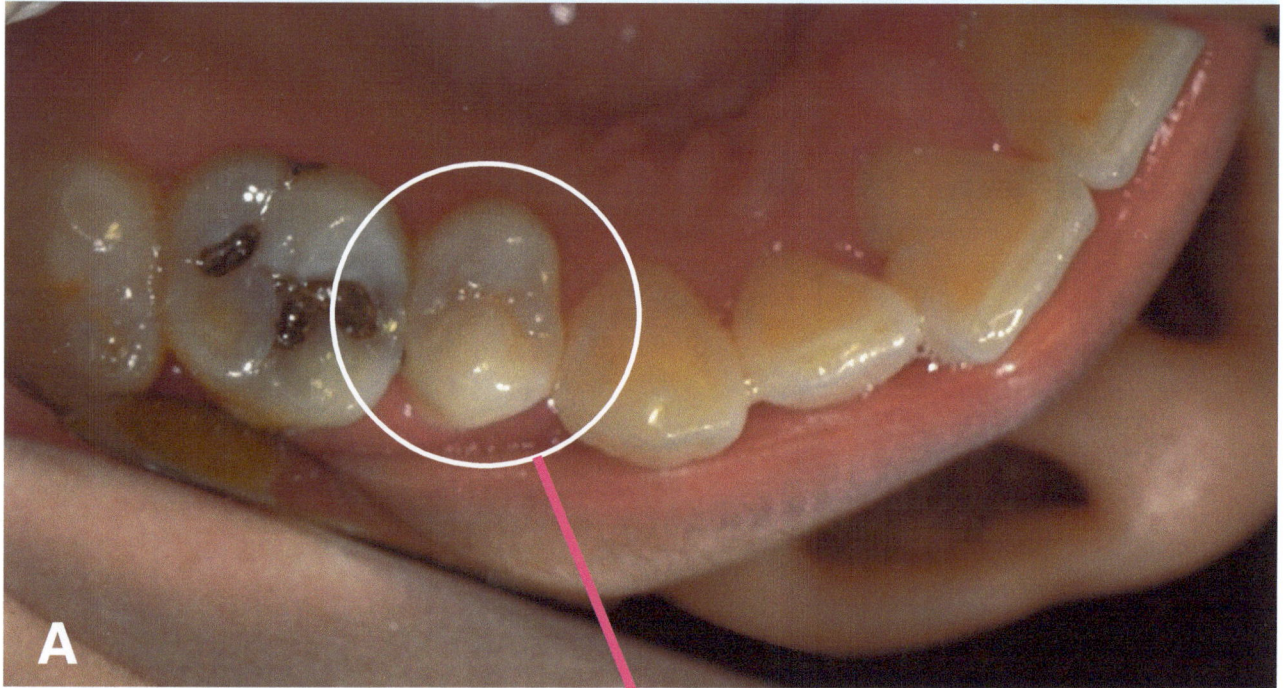

No obvious decay on this tooth.

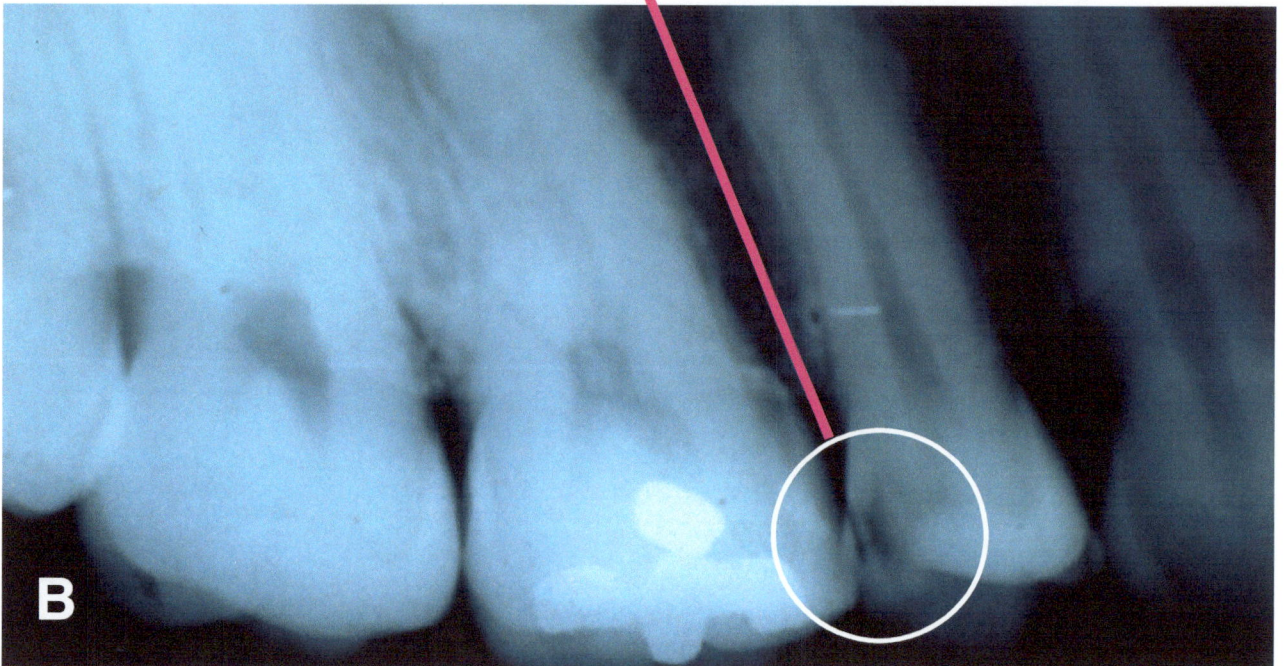

Radiograph shows radioluscency (dark area).

What you don't see can be harmful

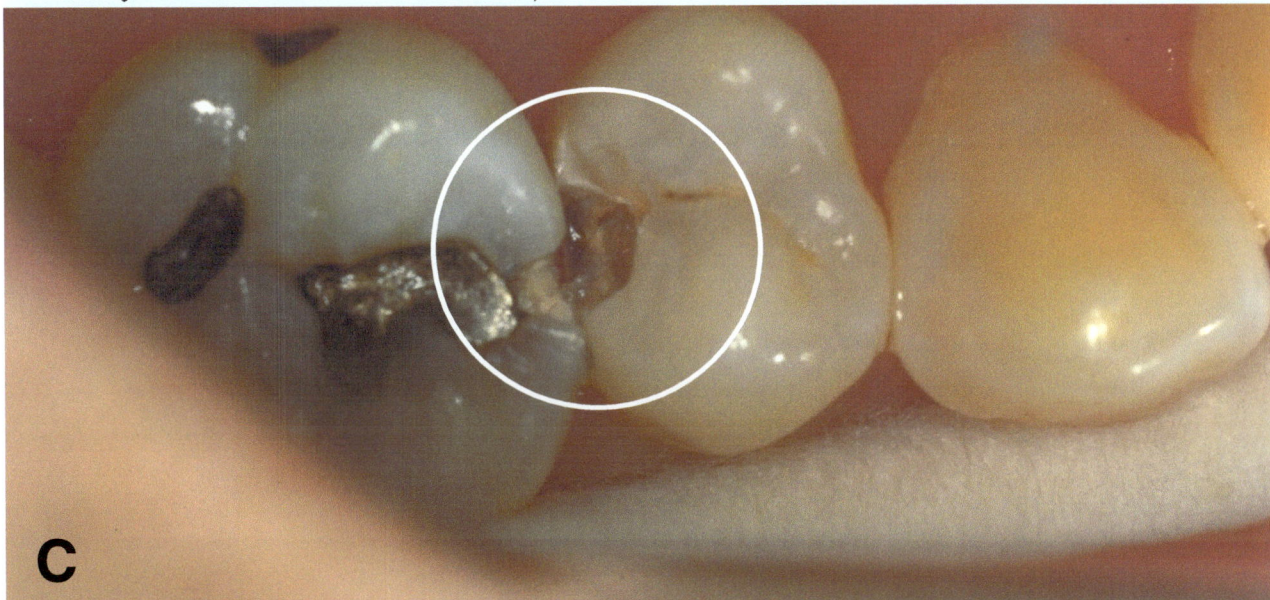

Penetration into suspect area shows decay. (Decay is also discovered on the adjacent tooth)

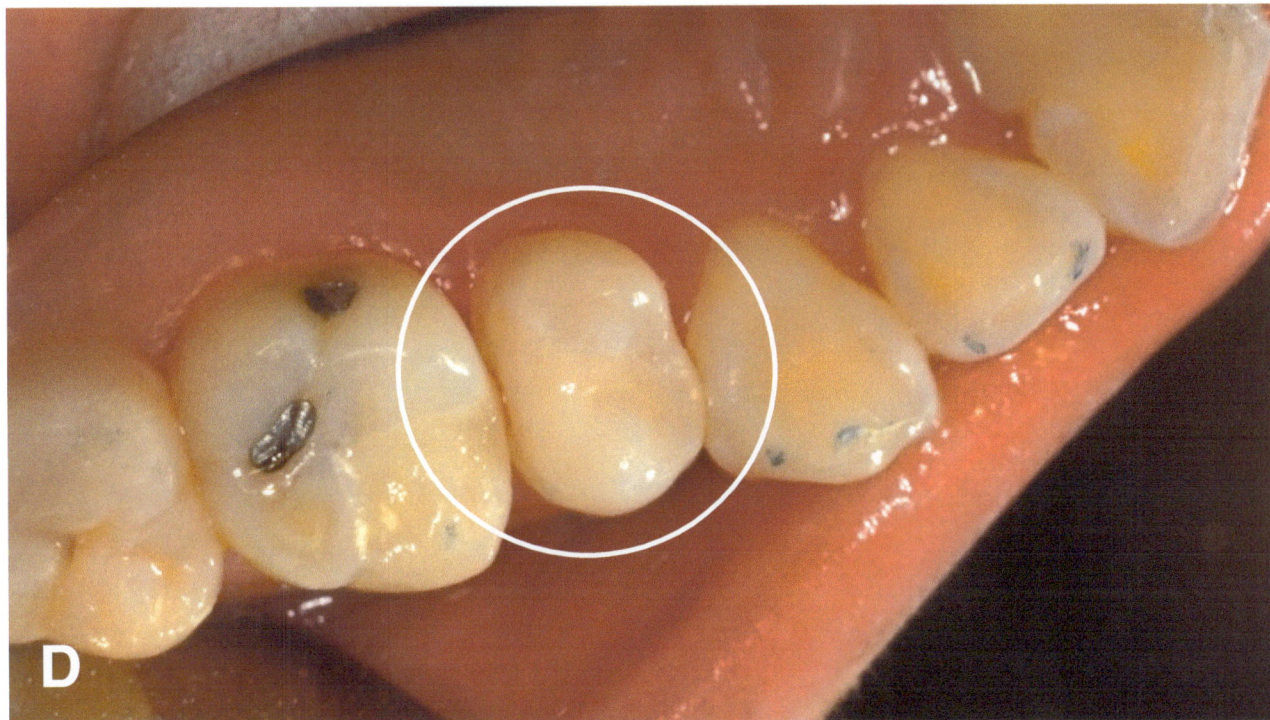

Decay has been removed and composite restorations (white filling) have been placed.

DISEASE (PATHOLOGY)

To understand disease and its effect on humans, you must understand health. In dental school, we spent four years studying the structure and function of the body, and more specifically, the oral cavity. Prior to dental school— during my undergraduate education—the general curriculum included courses in the humanities, sociology, and psychology. With all this knowledge regarding humanity and its environment, you would assume that arriving at a definition for health would be easy, and I guess you could say that a body without disease and one that hasn't sustained too much trauma is in good health.

But a body is subject to irritants and stress factors that tend to lower its resistance to the disease process. If one ate perfect foods, lived in a perfect environment, and constantly received proper love, friendship, and moral support, the body would function optimally, age gracefully, and eventually die (though I believe we will eventually find a way around death).

Back in the real world, we try our best to live and be happy. We overdo some things, learn (we hope) from our mistakes, and tend to stay relatively healthy. This is the civilization we were born into, and we do our best to cope.

Keep It Simple

The more complex your preventive program becomes, the less likely you are to pursue it for life. Fluoridated water systems have greatly reduced cavities. This additive, along with proper brushing at least twice a day is the basic preventive program.

To intelligently evaluate a hygiene program, consult with your dental professional. Periodic visits to the hygienist will allow you to implement the simplest and most effective hygiene procedures. Most people need to see a hygienist twice a year; however, this depends on your personal requirements. Different oral hygiene requirements occur because people have a variety of needs throughout their lives. I never used dental floss until about the age of 40, and my present condition is excellent.[14] For the past 11 years, I have used floss due to a change in my physiology that favored accumulation of plaque (Glide® Floss – it's easy to use... I love it. W. L. Gore & Associates, Inc. 1-800-645-4337). If you have undergone periodontal surgery or have had implants or other complex dental treatments performed, your visits should generally be more frequent.

Dental disease is related to two variables: 1) things you have control over, i.e., prevention, proper brushing (removal of plaque), professional cleanings (removal of tartar), periodic exams; and 2) things you don't control, i.e., bad dental treatment or a genetic predisposition to disease. Even with a predisposition you can compensate with a good exercise program, improved diet and proper use of vitamins and minerals.[15]

---

14. This should not be interpreted to mean that the use of floss is not beneficial. Patients need to discuss their individual needs with their dental professional.

15. Knowing when and how to dose vitamin and mineral supplements remains an overall difficult task. Until this area of therapeutics becomes scientifically verifiable and quantitatively accurate, its exact benefits will remain elusive.

Disease of the Mouth

Many diseases affect the mouth. Two that affect most people are cavities (carious lesions) and gum disease (periodontal disease). I will first discuss cavities.

Cavities (Carious Lesions)

In its simplest definition, a cavity is a hole in a tooth. As you explore the cause, or etiology, you find that a complex combination of pre-conditions needs to exist in order for a cavity to develop. It is generally believed that acid by-products produced by certain bacteria, which feed on sugar, are the culprits. However, this simple explanation doesn't explain differences in individual susceptibility. Two people can have generally the same diet, yet one may get numerous cavities and the other will remain healthy. So what other variables exist?

Genetic inheritance accounts for differences in such things as the exact chemical makeup of the saliva, the tooth anatomy, and the tooth's position in the mouth. As for saliva, its chemical make-up and cleansing actions promote health.   Situations whereby salivary flow is reduced (*xerostomia* or *dry mouth*)—such as in elderly patients taking certain medications or cancer patients subjected to radiation therapy—often result in increased susceptibility to tooth decay. Differences in tooth anatomy may make some individuals more prone to decay. The pits and fissures on certain molar teeth (back teeth) may make proper brushing more difficult, and bacteria may find these "dark caverns" an ideal living place to produce their acids. Similarly, a crowded or "twisted" tooth may make brushing difficult, allowing cavity-forming substances to remain on the teeth.

High stress levels have been shown to lower a person's resistance. This phenomenon has been related to a periodontal deterioration called acute necrotizing ulcerative gingivitis – or trench mouth

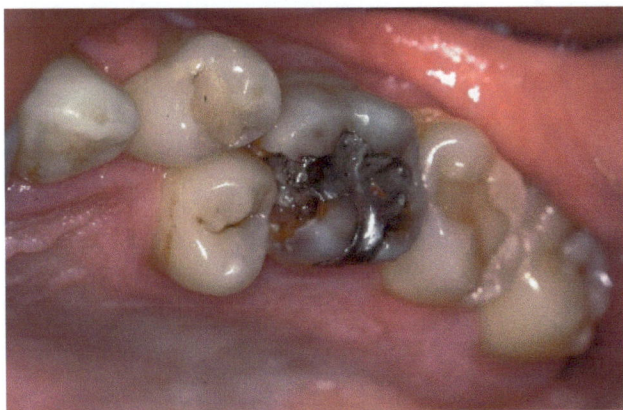

Pathologic eruption of this tooth has resulted in crowding. This created an area that was inaccessible to normal hygiene procedures, resulting in decay.

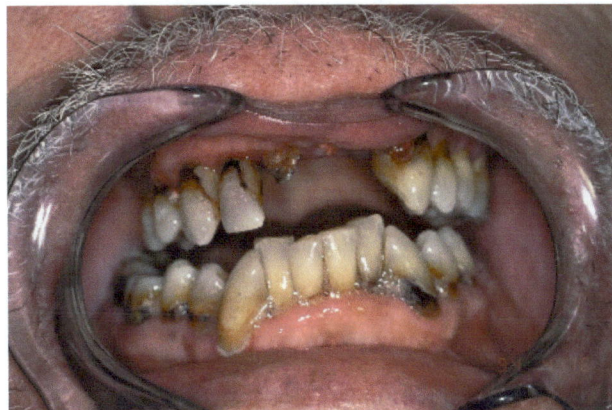

Rampant decay. Many medications reduce salivary flow which may result in dental deterioration.

(occurring among soldiers in the trenches or among college students at times of crucial exams). Stress may also be a contributing factor in the "cavity prone" adolescent years. This, along with hormonal changes, may influence a person's susceptibility to cavities.

A major contributing factor to tooth decay is iatrogenic dentistry, which occurs when the dentist, in some way, aids the development of tooth decay. Poorly executed fillings with open margins allow bacteria to leak into exposed tooth structure, causing recurrent decay. Poorly constructed crowns, bridges, and partial dentures[16] also contribute to this type of decay.

But why would a dentist do this to you? Probably, not on purpose. Most dentists are sincerely concerned with excellence and feel very bad when things don't always go

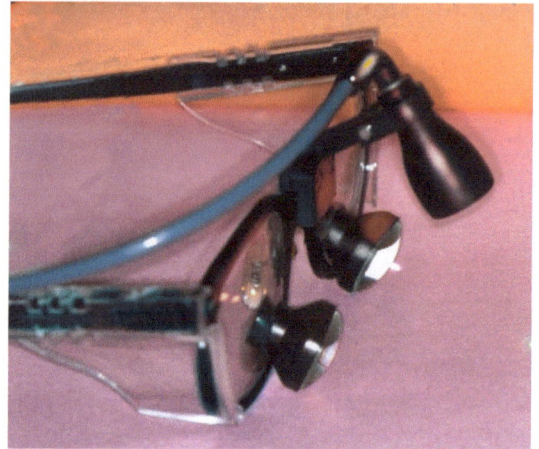

Custom lenses with magnification. Also a high powered light source allows a dentist to see much better. Designs for Vision, Inc. 1-800-345-4009

right. After all, their efforts need rewards other than money to add dignity and satisfaction to their job. But when financial constraints exist, or an inexperienced or anxious practitioner performs procedures, problems develop.

Dental procedures should always be performed with high-powered lenses, good illumination and a quiet atmosphere. Dentistry requires precise, intricate operations. If a dentist is rushed or running between treatment rooms or is just agitated, results can be compromised. Other factors that hinder results are the quality of the materials (using inferior materials to save costs) and the quality of the laboratory technician. Compromises ultimately cost the patient more time and money—and possibly the loss of teeth.

A dentist friend of mine (Dr. Steven Green of Miami, Florida) is actively involved in vitamin and mineral therapy in his general dental practice. He is quite knowledgeable regarding biochemistry and its clinical relevance. He told me that tooth sensitivity and decay are often related to a complex chemical process, and said he has successfully reversed some of these clinical inflammatory episodes with counseling of these stressed patients as well as with specific vitamins and minerals. Though I am not a biochemist, nor am I a researcher in the academic sense, his philosophy of treatment intrigues me. This is an area of dentistry that was not discussed in dental school and, even today, it is rarely mentioned in journals and dental meetings. Dr. Green's biochemical analysis relates the deterioration in the mouth to inflammatory and degenerative changes in other areas of the body. He also talks of vitamin therapies, antioxidants, and how such ailments as arthritis, heart disease, and numerous other systemic conditions have more of a common whole system interrelationship. This "whole" concept is interesting because it places "dental disease" in perspective with a patient's other inflammatory conditions.

As research in these areas continues, developments will, we hope, make sense of these diverse relationships, and specific tests will lead to improved preventive therapies.

16. Partial dentures have clasps that attach to teeth, as compared to full dentures where no teeth are present—refer to the chapter on Prosthetics.

Cavity Diagnosis

Cavities are discovered by either visual probing of the area and/or with radiography (x-rays). When examination reveals a large, obvious cavity, diagnosis is easy; however, some cavities are quite small when first discovered or hidden beneath a previous filling or other type of restoration. Cavities can also appear slightly beneath the gum line, making visual diagnosis difficult.

Many times a small cavity may be diagnosed as arrested decay—meaning the lesion has stopped progressing and treatment may not be necessary. If a dentist is in doubt, future periodic exams will help determine the status—in other words, leave it alone and check it later.

Radiographically, cavities appear as dark areas. An experienced dentist can usually detect these lesions. Improvements in dental radiography—use of digital and computer devices—have greatly aided diagnosis. Once a dentist discovers a cavity, its position and size are registered in a dental examination chart. This, along with all other information, forms the basis for a plan of treatment.

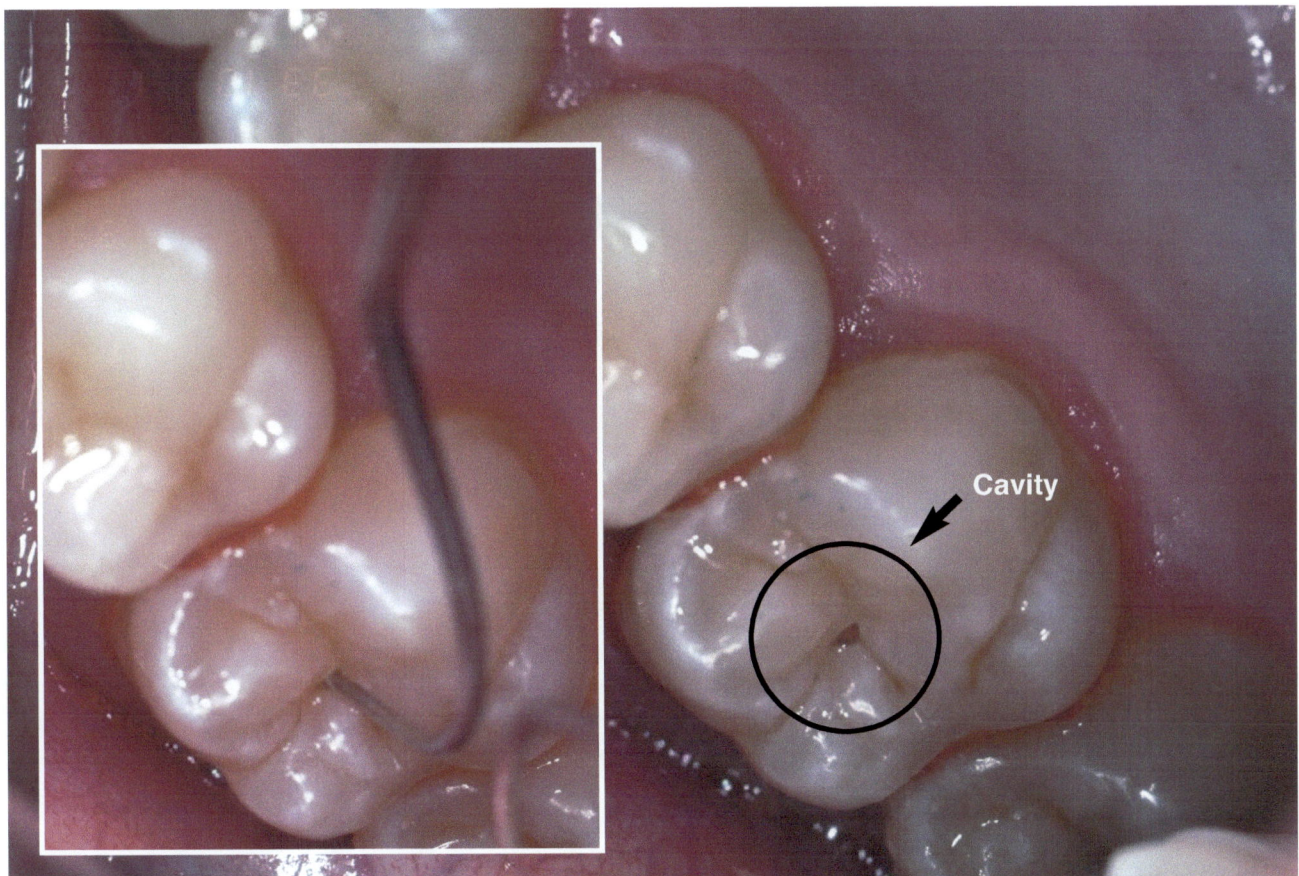

Cavity

A small pit is initially probed with an explorer.

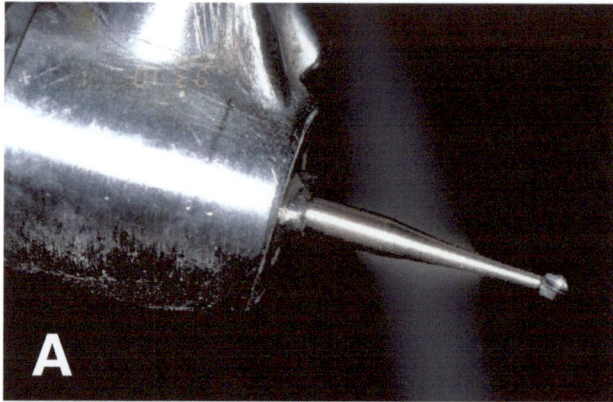

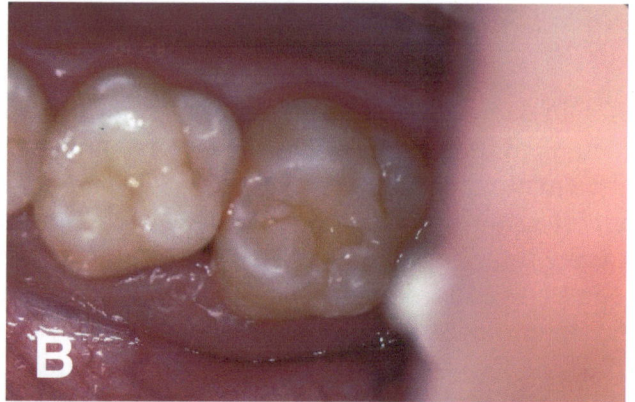

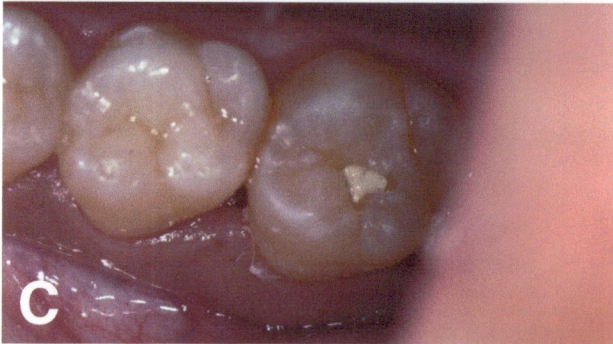

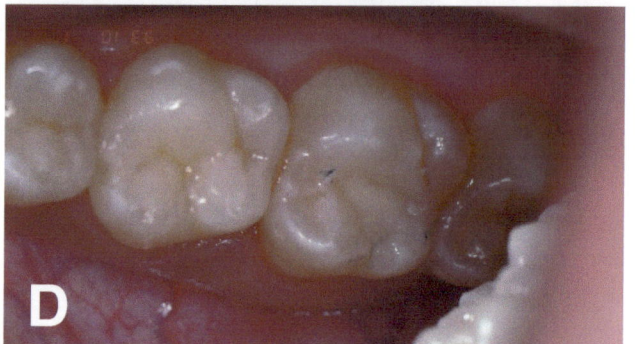

Conservative cavity excavation preserves healthy tooth structure.

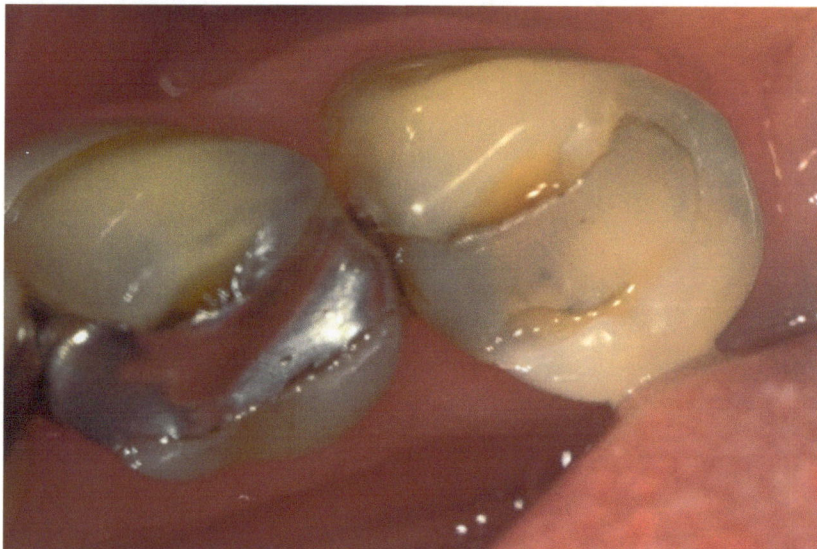

Defective restorations / recurrent decay.

Cavity Diagnosis and Restoration

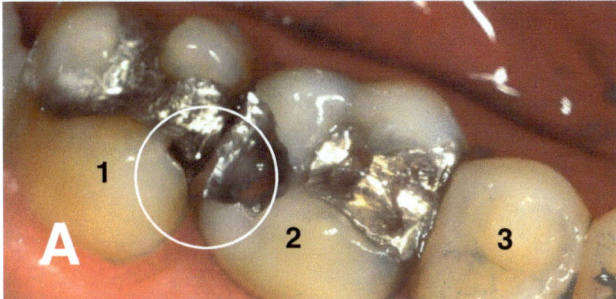

Recurrent decay adjacent to an amalgam restoration.

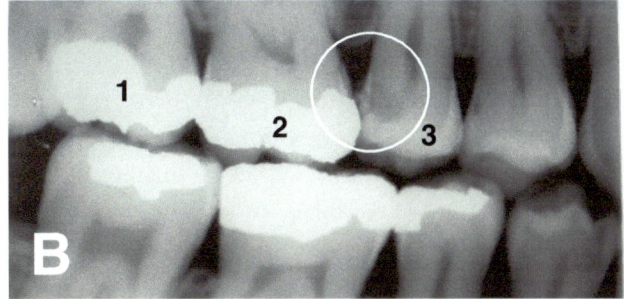

Radiographic appearance of decay on an adjacent tooth.

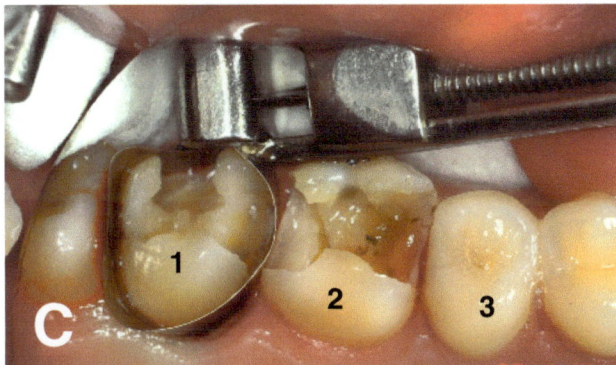

Removal of all amalgam, decay and soft tooth structure.

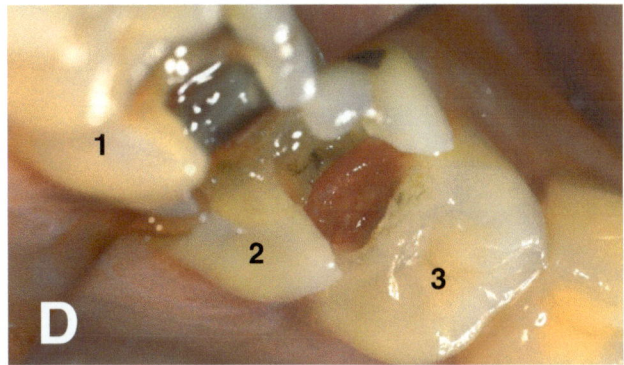

Hidden decay becomes obvious on this bicuspid tooth

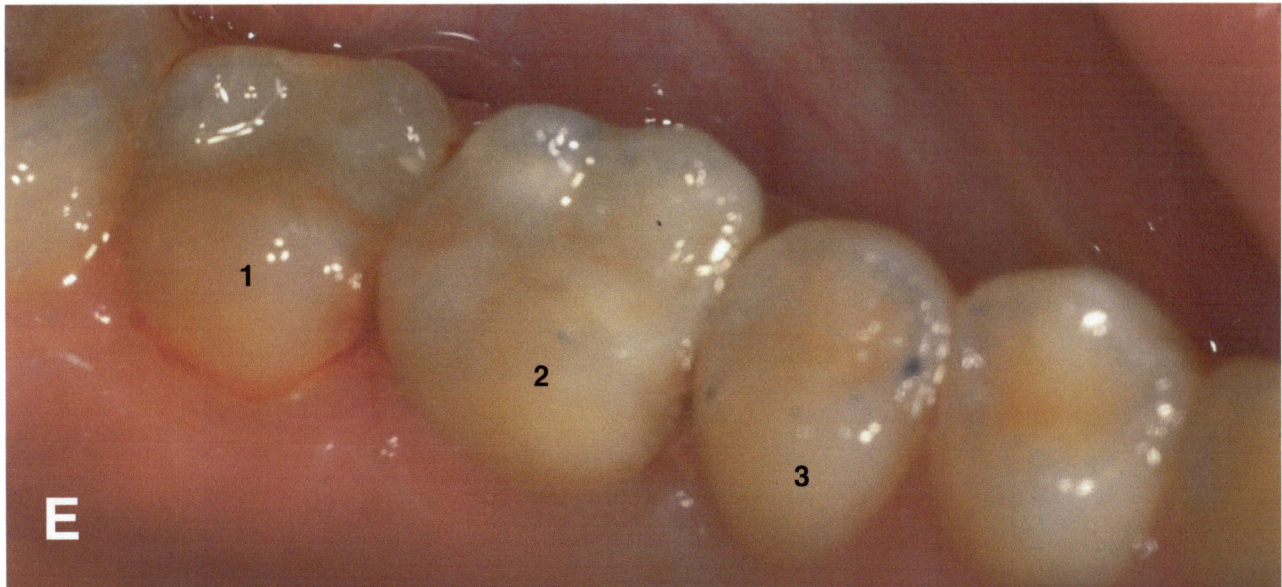

Routine operative procedures are performed and final composite restorations are placed.

Treatment Options

Treatment of cavities usually involves removal of all decay and placement of a filling. If the decay is small, anesthesia is often unnecessary. There are many types of filling materials. In the past, the filling most often used for the back teeth was a material called amalgam—

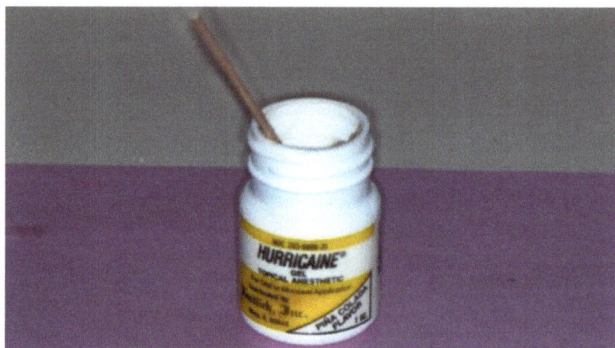

When anesthesia is necessary, topical anesthesia placed prior to the injection helps reduce patient discomfort.

a combination of silver, mercury, and other elements. I have had these types of fillings in my mouth for over 35 years with few problems. There is controversy today, however, regarding possible toxic effects caused by mercury in the amalgams.[17]

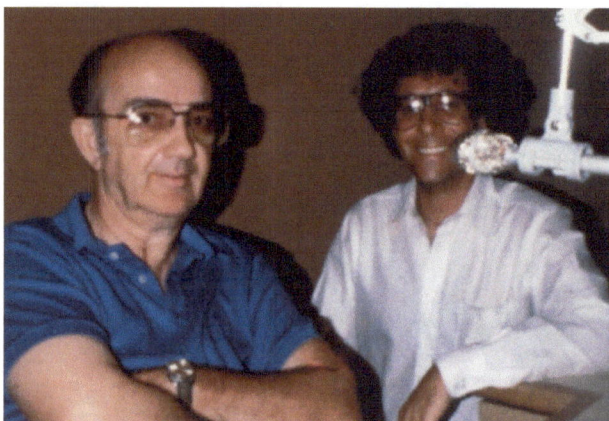

Defective amalgam restorations replaced with new ones. Polishing of these amalgams makes a smooth surface that is less susceptible to the accumulation of plaque buildup.

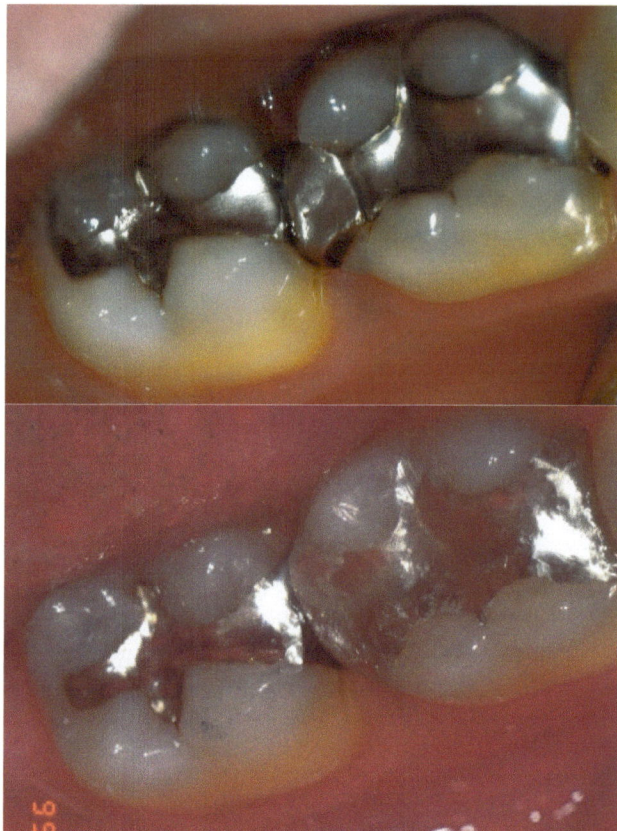

17. Though some patients may be sensitive to different materials and respond with different clinical symptoms, I believe the majority are not affected. About 10 years ago, when my friend Bill Calder hosted his fantastic Miami radio show (he used to do bits with Larry King), he regularly invited me as a guest to talk about music and dentistry (He called me the singing dentist. When I asked him how many singing dentists there were, he responded straight faced and said ten.). Since I was asked so many questions about the mercury filling issue, I investigated the facts and opinions of various opposing dental groups. The American Dental Association indicated that these fillings were safe; the opposing dental association called the fillings poison. When I personally called the deans of a number of dental schools to see if they had these silver mercury fillings in their mouths, 100% of them informed me they did and believed there was no danger.

These gold restorations, called onlays have been in good shape for about 40 years.

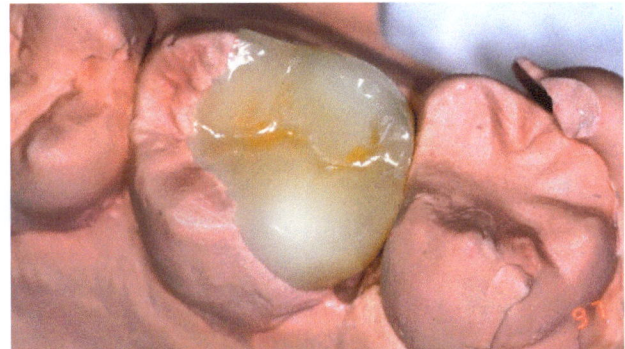

A laboratory processed restoration made on a model of an impression of the cavity preparation. This reinforced indirect "filling" is bonded into the tooth.

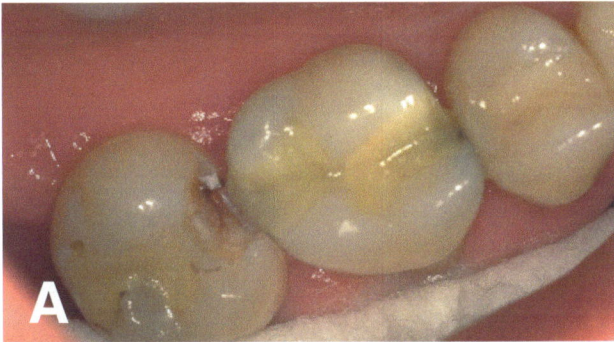

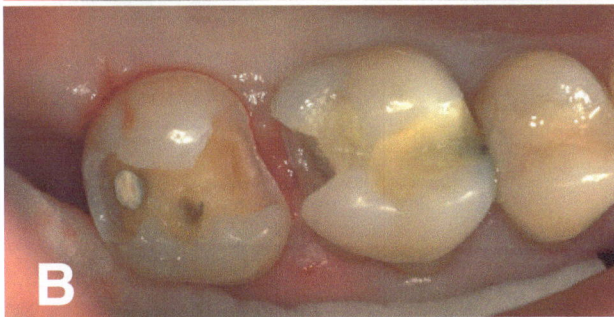

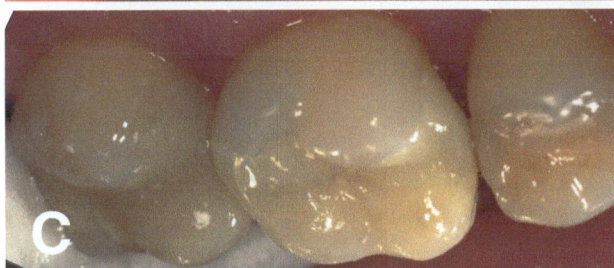

Replacement of worn/defective "plastic" restorations with an improved, more durable "composite".

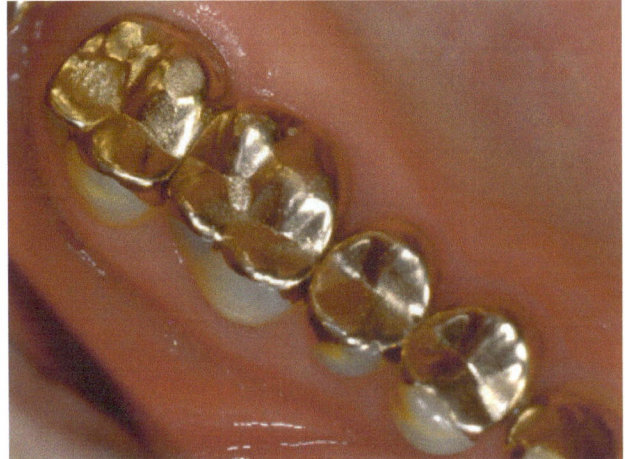

Today's trend, though, is to avoid these mercury-containing fillings and use tooth-colored, bonded composite restorations. The problem is that these reinforced plastic fillings don't necessarily hold up long term. (As their popularity and usage have increased, improvements have been made). Alternative restorations for back (posterior) teeth are bonded porcelain, gold fillings, or crowns. I have seen gold restorations in good shape 40 years after their placement. Hopefully, research in re-growing natural enamel will someday lead to the ultimate restoration.

Front teeth obviously need natural tooth-colored fillings. Bonded composites work well here. Though porcelain restorations tend to be superior, they do require the services of a good laboratory. The extra time and material make these procedures much more costly.

I will discuss prevention in greater detail later. For now, let me say that early decay detection is crucial, not only in terms of saving teeth, but also in saving time, money, and dental discomfort.

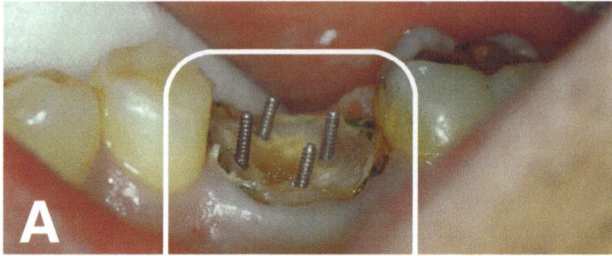

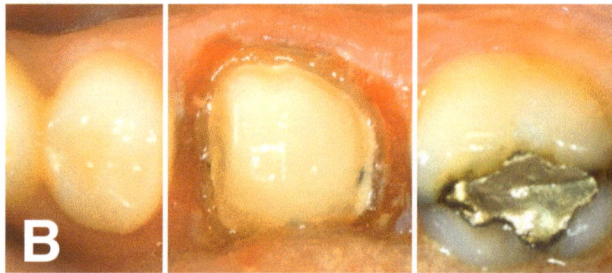

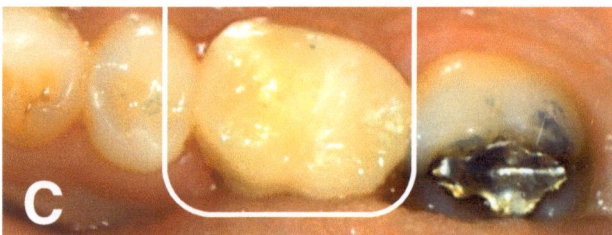

Severely damaged teeth can be restored with the utilization of titanium pins which help retain a bonded core. A porcelain fused to gold crown is then fabricated and cemented over the core.

Small cavities are easier to restore.

Larger areas of decay destroy more tooth structure and necessitate operative procedures closer to the pulp chamber, which houses the nerves and blood vessels. Not only are these teeth more difficult to restore, but nerve damage may also occur due to infection and trauma. The ability to bond the newer composite fillings in these situations allows the dentist to preserve more natural tooth structure. However, when a more substantial restoration becomes necessary, a crown is the preferred restoration.

A crown is an artificial tooth, fabricated by the dental laboratory, which is cemented onto the prepared remains of a natural tooth. Crowns can be made of gold, porcelain fused to gold, all porcelain or be constructed of other materials. If they are made properly, they will function well for years; if they are poorly made, or if inferior materials are used, they tend to do more damage than good (this applies to all dental restorations).

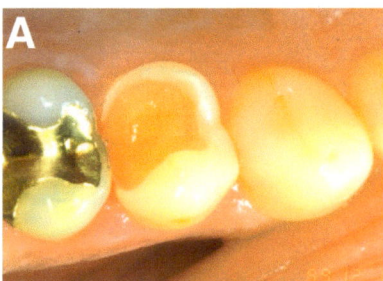

Very deep decay has been delicately dissected from this tooth.

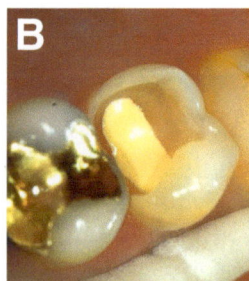

An anti microbial dressing has been placed. There is a good chance that the nerve tissue will survive and not require root canal therapy. This procedure is called an indirect pulp cap (as compared to a direct pulp cap where the nerve tissue is actually exposed).

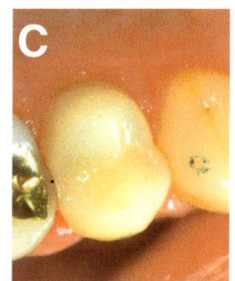

A composite restoration is placed.

"Fixing a Broken Filling"

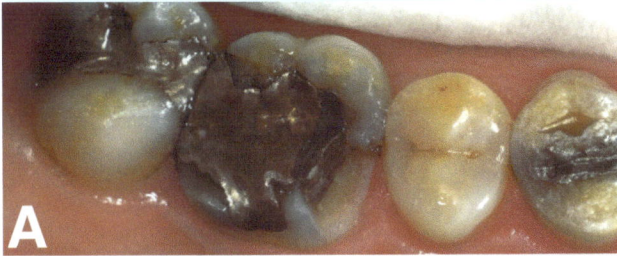

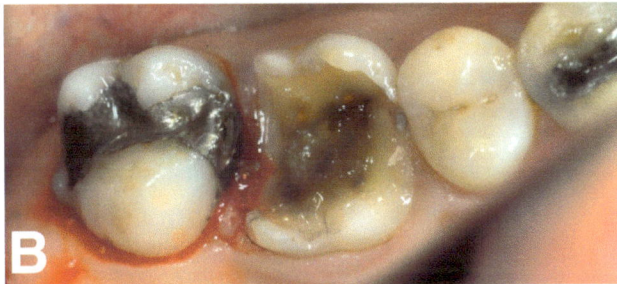

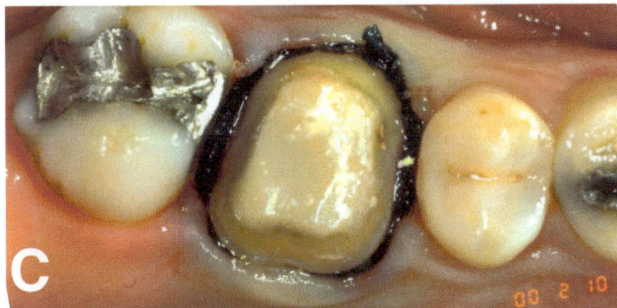

A

B

C

D

Crown cemented in patient's mouth

E

F

This patient presented to my office with a large fractured amalgam restoration. Following removal of all the amalgam and all soft tooth structure, a core material was placed. Tissue retraction cord is utilized to separate the gum from the margin of the preparation prior to taking an impression. (A, B and C).

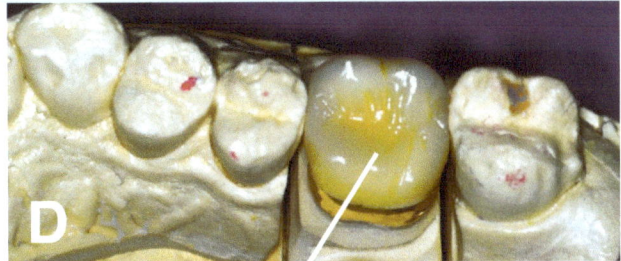

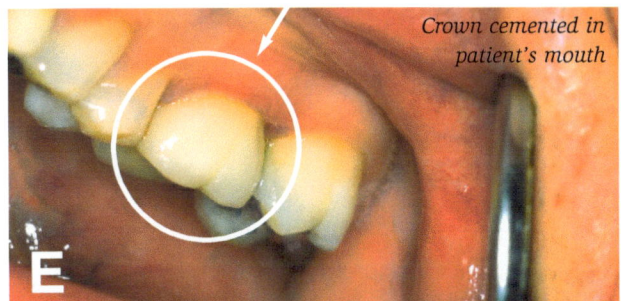

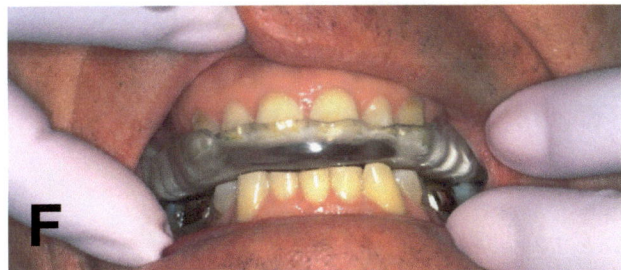

The impression is taken and sent to the laboratory for the fabrication of an artificial crown. Since this patient had a habit of grinding his teeth, we felt that a porcelain surface would be too fragile and therefore utilized a reinforced composite (plastic derivative) bonded to a gold core (fibercore crown, by Jeneric Pentron Co. 1-800-551-0283) (D and E).

We also made a bite appliance that the patient will wear in order to prevent damage to his teeth when grinding. (F)

Nerve Damage

Damage to the nerve of a tooth may occur due to physical trauma, deep decay, or any other aggravating circumstance that causes inflammation within the pulp chamber. This tissue has the ability to heal if the trauma is below a certain threshold or is of short duration. However, in a typical deep decay situation where there is chronic bacterial contamination, the nerve tissue eventually is destroyed and becomes what is called necrotic, or dead. Sometimes this occurs gradually, without the patient even experiencing a "toothache". Other times, there is acute[18] infection resulting in a toothache.

Treatment involves removing all debris from the pulp chamber and root canals, cleaning and disinfecting these areas as well as possible, and finally, placing a filling material called gutta percha. Welcome to the world of Root Canal Therapy.

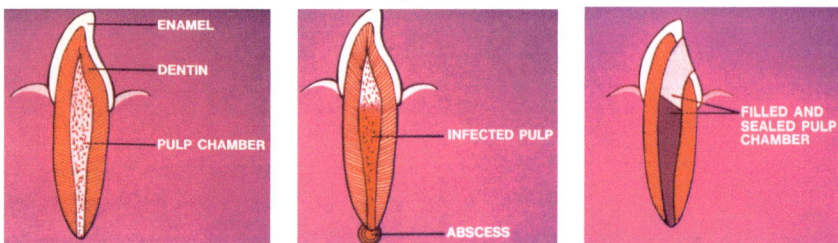

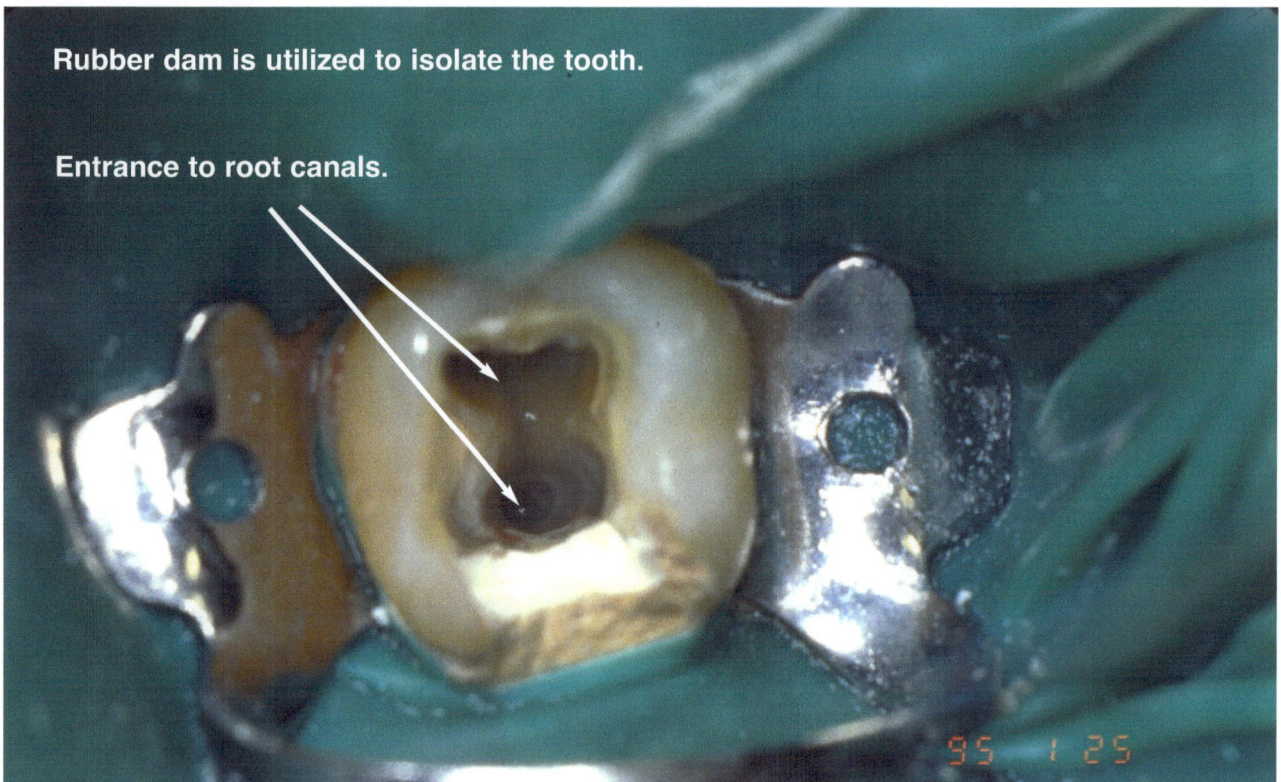

Rubber dam is utilized to isolate the tooth.

Entrance to root canals.

95 1 25

---

18. Acute: Immediate as compared to chronic—which is long term.

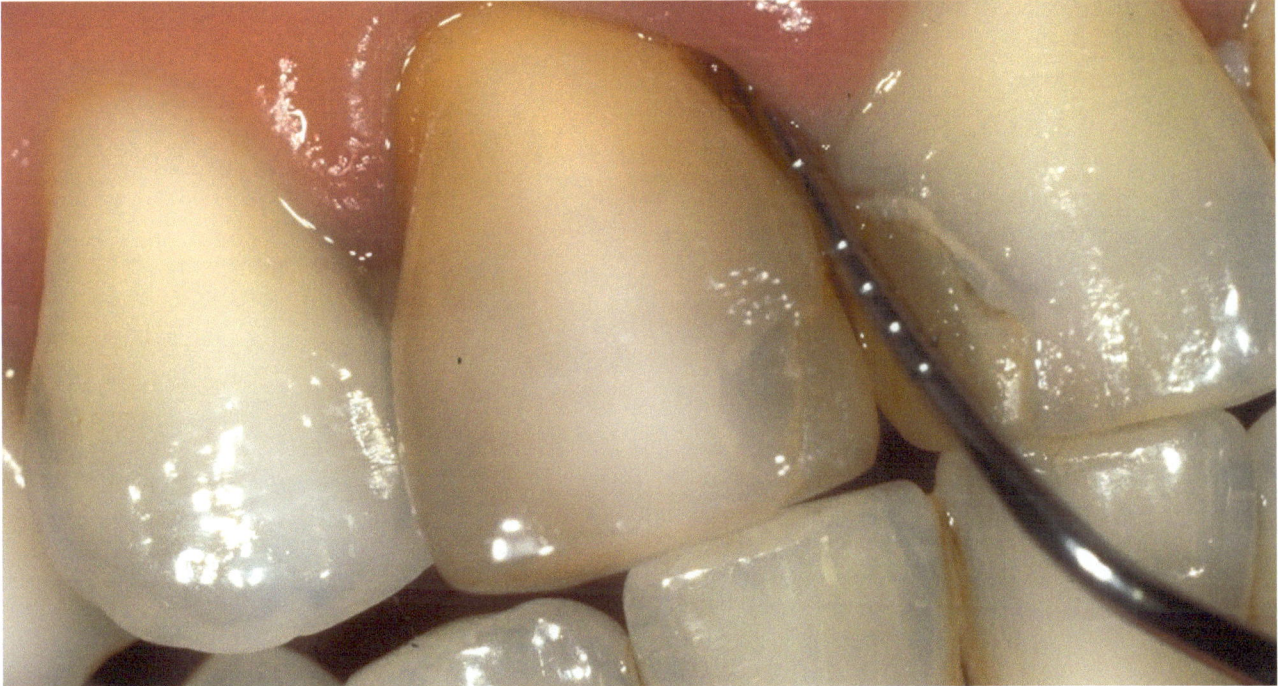

Dead (necrotic) nerve tissue along with other deteriorated blood components have diffused into this tooth and has caused this type discoloration. In this particular case the problem is compounded by a deep periodontal pocket.

Recently, I ran into Holly, the office manager who works for the dermatologists downstairs. Holly is not only a very nice person, but also a great administrator. I told her I was running a special on root canals this week—two for the price of one—and we laughed. She then reminded me about the time when I saved her from having root canal therapy. A general dentist had referred her to a root canal specialist (endodontist) to evaluate a sensitive tooth. The endodontist told her that root canal therapy was necessary. Holly opted for another opinion and visited my office. I remember not seeing an obvious reason for root canal therapy. I did, however, see a somewhat traumatic "bite," so I adjusted her occlusion. Years later, she's still doing fine.[19]

Nerve Damage Diagnosis

Nerve damage severe enough to require root canal therapy can be diagnosed most often without a problem. When a patient has a toothache or deep decay, the dentist will evaluate a radiograph[20], anesthetize the tooth,[21] and remove all decay. If, in this process, the nerve becomes exposed, several options exist.

---

19. I believe most dentists render honest opinions, yet differences in diagnoses will occur. A nerve may "appear" normal yet slowly deteriorate over time. Honest differences in diagnosis should be differentiated from a blatantly fraudulent diagnosis.

20. A radiographic evaluation of a tooth in need of root canal therapy will generally show deep decay or a dark area at the end of the root (peri-apical radioluscency—indicating some bone destruction).

21. Sometimes drilling is done without anesthesia —slowly— to determine if the nerve has died. This is one of several diagnostic methods.

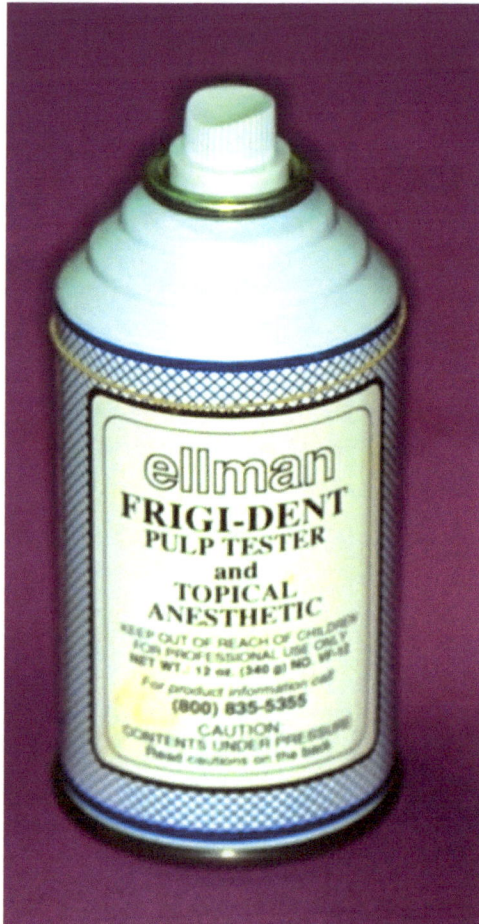

One of the ways to test tooth status is by placing a cotton pledget saturated with a freezing agent on the tooth. This tests for sensitivity to cold.

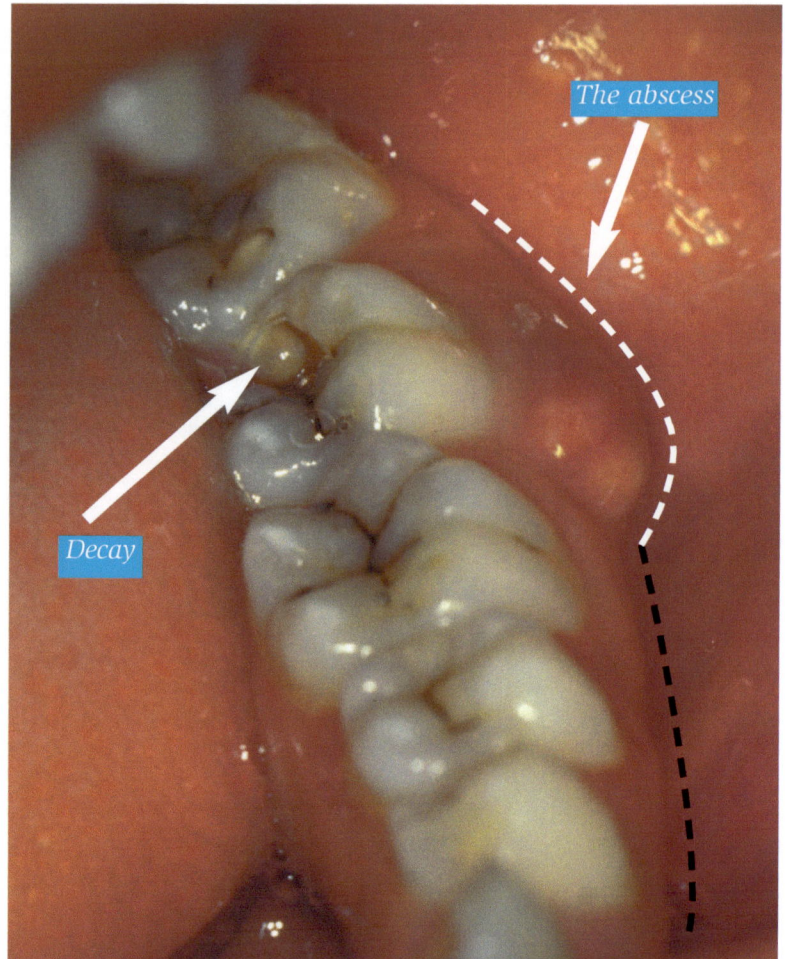

A badly decayed molar tooth shows signs of irreversible nerve damage resulting in an abscess.

If the exposure is small, a layer of medication can cover this area (pulp cap) and a filling can be placed. The tooth may be able to heal itself with no further problems. A larger exposure will generally require immediate removal of nerve tissue, irrigation with antiseptic solutions, and placement of a temporary filling. The stage is now set for future appointments to proceed with definitive root canal therapy. Sometimes infection travels down the root canal and destroys bone. This bone destruction can progress and forge passage exiting into the mouth. This results in drainage and is called a fistula (often accompanied by relief of pressure and pain). Another means of diagnosis is made based on a darkening of a tooth—especially if the patient has a history of trauma. A pulp test, whereby a mild electrical current is applied to the tooth, will often elicit a negative response, indicating a dead or dying nerve.

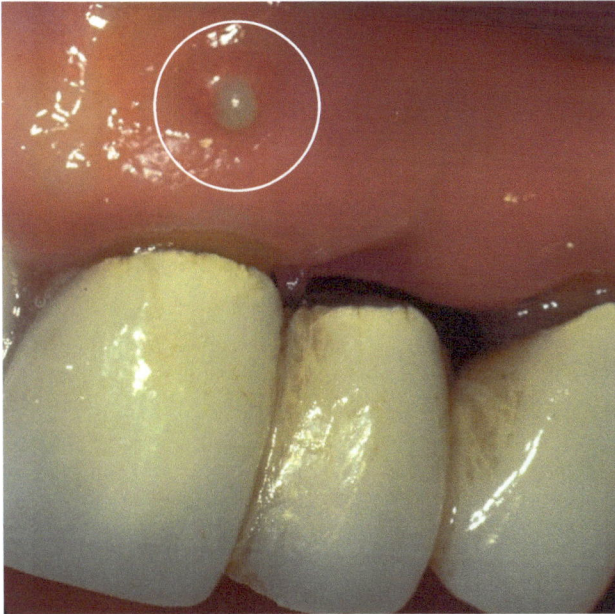

Once a painful abscess exits the tissue, the patient usually experiences relief from the discomfort of pressure. This exit tunnel is called a fistula.

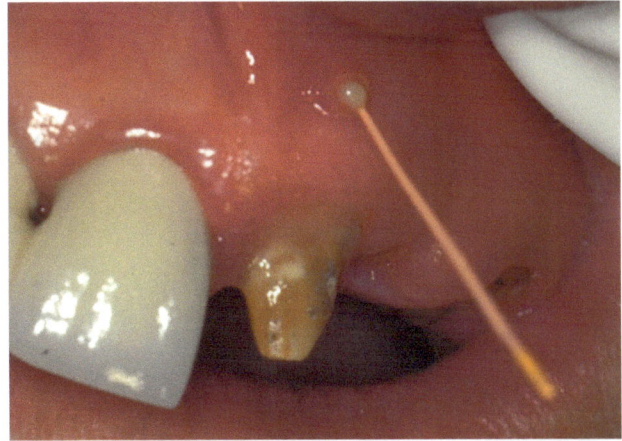

A gutta percha point besides being utilized to fill the root canal can also be used as a diagnostic pointer. When placed in the exit of an abscess it usually identifies the tooth origin of the infection when seen on an x-ray.

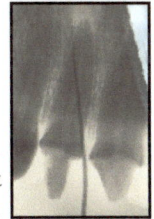

Radiographic appearance of gutta percha on another patient.

Sometimes obvious diagnostic signs—such as deep decay, radiographic evidence, a fistula, or change in color—are not present. An experienced dentist will excel in his or her diagnostic abilities and hopefully save the patient the time and expense of unnecessary treatment.

Drug Abuse And Dental Care Don't Mix

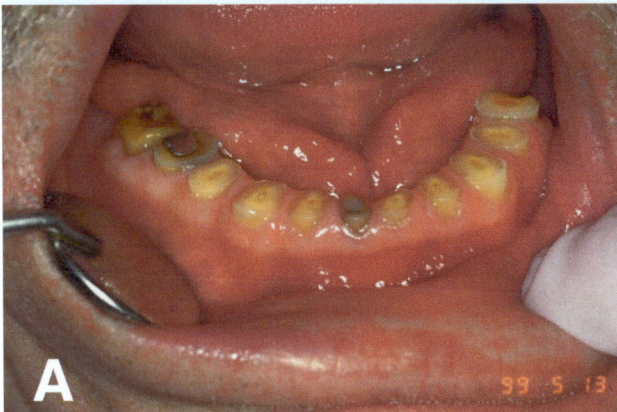

A

Before root canal therapy

B

After root canal therapy

C

A stoned (intoxicated) dentist destroyed all of my patient's lower teeth.

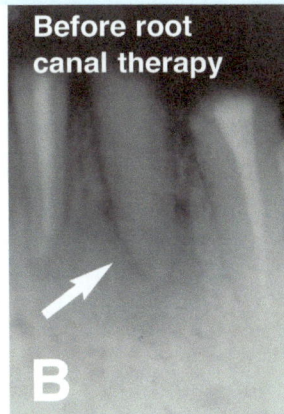

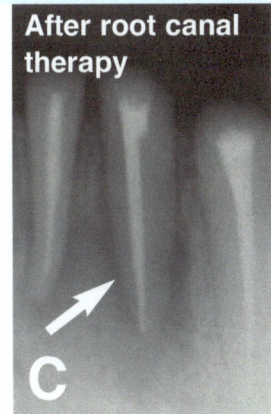

Root canal therapy became necessary.

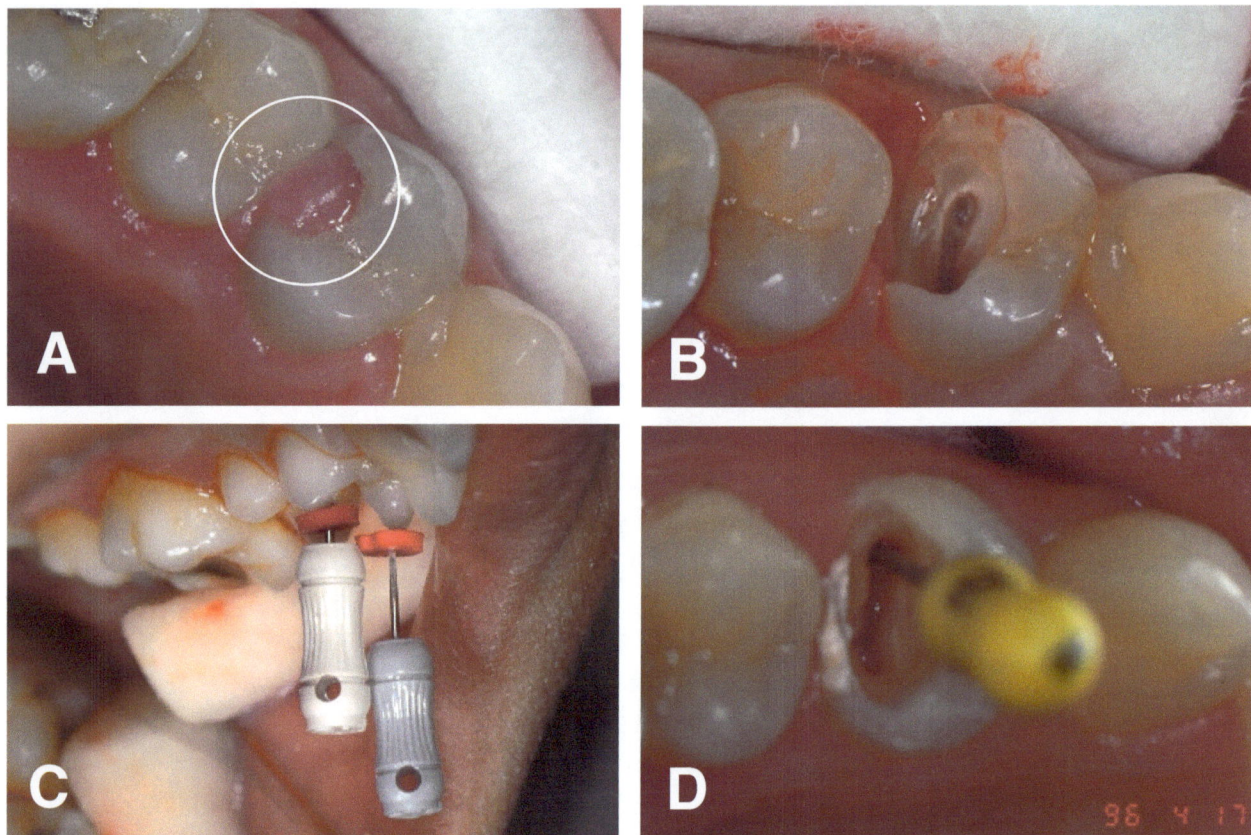

A- Overgrowth of inflamed tissue within a cavity.
B- Excavation of all soft tooth structure reveals necrotic debris within the root canals.
C- Two root canal files placed in two canals.
D- These instruments are utilized to clean and shape the canals.

Root Canal Therapy

Once a diagnosis is established and root canal treatment is indicated, therapy can begin. Whether a general dentist or an endodontist (root canal specialist) renders this therapy depends on the patient's decision after consulting with their general dentist. If the general dentist feels capable of performing the treatment, has good experience, and is honestly aware of his or her limitations, and if the patient is properly informed of the options and possible outcomes, then this educated patient can give an "informed consent."

In my practice, I perform most endodontic procedures—but after years of experience and a policy of accompanying my patients to specialists and observing procedures first hand—my background is solid. When I occasionally run into a problem, I again accompany the patient to a specialist.

Accessing The Root Canal

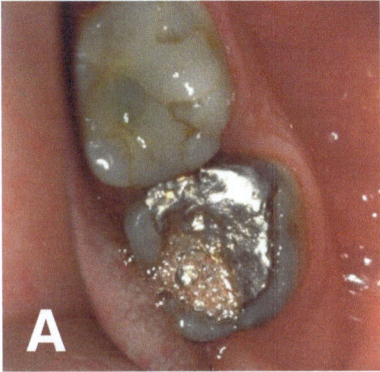

Old, leaking silver amalgam restoration.

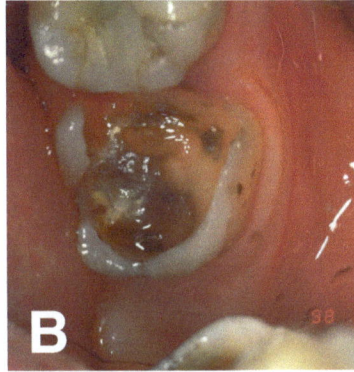

Following removal of the restoration dark, decayed tooth structure is evident.

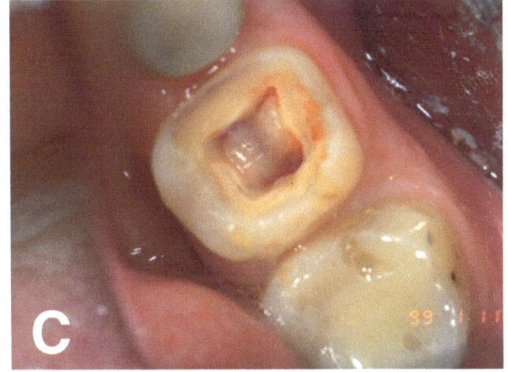

Upon careful dissection and removal of all infected debris exposure of the canals becomes evident. Inexperienced dentists sometimes fail to expose the total canal access for proper root canal therapy.

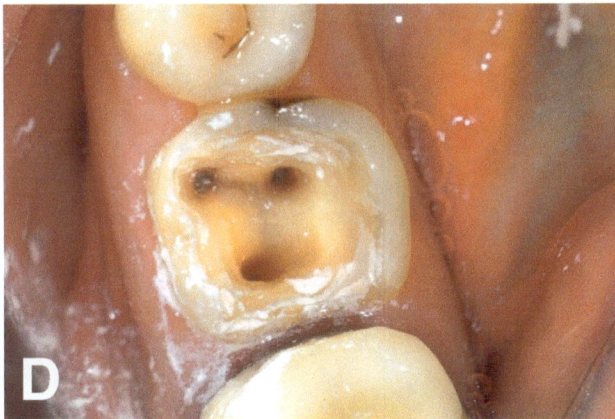

Proper access is achieved.

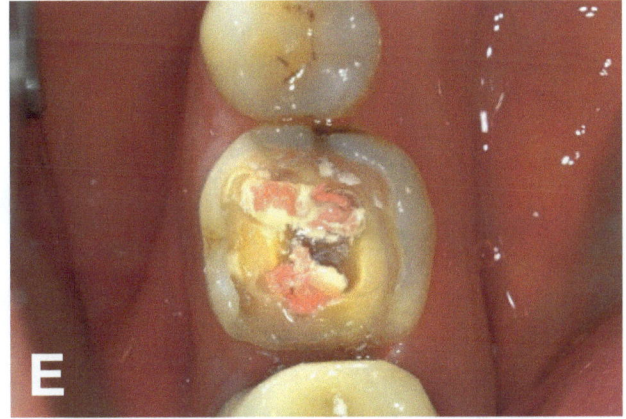

Once canals are cleaned, gutta percha points are cemented in the canals completing root canal therapy. Now the tooth needs to be restored.

Root canal therapy is often not as bad as its general reputation. Many times it can be completed in one appointment and in a painless manner. Patients can relax with headphones or watch virtual reality or movies.

The complexity and cost of the treatment depends on the tooth anatomy. Front teeth are easier not only in terms of accessibility but because they generally have single, larger roots. Back teeth are naturally more difficult for the opposite reasons. When a dentist takes the necessary time to properly evaluate the radiograph and anatomy and performs treatment with magnification and a good light source, successful treatment usually occurs.

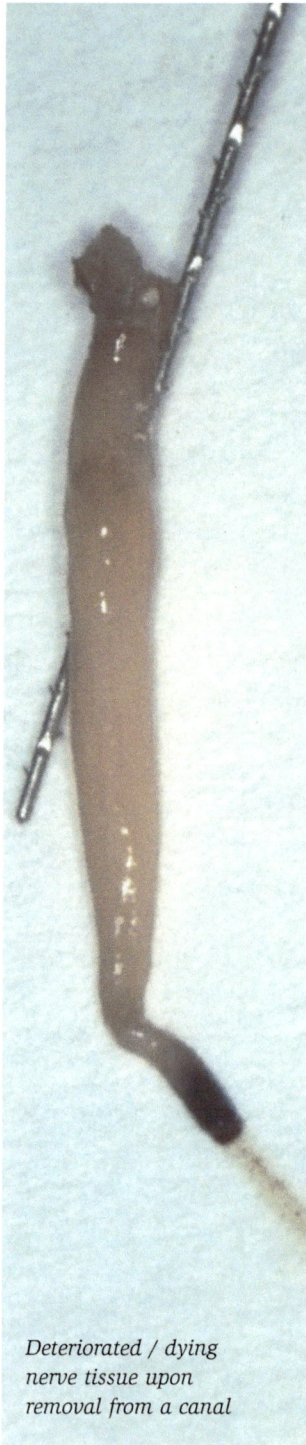

Root Canal Therapy and the Restoration　　　(Photos A – H)

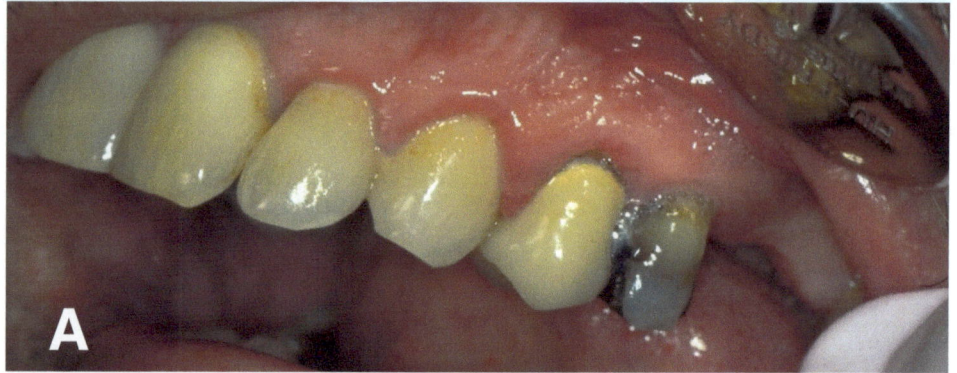

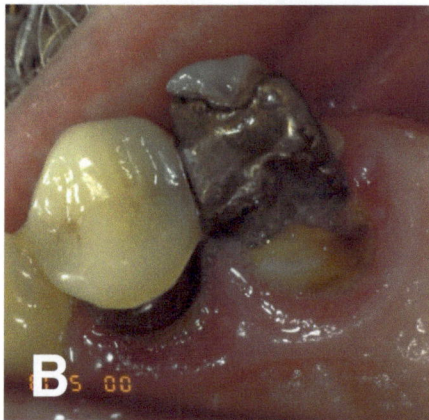

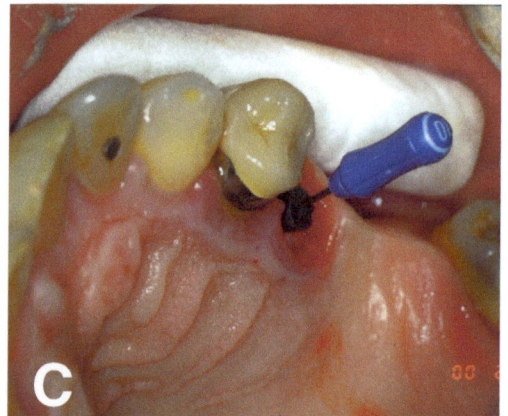

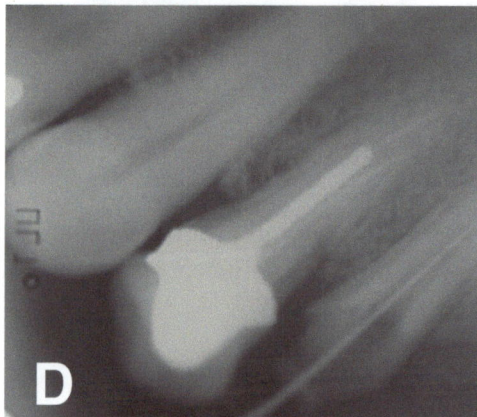

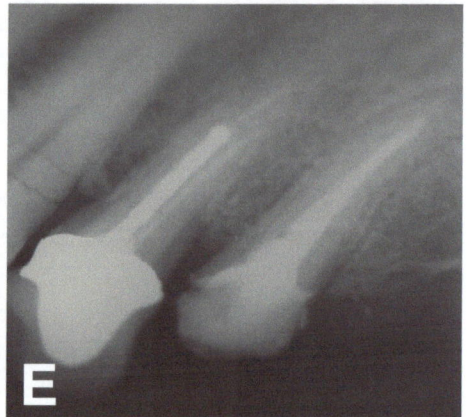

Deteriorated / dying nerve tissue upon removal from a canal

A and B - Initial appearance of a necrotic tooth with an old, fractured and unaesthetic amalgam restoration.

C, D and E - Following removal of the amalgam and all soft tooth structure, endodontic (root canal) therapy is initiated and completed.

Root Canal Therapy and the Restoration (Continued)

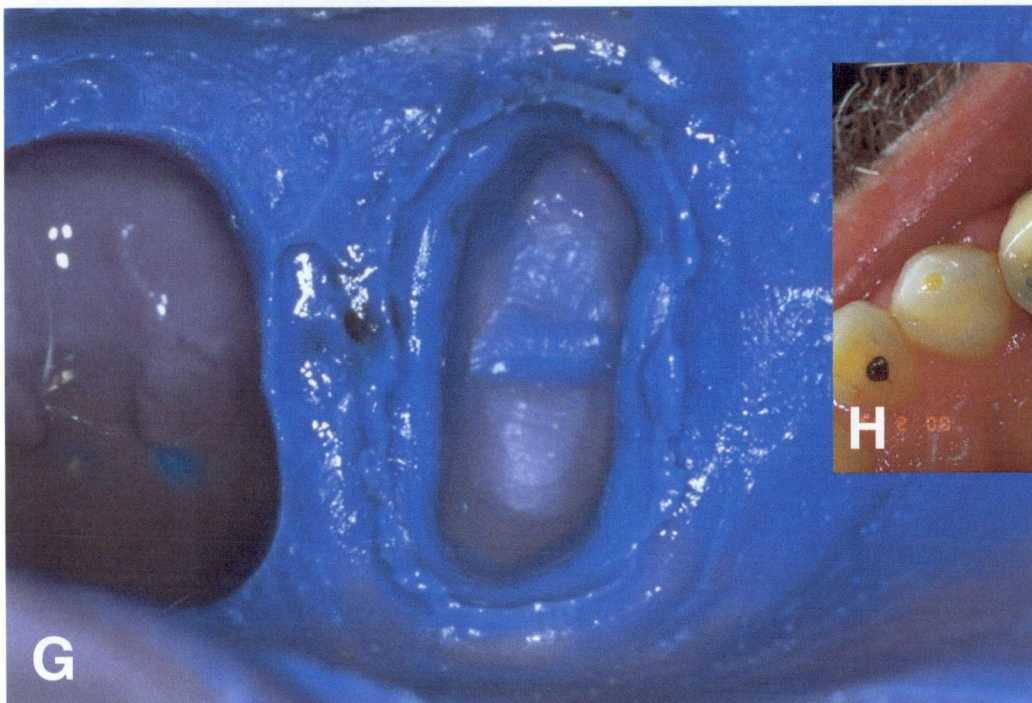

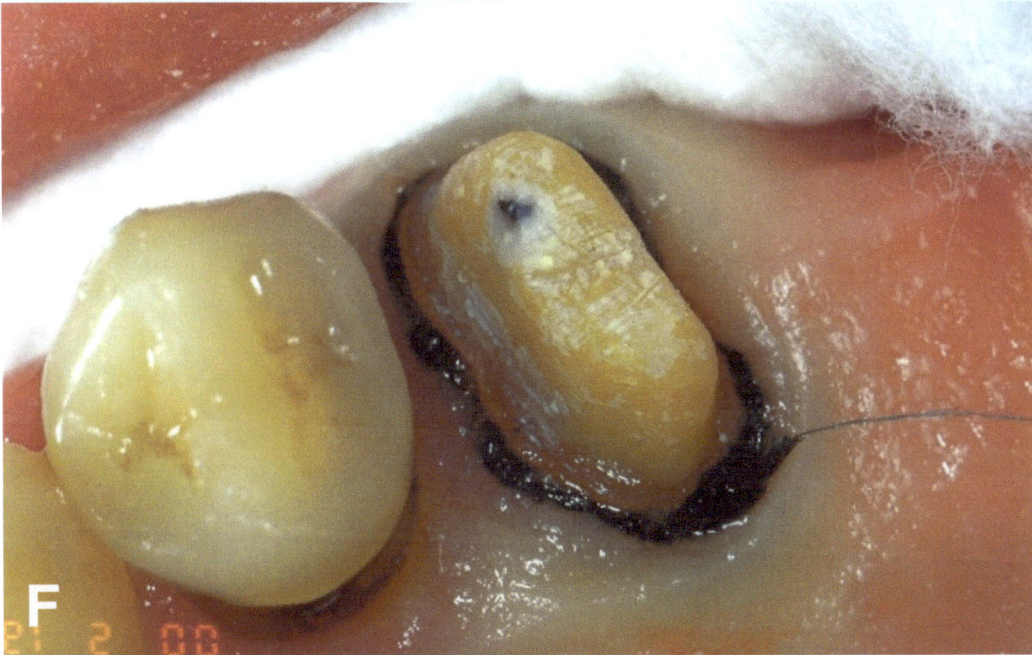

F -   A carbon fiber post and core (C-Post System, Bisco Dental Products 1-800-247-3368) is placed and gingival retraction cord is inserted. (This cord is removed just before the impression is taken – this allows the impression material to record the margins of the preparation while the adjacent gum tissue is temporarily displaced)

G - The success of the final crown is dependent upon the dentist spending the appropriate time necessary to take an accurate impression.

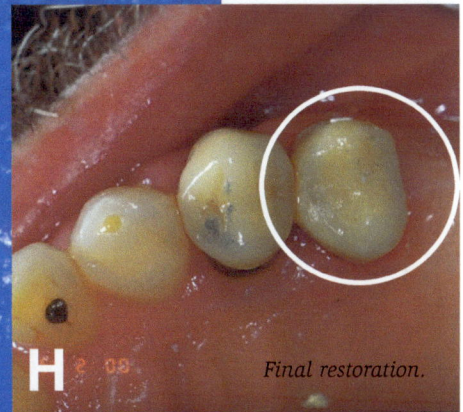

Final restoration.

Computer generated "optical impressions" are now being marketed. This technology may replace the present impression techniques.

Endodontic Surgery: The Apicoectomy

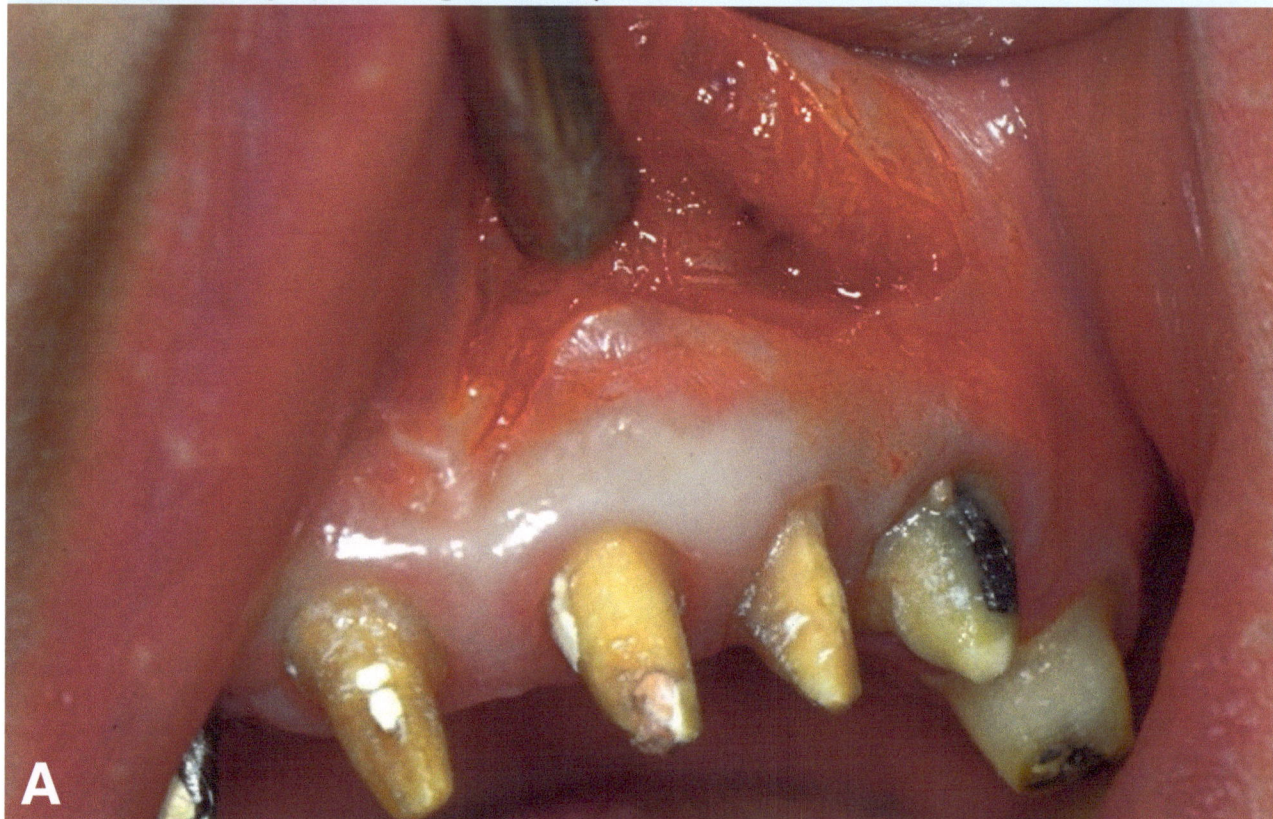

Chronic infection sometimes requires surgery. An apicoectomy is performed. This involves removal of chronic debris along with cutting off the end of the root and sealing the root canal.

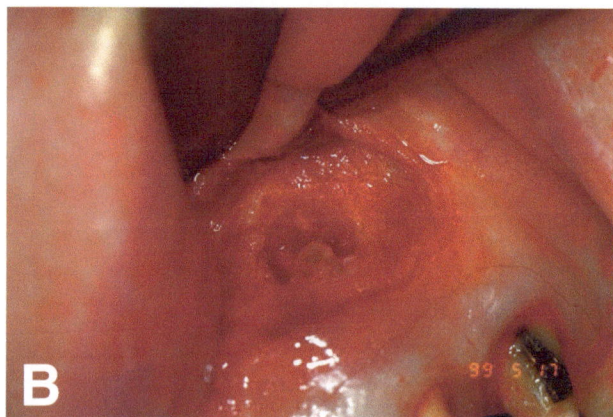

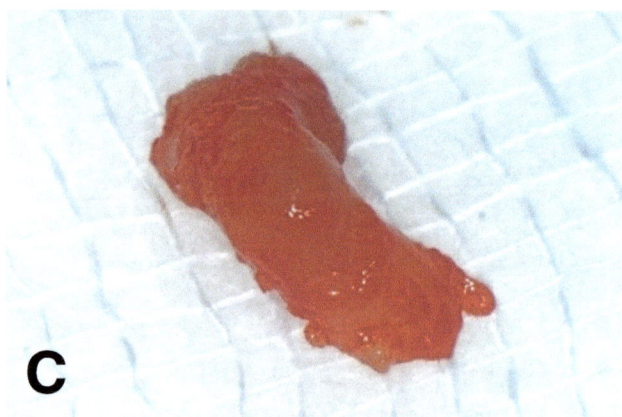

Tissue removed is often sent to the pathology lab for microscopic evaluation and definitive diagnosis.

Simultaneous Root Canal Therapy And Endodontic Surgery

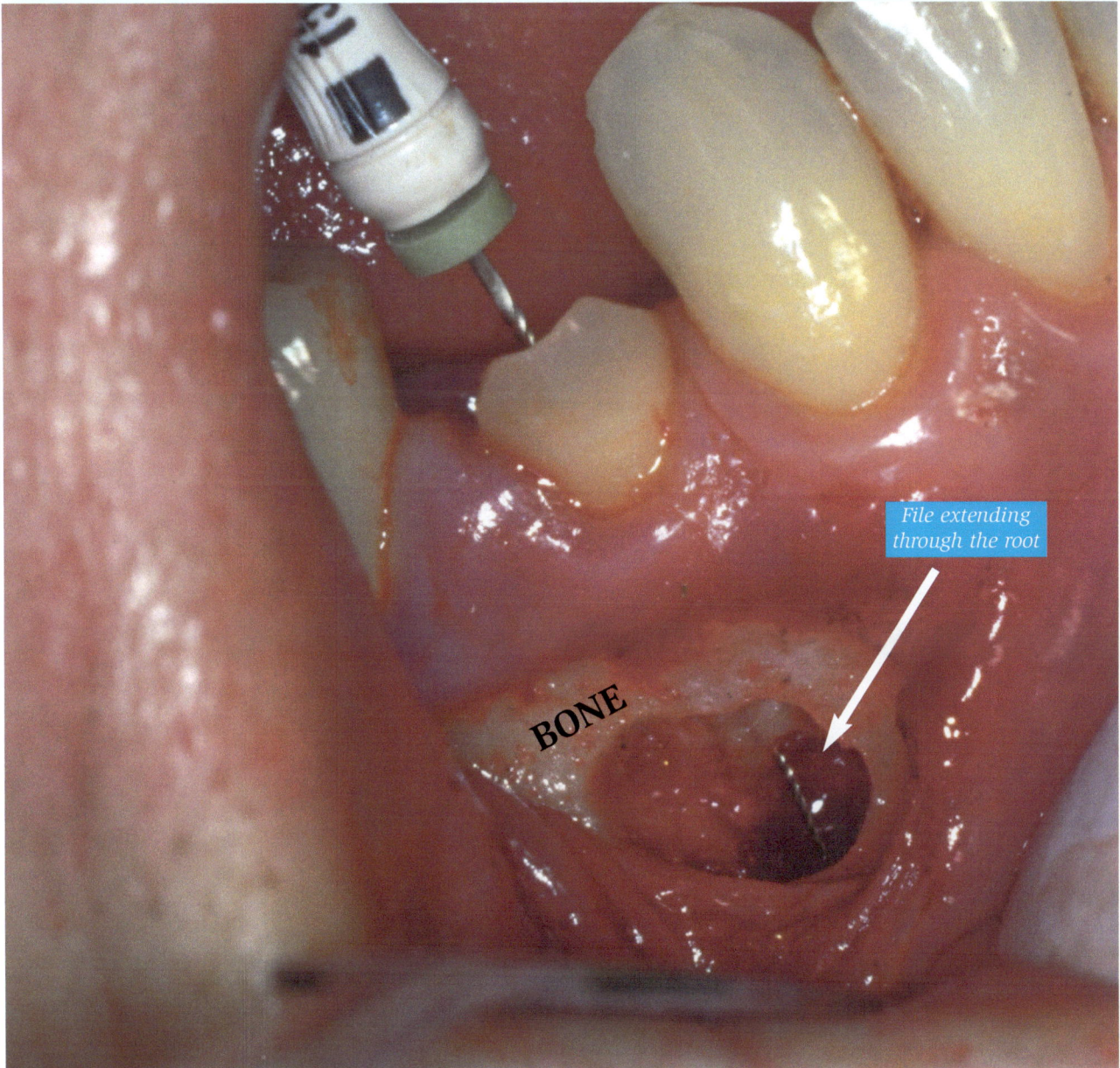

File extending through the root

BONE

An apicoectomy is sometimes performed along with standard root canal therapy. Here a file can be seen penetrating out of the canal into the abscessed area where bone destruction has occurred. Following these procedures bone re-growth usually occurs as a natural healing process.

After the Root Canal Therapy Is Completed

Now it's time to rebuild the tooth. The type of restoration depends on what is left of the tooth. In extreme situations, all that remains is a root. In this case, it is necessary to place a post into this root and build up the tooth around this supporting structure. Later, an artificial crown can be fabricated. When less tooth destruction has occurred, a post may not be necessary; bonding of composite material to rebuild the tooth can often suffice or act as a core buildup to support an artificial crown.

Often a patient questions if saving the tooth is worth the time and expense, especially one that is badly broken down. To answer this question, I use the analogy of a brick wall. Your teeth are like the bricks, each supporting the structural integrity of the wall. As bricks are lost, the wall gradually loses strength, and if enough bricks are lost, the wall collapses. When a tooth is lost, a shifting of adjacent teeth can also occur, creating unfavorable traumatic biting forces and difficult access for proper hygiene.

Tooth loss is fortunately not a life or death situation. As a matter of fact, dental services for some people are elective procedures. If you can afford the time and expense of saving a tooth, however, it is best to do so. Dentists sometimes make decisions based on the strategic significance of saving a particular tooth. A third molar (wisdom tooth) is best extracted. A front tooth loss would obviously leave a cosmetic problem. A tooth with a poor endodontic prognosis due to a difficult anatomical picture or some other technical hindrance might best be extracted.[22]

If the dentist decides to extract a tooth, the question then arises as to the necessity of artificially replacing this tooth with a bridge, implant, or other prosthetic appliance (or to leave the empty space as is—not all teeth need be replaced). The chapter on prosthetics will explain these options.

Fabrication Of Posts

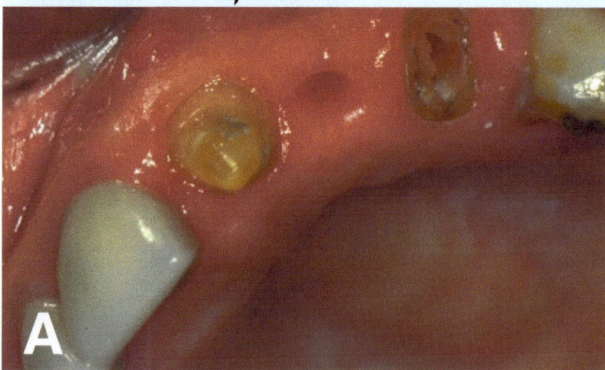

A

In this particular case, following root canal therapy only the roots are left to restore. In order to restore these roots it is necessary to fabricate posts.

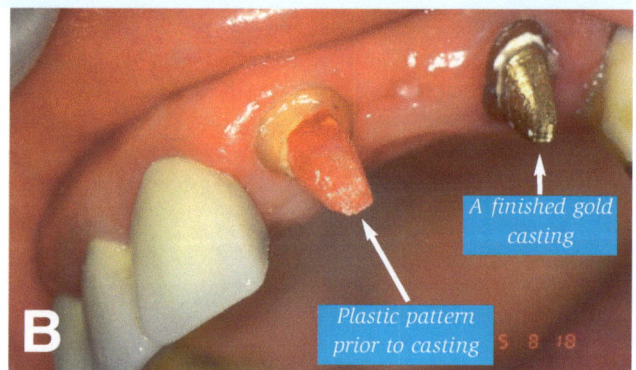

B

A finished gold casting

Plastic pattern prior to casting

A plastic pattern is fabricated and cast in gold. This is then cemented into the root canal. Artificial crowns or bridges are cemented onto these posts.

22. However, surgical procedures are sometimes used whereby the end of the root is cut off and a filling material seals this area. This is called an apicoetomy.

The Restoration Of An Endodontically Treated Tooth

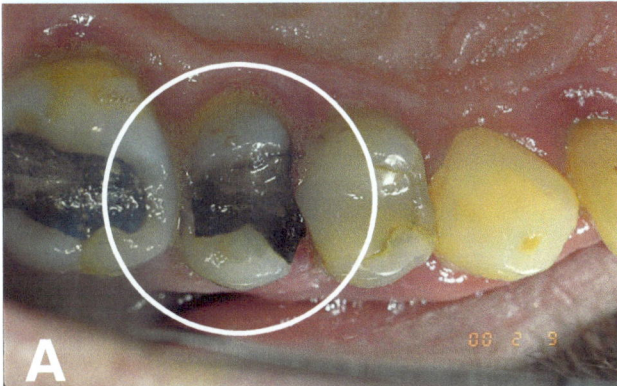

This patient presented with a necrotic tooth and large, old amalgam restoration.

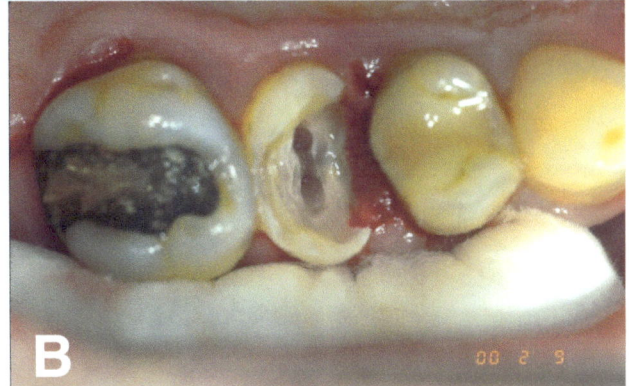

Following removal of the amalgam and meticulous dissection of all soft tooth structure, the canals are located.

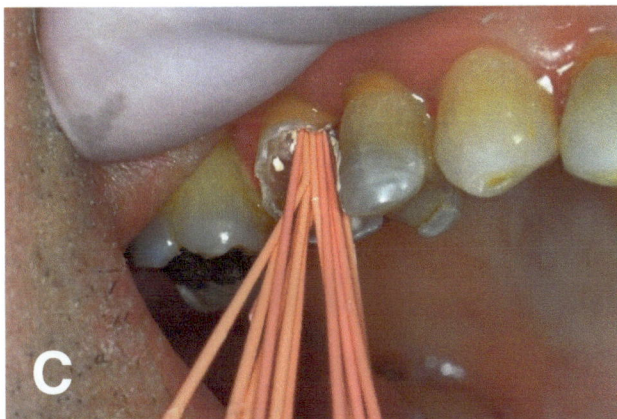

Root canal therapy is completed.

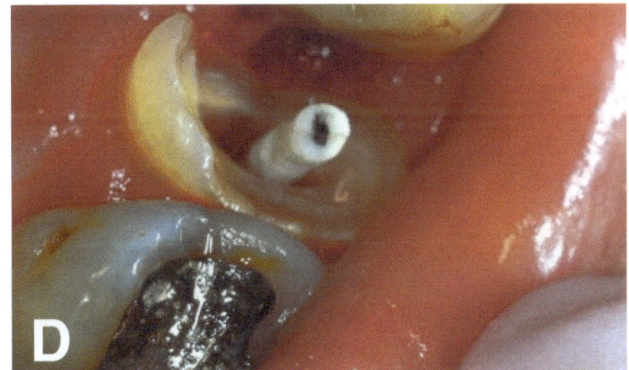

A carbon fiber post (C-Post) is bonded into the canal. These synthetic post systems seem to be replacing the gold cast posts in terms of their less complicated and more effective utilization.

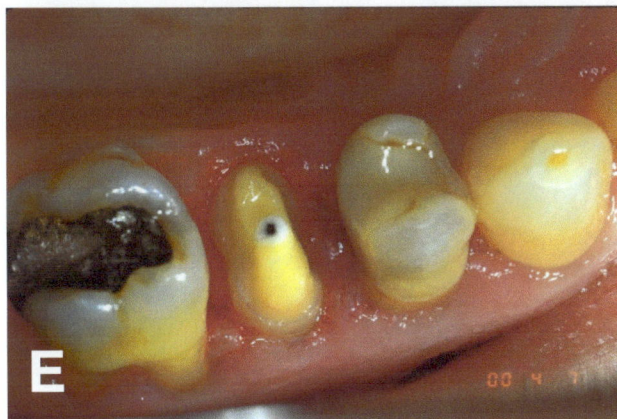

C-Post core material is then bonded to place.
C-Post system, Bisco Inc., Itasca, Illinois 1-800-247-3368

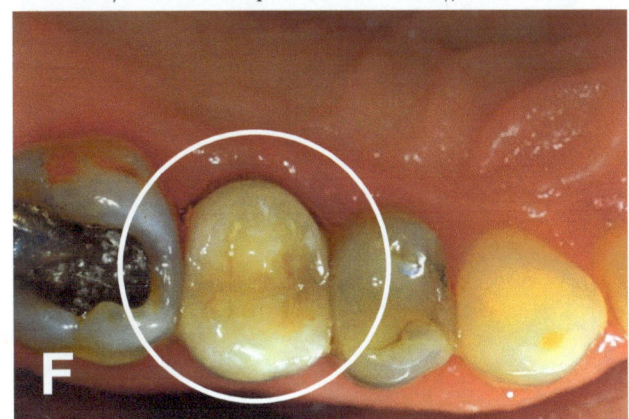

The final artificial crown cemented in place (porcelain fused to gold).

The Restoration After The Root Canal Therapy

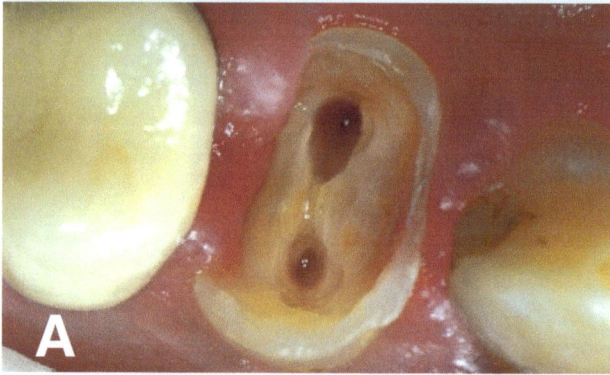

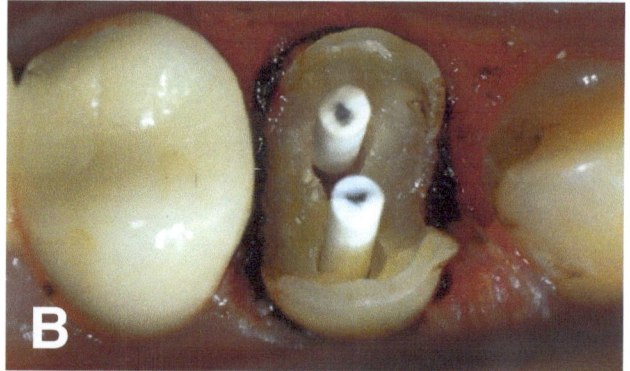

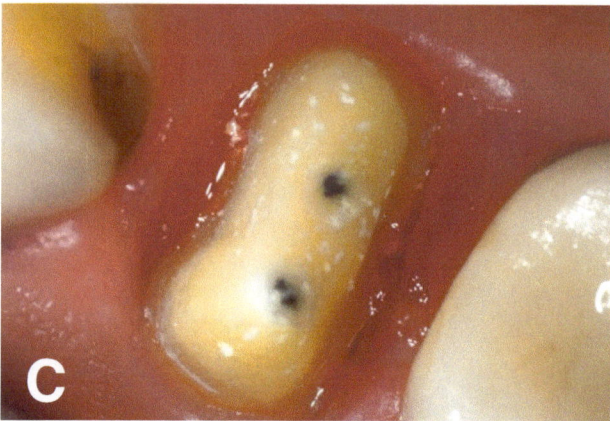

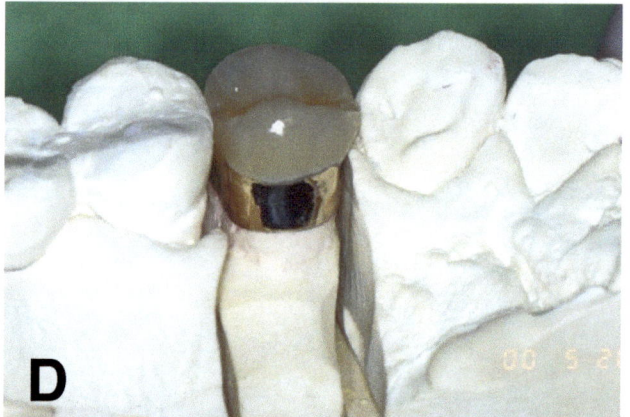

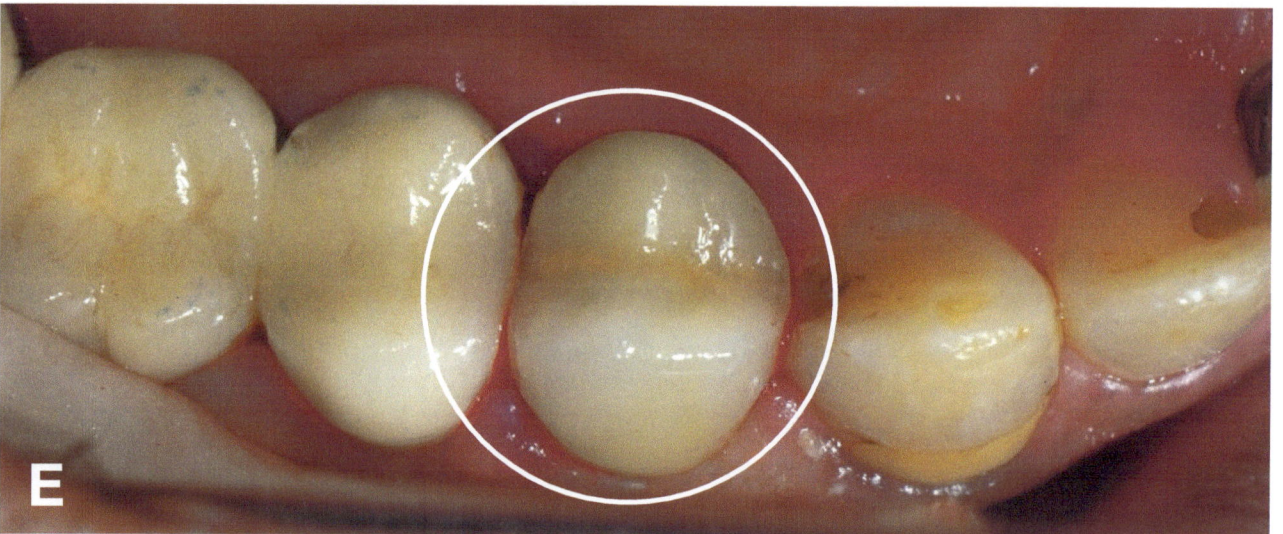

A - Remaining root (after root canal therapy).
B - Two carbon fiber posts bonded to place.
C - C-Post core bonded to place.

D - porcelain fused to gold crown on model.
E - Final crown cemented in place.

The All Gold Crown

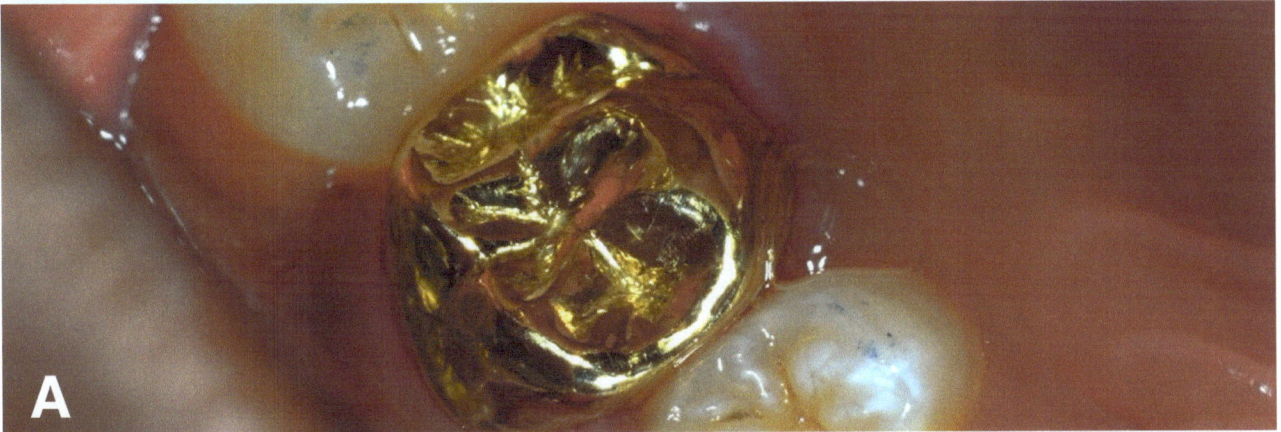

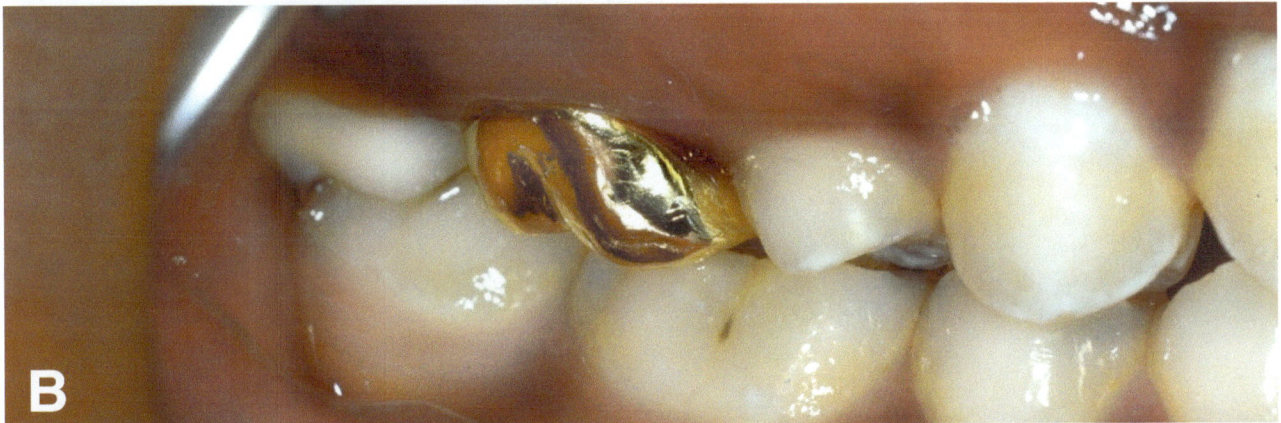

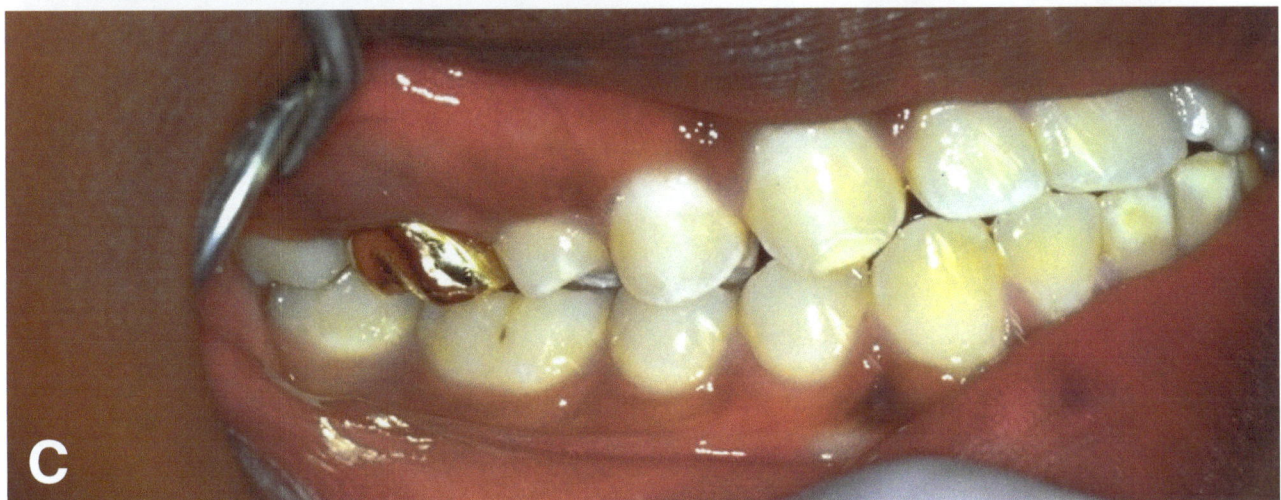

Following root canal therapy, and placement of a post and core, an all gold crown is an excellent restoration in terms of durability. I have one in my mouth, on a lower back tooth. It has been functioning perfectly for years.

An Emergency Restoration

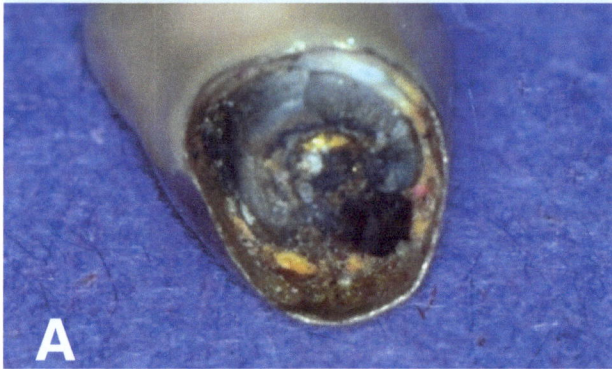

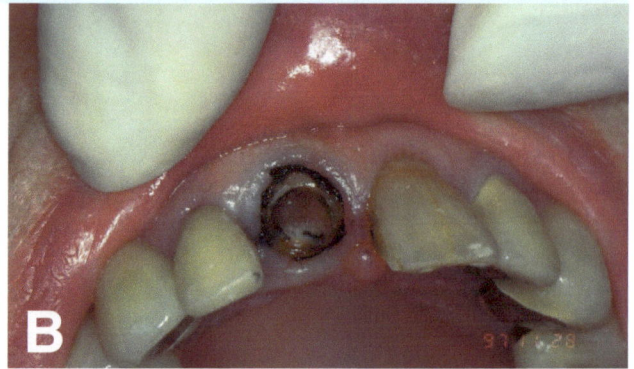

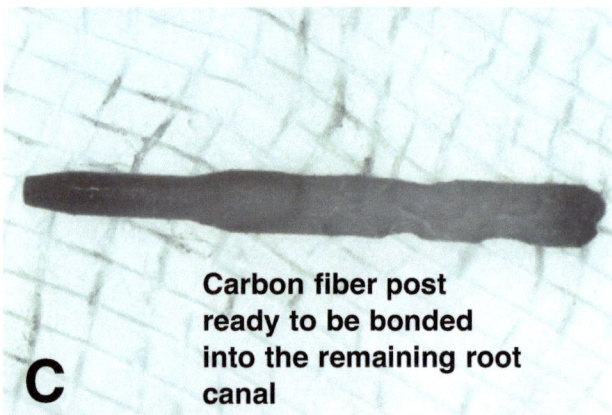

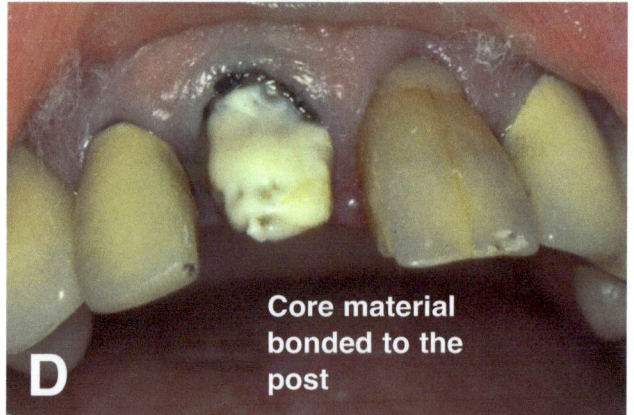

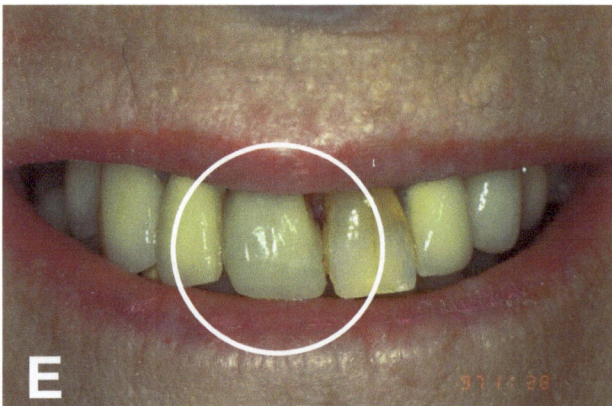

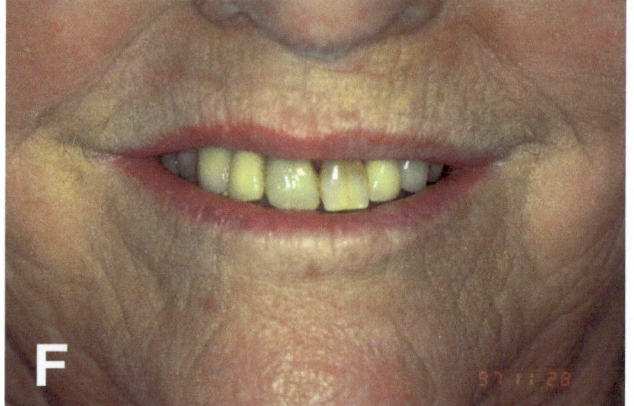

Carbon fiber post ready to be bonded into the remaining root canal

Core material bonded to the post

Several years back this emergency patient appeared in my office with a dislodged front artificial crown. Since she was about to leave on a seven day Caribbean cruise she needed an immediate restoration. Following placement of a carbon fiber post and core, I utilized composite material (Prodigy by Kerr Corp., Orange, CA 1-800-537-7123) to directly sculpture an artificial crown onto the core. This eliminated the need for a laboratory fabricated crown. (Hopefully, improvements in these composites will prolong their durability)

Prevention

If no one got cavities or periodontal disease or suffered dental trauma, I'd probably be playing and writing my music full time. I'd be happier[23], my ex-patients would be happier, and Nerida, my dental assistant—I wonder what Nerida would be doing? Oh, I know, she'd be a music publisher working with her husband Gino's catalogue of fantastic songs.

Preventing or reducing the need for dental treatment is a goal that can be accomplished. Unfortunately, however, you are presently stuck with what you have. If you managed to get through your childhood and early adolescent years without the ravages of dental decay or poor dental treatment, you're probably in decent shape.

Presently, there is no available man-made substitute that equals a healthy tooth in terms of form, function, and durability. So from a preventive point of view, good periodic exams and competent preventive advice can help avoid destructive processes and the necessity for restorative procedures using artificial materials. This care needs to begin in early childhood.

Periodontal Disease

This disease process involves inflammation of the tissues surrounding the teeth. Initially, when the inflammation is confined to the gums (gingiva) it is called *gingivitis*. If it progresses deeper and affects the bone it is called *periodontitis*. The usual cause for this inflammation is the accumulation of plaque and tartar along the gum line. Plaque is a soft, sticky substance that harbors bacteria. It can be easily removed with proper brushing. When it remains on the tissues for an extended period of time it can calcify into tartar (calculus). This material is more difficult to remove. The progression of the disease varies and is dependent on a number of factors including the genetic susceptibility of the patient. Sometimes there is no clearly identifiable cause (etiology) for periodontal disease.

Deterioration initially begins with a separation of the gum from the tooth. This is called a *periodontal pocket*. As this pocket gets deeper, it becomes more difficult for a toothbrush to clean the area. Bleeding may occur and the inflammatory process may eventually cause bone destruction, loosening of the tooth, and possibly, tooth loss. Depending on a number of factors, the destructive process may remain localized (generalized light bleeding of the gums when brushing may be a sign of this status), or it may progress at differing rates.

Prevention is best accomplished by early detection via a thorough examination. In minor cases, treatment involves a few good hygiene appointments—thorough cleaning of all the tissues to remove plaque and tartar along with a few lessons in home hygiene procedures.

---

23. This is not necessarily so. Our destiny is sometimes beyond our control. Besides, I've grown to appreciate the results of performing fine dentistry.

Tartar Plaque And Stain (Photos A — C)

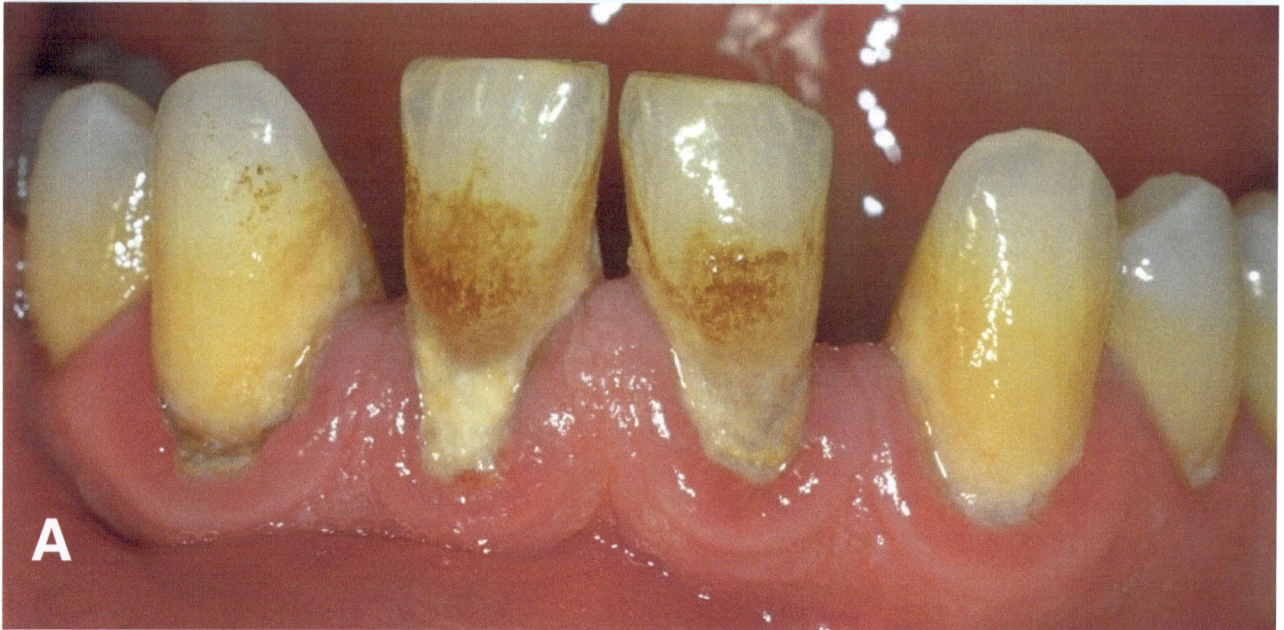

Heavy tartar accumulation and staining from poor oral hygiene and excessive coffee and cigarette consumption.

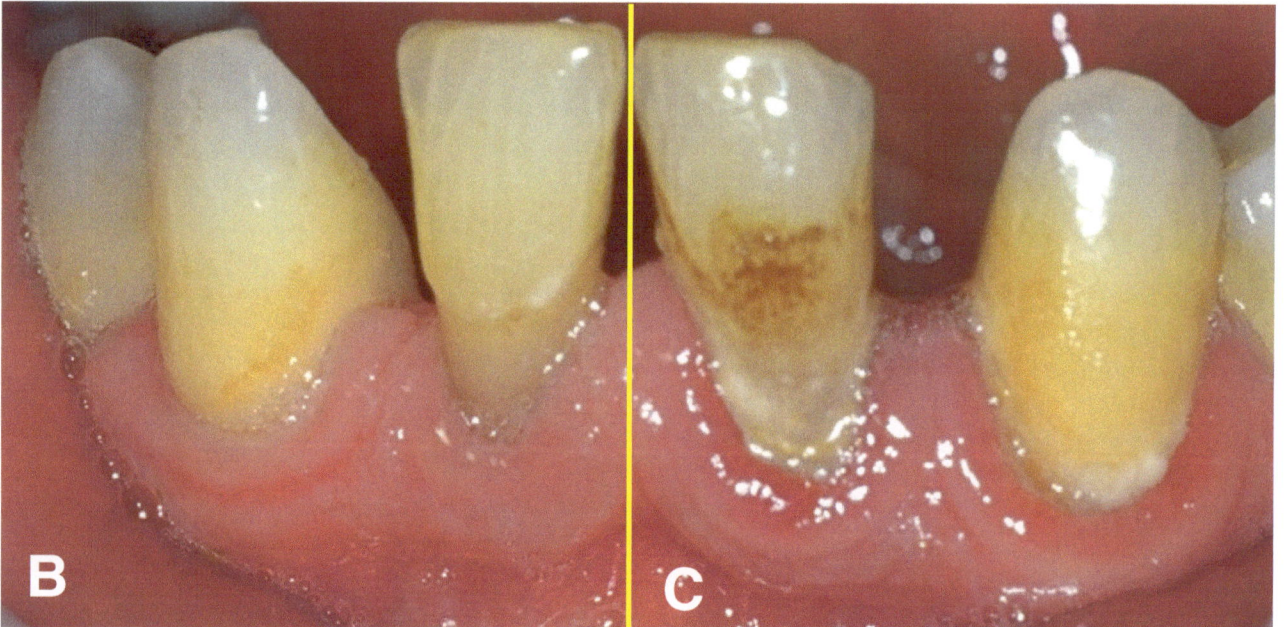

One week following removal all tartar and plaque .
Tissues (gingiva) now appear pink, non-inflamed and healthy.

Red and inflamed tissues on untreated side.

Most Prevalent Area Of Tartar Accumulation

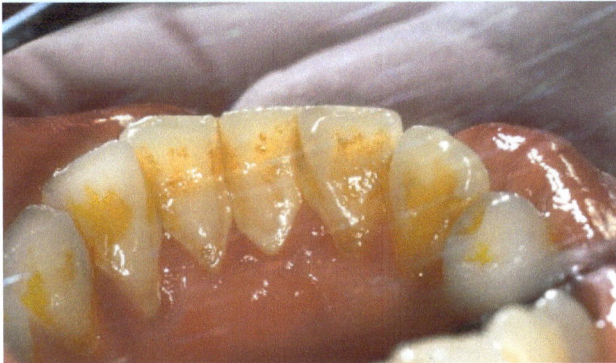

Most prevalent area of tartar and plaque accumulation – on the inside (lingual surfaces) of the lower front (anterior) teeth.

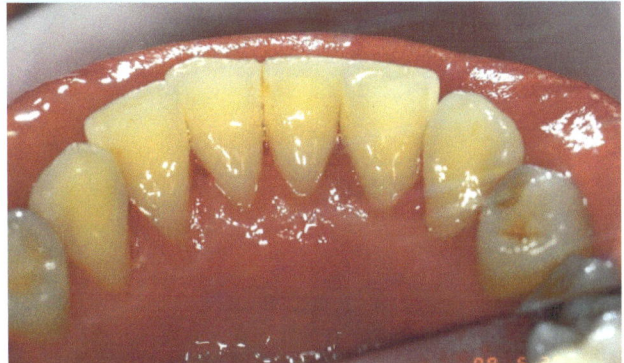

Following scaling, note clean teeth and healthier gums.

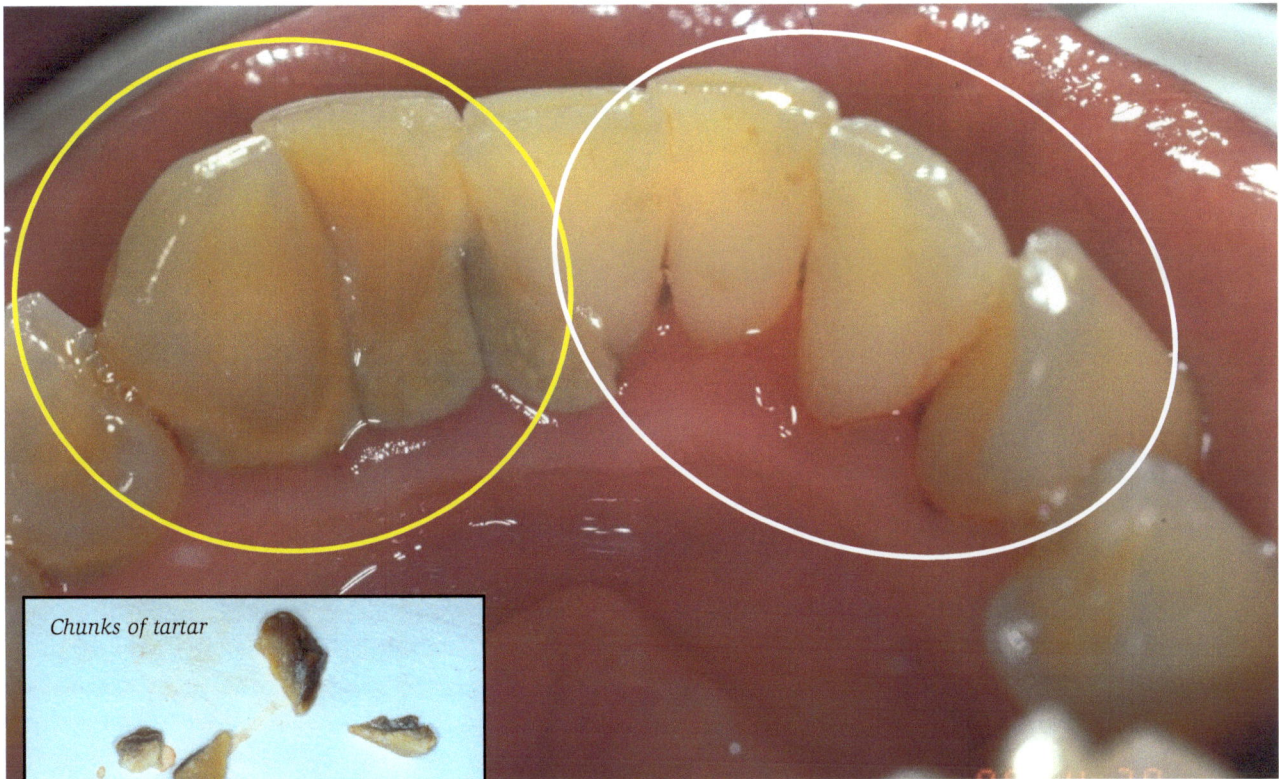

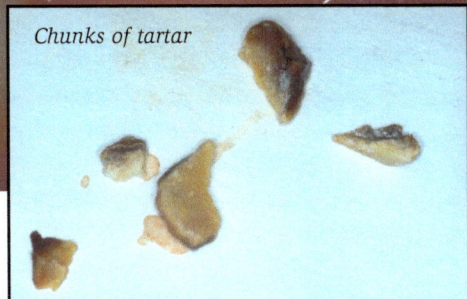

Chunks of tartar

Excessive tartar covering almost the entire tooth surface —removed on one side.

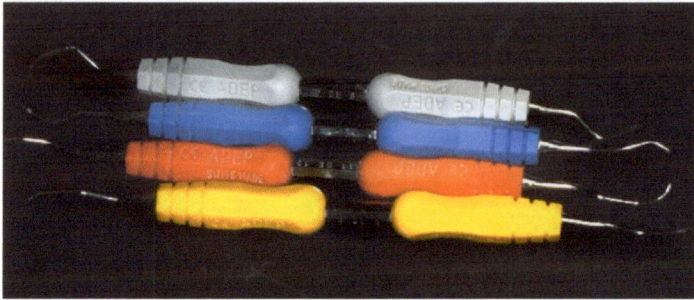

Besides utilizing an ultrasonic cleaner, these Swiss hand instruments will remove most debris and smooth the tooth structure, provided they are kept very sharp.

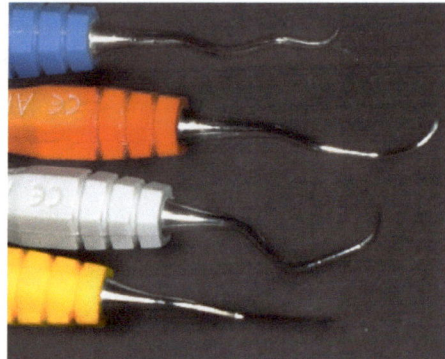

A. Deppeler Dental Instruments of Switzerland. Téléphone + 41 (0) 21 825 17 31

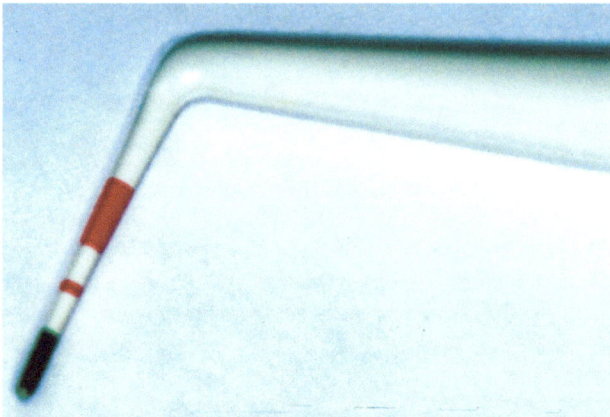

A periodontal probe will detect pockets and defects.

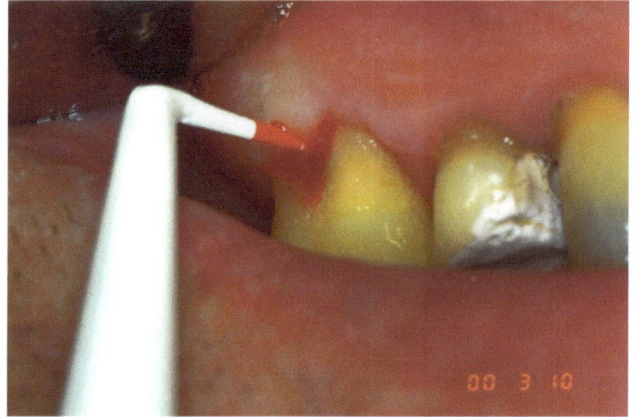

Bleeding on gentle probing indicates inflammation.

Advanced Cases

In more advanced cases of periodontal disease, initial therapy involves anesthetized deep cleanings over a period of four or five appointments. These cleanings are known as deep scaling and curettage. Scaling is the process of removing tartar from the teeth and root surfaces, and curettage is the removal of diseased soft tissues on the inside of the periodontal pocket. Once this is performed, the inflammation usually subsides, the pockets tend to shrink, and the gums regain a healthier, pink appearance. In some situations, antibiotics are administered along with a prescription mouth rinse such as chlorhexadrine.

The dentist then re-evaluates the situation. If deep pockets still exist or if there is radiographic evidence of bone destruction, surgical procedures may be indicated.

My Personal Experience

At age 53, I have pretty good dental health. Other than having had my four wisdom teeth removed when I was 25, I have all my teeth. My teenage cavities were restored with silver amalgam. Though these mercury-containing alloys are presently viewed as toxic by a contingent of dentists, I have been well served by them for the past 35 years.[24] I do appreciate, however, the concerns and possible ill effects that this metal may have on certain sensitive patients.

My personal periodontal experience began two years ago with a slightly painful pressure around the gum of a tooth. The following day, I took a radiograph of the area and measured a deep pocket with a periodontal probe. The radiograph revealed some bone destruction, though minimal and not enough to make the tooth loose or movable. My dental hygienist, scheduled me for an appointment to clean the defect. I administered Novocaine to myself since the area was in the front of my mouth and easily accessible (This allowed my hygienist to reach the bottom of the defect for appropriate cleaning without my jumping through the ceiling). Following the procedure, the discomfort was resolved; I was concerned, however, that radiographic evidence indicated damage had occurred. I made an appointment with my friend, the periodontist.

His treatment began with a thorough periodontal examination. This exam differs from the screening examination I perform as a general dentist in that it is more comprehensive —pocket depths are measured along with other indicators of the present status.

His exam was followed by another appointment to review the results and discuss the treatment. Fortunately, my disease status was minimal. It was caused by accumulations of tartar that routine cleanings had not removed. This is an interesting situation because, generally, dental hygienists avoid instrumenting too deeply into a patient's gum tissue to avoid discomfort. Over the years, this type of conservative therapy may result in the necessity for a few anesthetized deep scalings.[25]

Four appointments were arranged for my therapy. Since this particular periodontist had at least four dental hygienists on staff, I elected to receive therapy by each hygienist in order to evaluate the differences.

During these appointments, the hygienist placed a topical anesthetic on my gum, after which the periodontist administered the injectable anesthesia. None of this was fun, though the discomfort was within an acceptable level. Listening to music with headphones greatly diminished my anxiety.

Overall, I found few differences in the touch of the four hygienists, and they were all very nice and empathetic. During my re-evaluation appointment with the periodontist, the results were good. Besides being taught and encouraged to practice better at-home oral hygiene procedures—brushing with a good brush and properly using dental floss—further treatment was not necessary. I was relieved!

My mouth felt very clean, and as I mentioned to the periodontist, the therapeutic tightening of my gum tissue felt like a face-lift. I just felt better and knew this was necessary and beneficial in terms of long-term dental health.

---

24. A few years ago one of these amalgams fractured, and I eventually had this tooth restored with an all gold crown.
25. It is unfortunate that dental hygienists, who are highly-trained professionals, are not allowed by Florida law to administer injectable anesthetics.

Periodontal Surgery

Advanced periodontal disease leads to destruction of the bone that supports the teeth. If I had deteriorated to this degree, my initial deep cleanings would have been only the first step in a treatment plan. The goal of periodontal surgery is to reduce periodontal pocket depths and to re-contour, and in certain situations, encourage the re-growth of supporting tissues. This altered anatomy should allow patients to perform more effective hygiene procedures. Of course, if the initial factors responsible for periodontal disease are not corrected, problems usually recur. So before undergoing surgery, it is important for patients to demonstrate an ability and willingness to improve hygiene procedures (stop smoking,[26] and try to improve their overall health with proper diet and exercise).

In many cases, the end result of advanced periodontal disease is tooth loss. There is only so much that can be done to save teeth once the destructive process has reached a point where practically no bone remains. Weakened teeth, however, may be supported and splinted together with stronger teeth, and lost teeth can be replaced with artificial teeth—which leads us to the next chapter—Prosthetics.

Surgery   *(Photos A - H)*

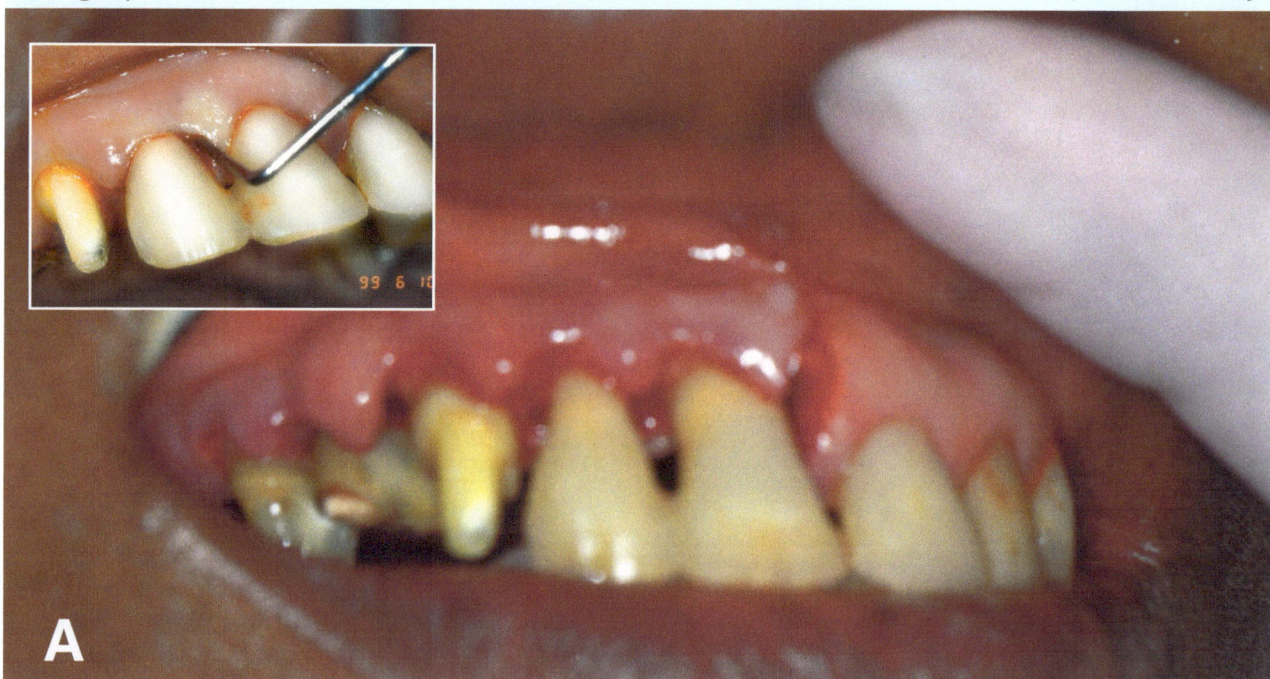

A

Advanced periodontal disease (periodontitis). Probing depth is measured. Surgery is required in order to eliminate these deep pockets, and also recontour bone, and expose roots so that these teeth can be restored.

26. Cigarette consumption retards healing. I quit smoking cigarettes about 10 years ago with the help of a nicotine reduction system called *"One Step at a Time Withdrawal System"* made by *Newmark Laboratories (800-338- 8079).*

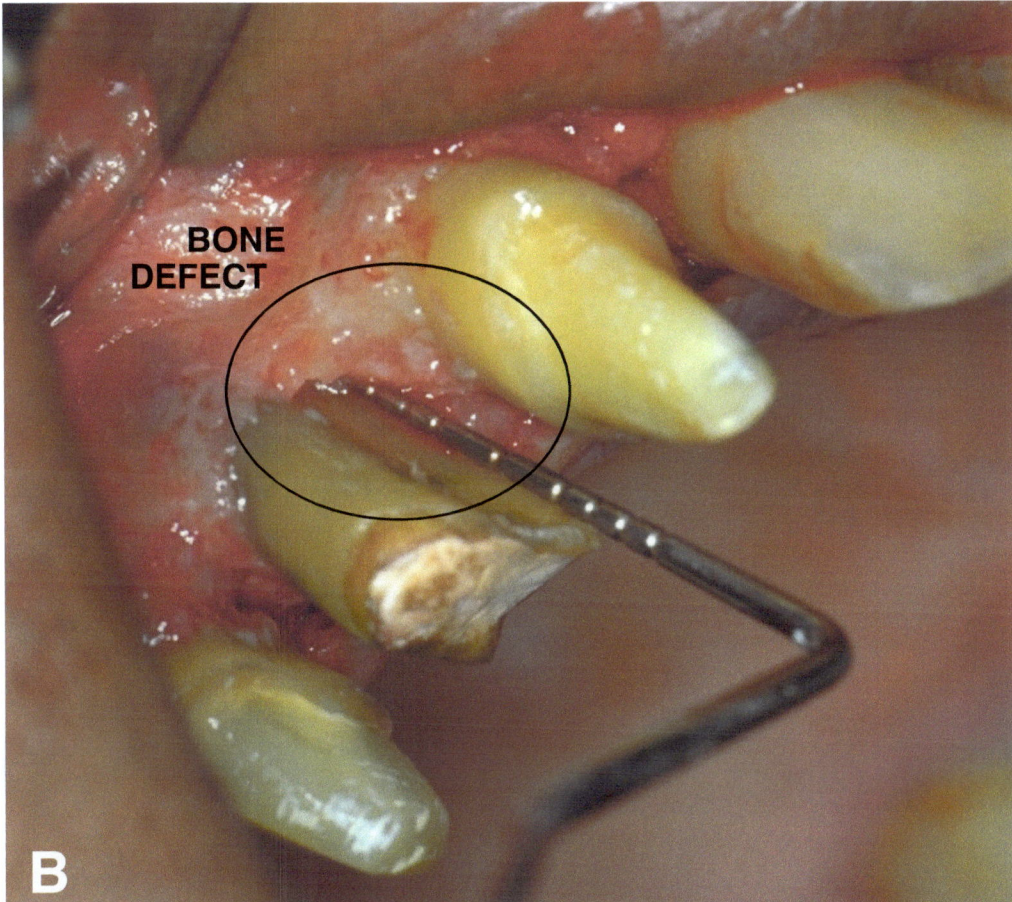

B

*Bone defects
are analyzed
and treated.*

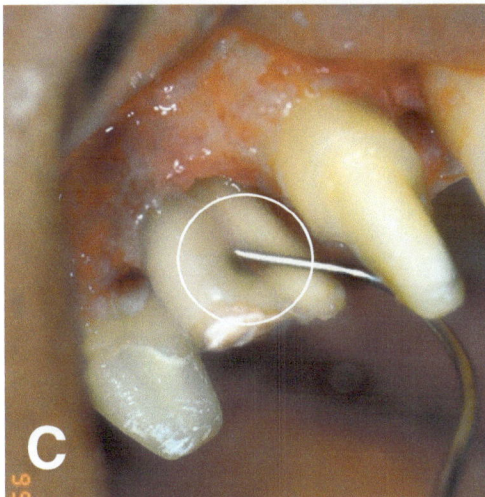

C

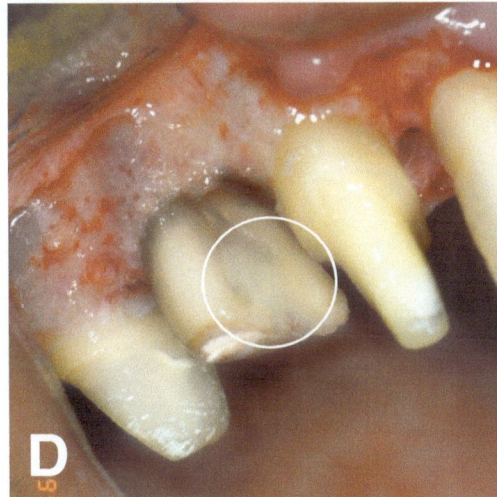

D

*Decay or other
perforations are
discovered and
sealed.*

Surgery *(Continued)*

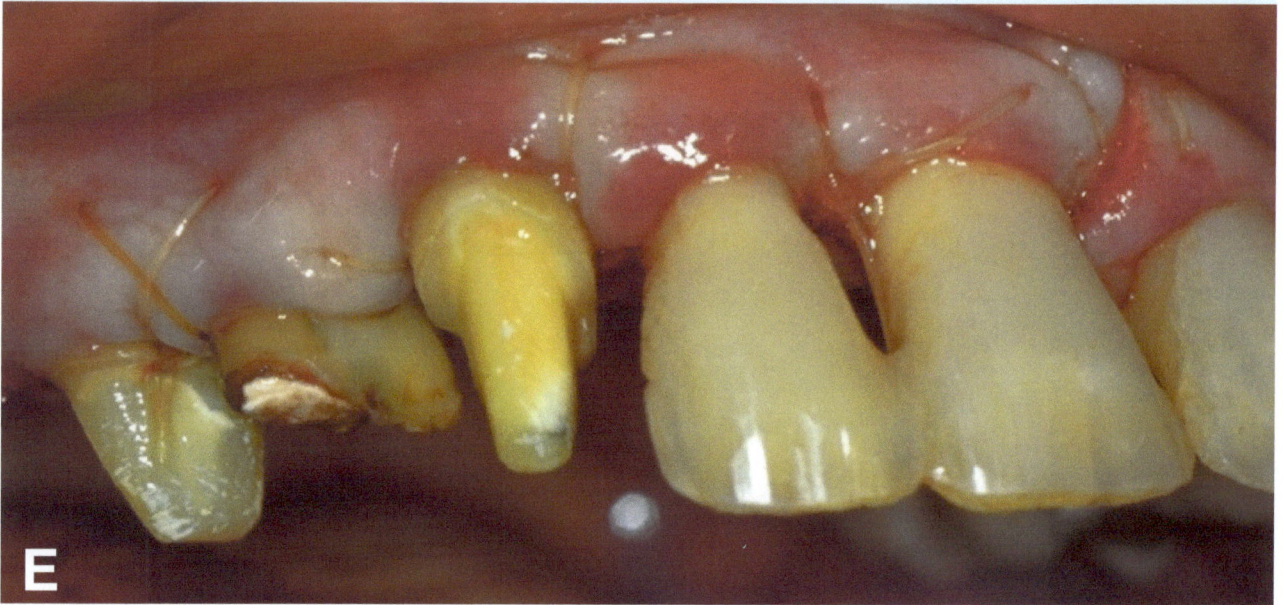

Suturing readapts tissues to the bone and teeth.

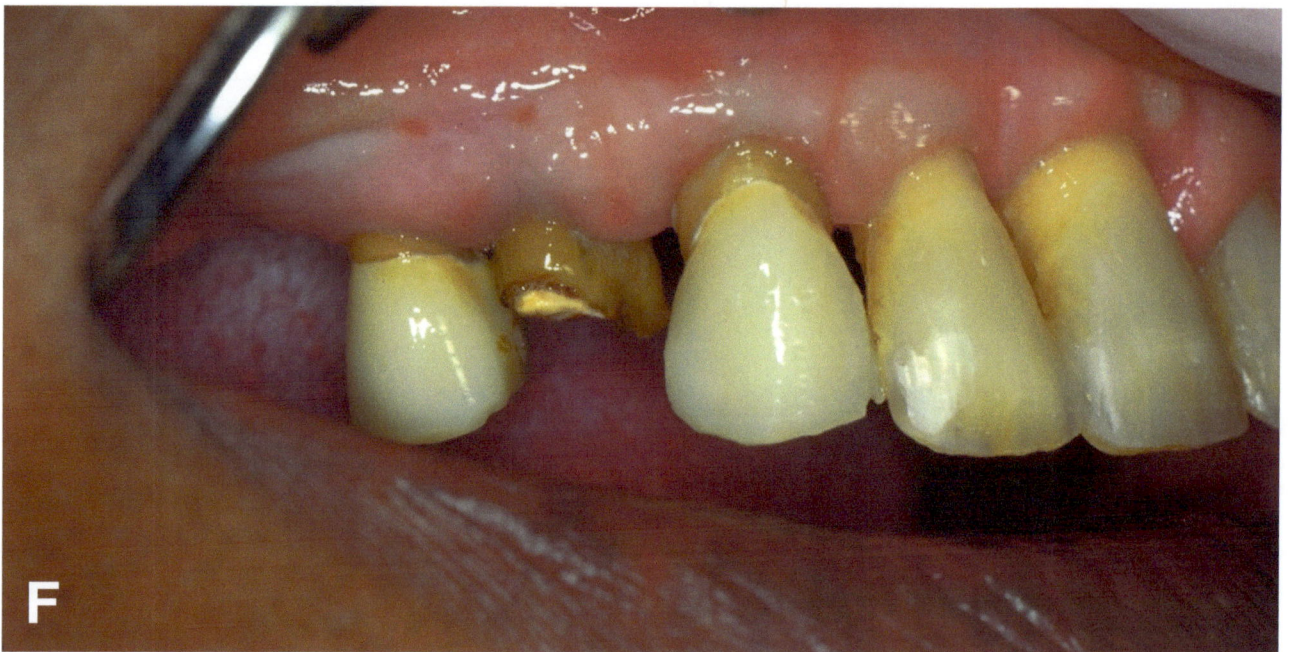

Healing at three weeks shows healthier, non-inflamed tissues with elimination of deep pockets.

Surgery (Continued)

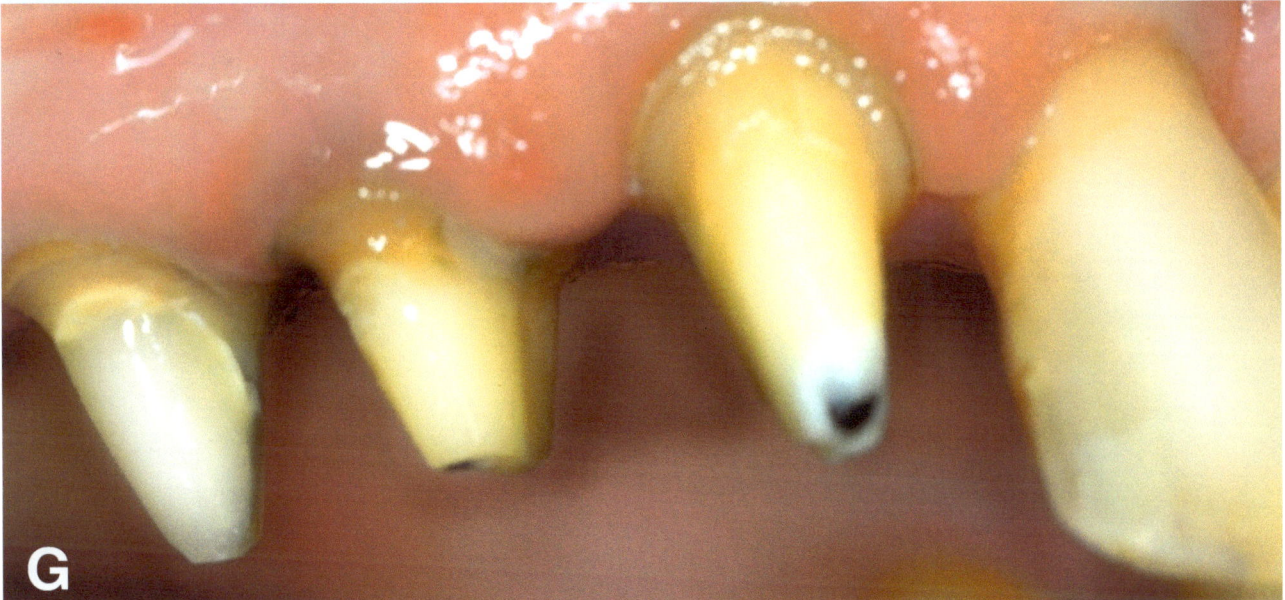

Carbon fiber posts and composite cores are utilized to rebuild on the roots.

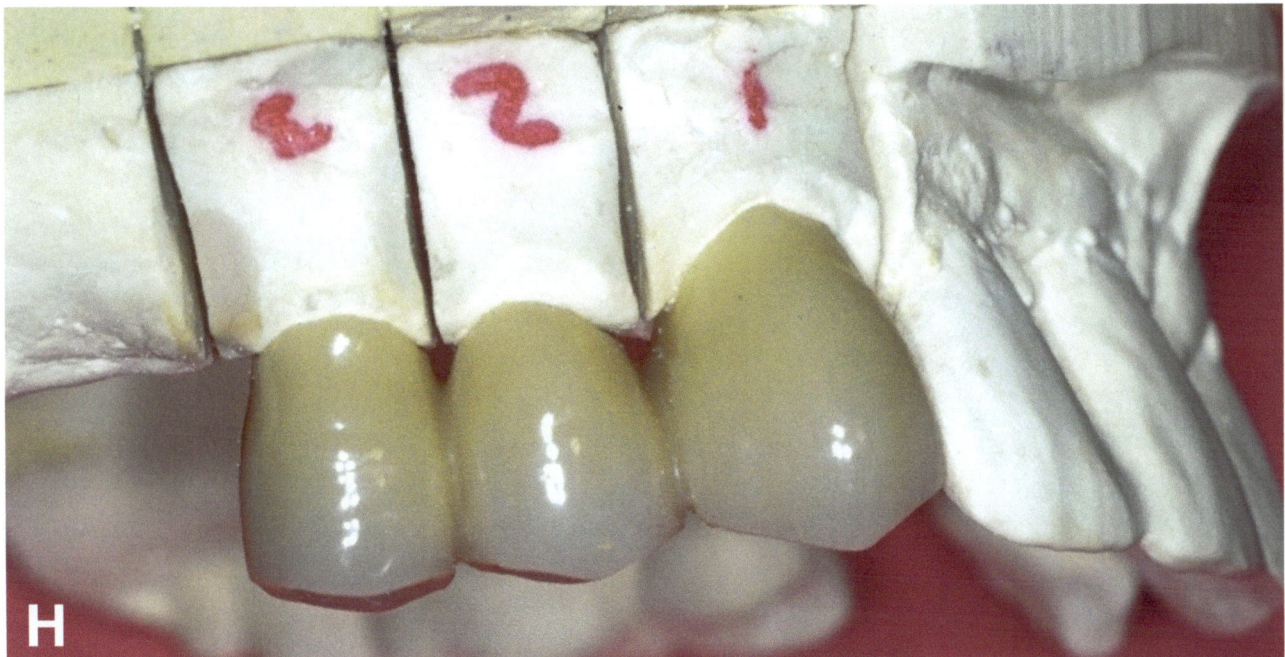

A temporary splint is fabricated. This will restore function and aesthetics, and support the teeth during healing before a final porcelain fused to gold prosthesis is made.

Periodontal Surgery And Guided Tissue Regeneration   (Photos A - G)

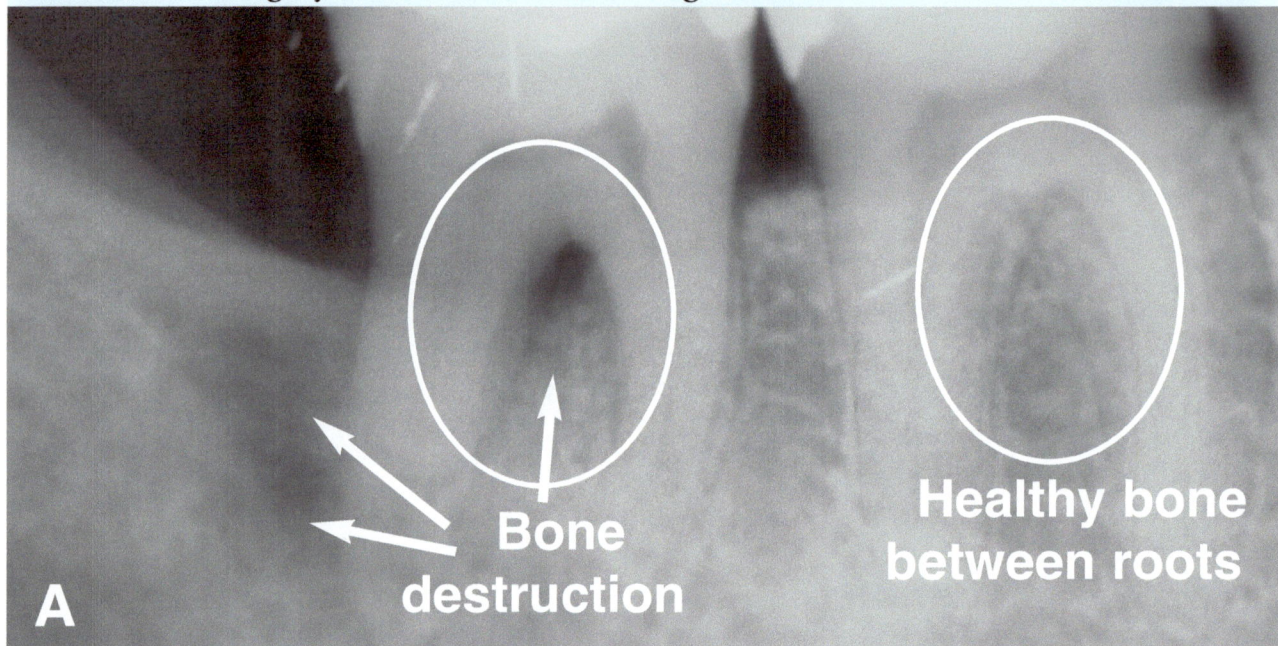

Bone destruction

Healthy bone between roots

A

Periodontal disease can be diagnosed radiographically when bone destruction has occurred.

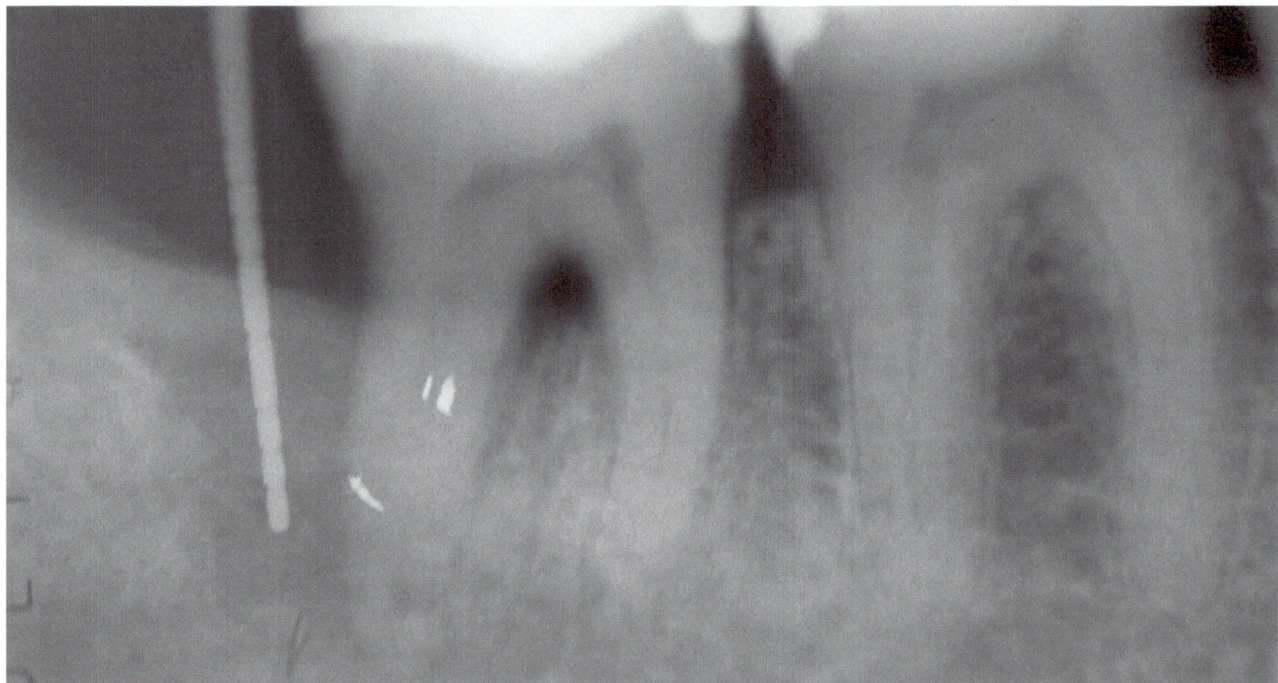

A dark area on an X-ray (radioluscency) with a probe in a deep pocket.

Periodontal Surgery And Guided Tissue Regeneration   **(Continued)**

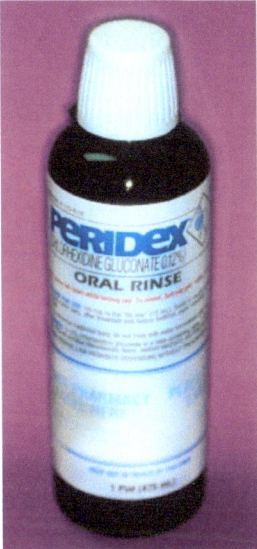

Prior to surgery an anti-septic rinse is utilized.

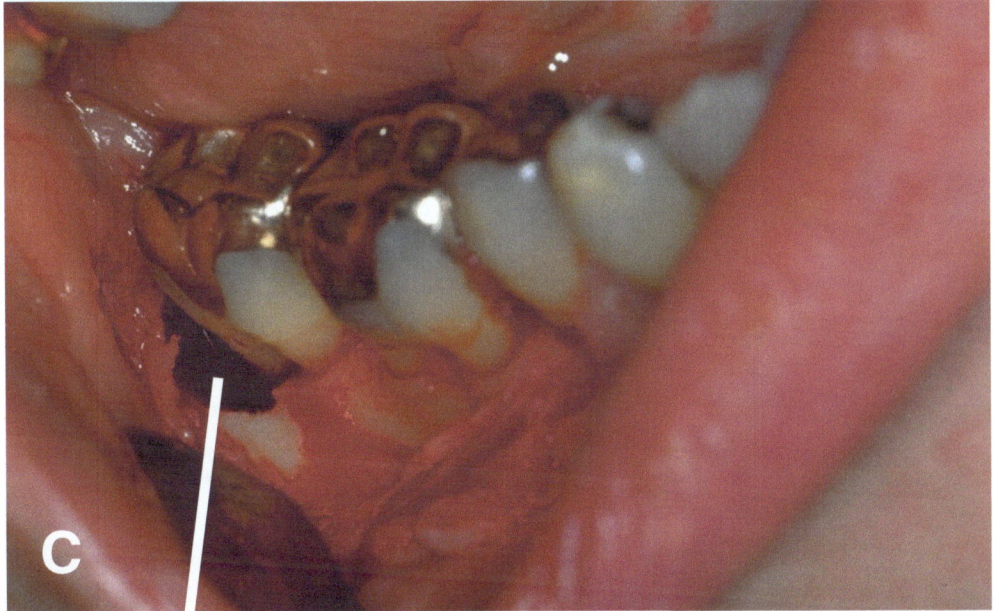

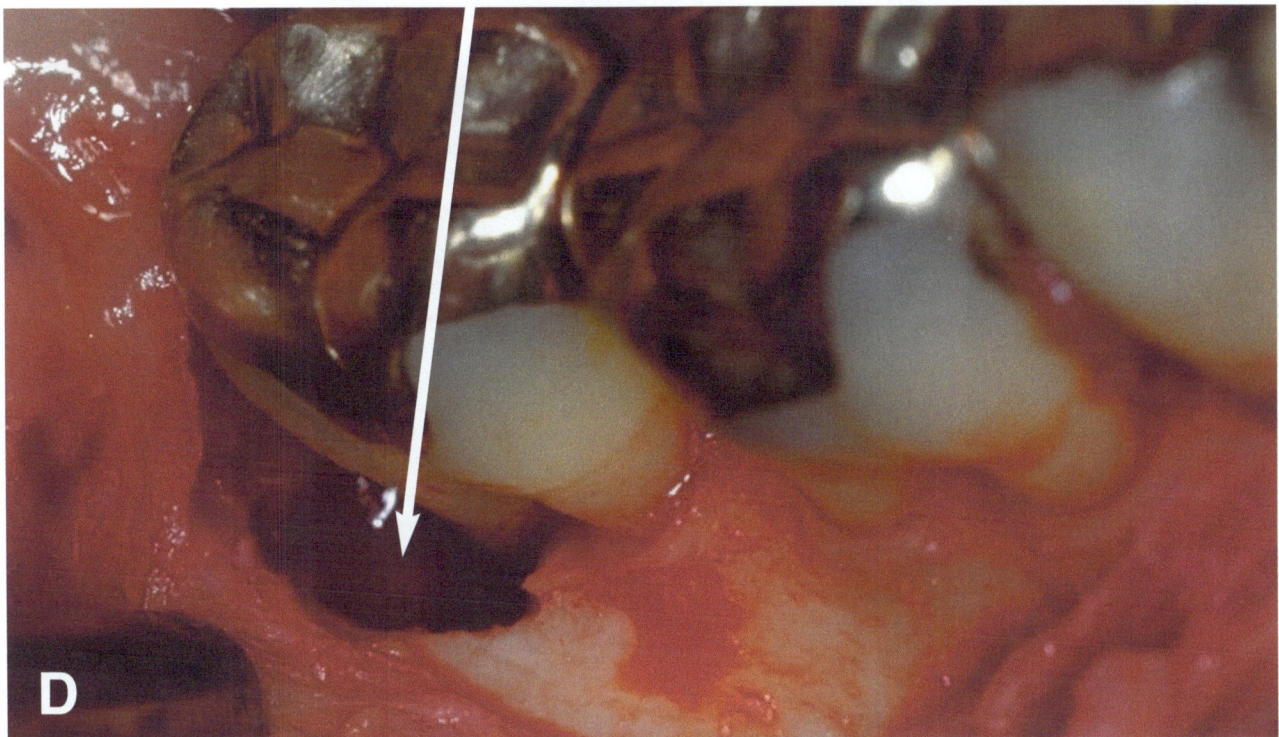

The bone defect is discovered and cleaned out (debrided).

Periodontal Surgery And Guided Tissue Regeneration   (Continued)

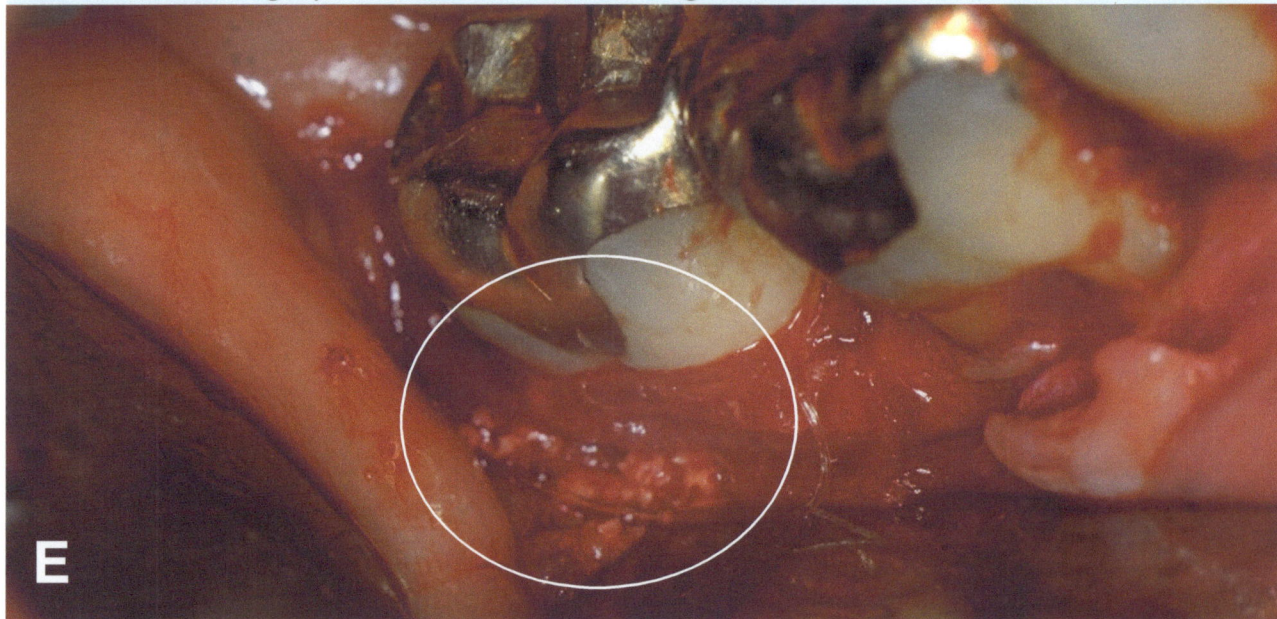

A bone graft is placed and covered by a membrane (membrane is not visible). This surgical procedure is based on the advent of "guided tissue regeneration" — a result of research efforts developed to re-grow bone and adjacent tissues.

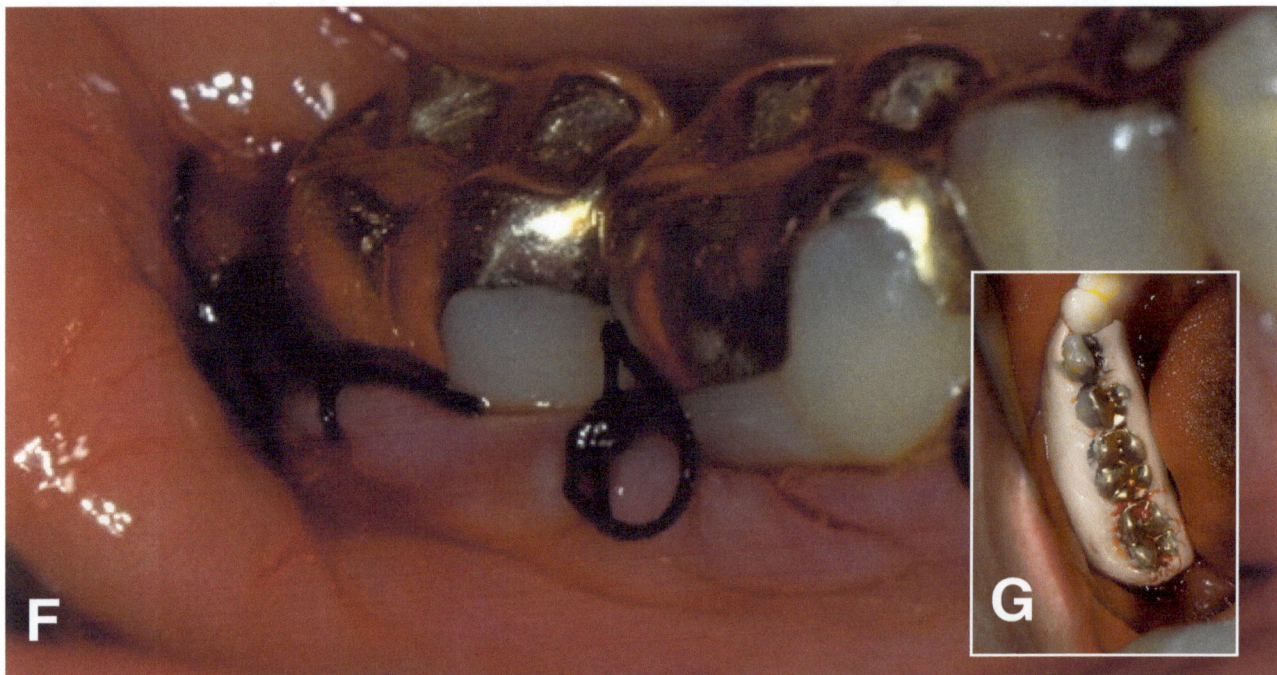

Closure with sutures and placement of a dressing.

BIO-OSS® ≡ BIO-OSS®

A sterile, biocompatible natural porous bone mineral for use in periodontal and maxillofacial surgery.

DESCRIPTION:

Bio-Oss® is a natural, non-antigenic, porous bone mineral matrix. It is produced by removal of all organic components from bovine bone. Due to its natural structure Bio-Oss® is physically and chemically comparable to the mineralized matrix of human bone. It is available in cancellous (spongiosa) and cortical granules and blocks.

PROPERTIES/ACTIONS:

Bio-Oss®: The anorganic bone matrix of Bio-Oss® has macro- and microscopic structures similar to human bone. The formation and ingrowth of new bone at the implantation site of Bio-Oss® is favored, due to its trabecular architecture, interconnecting macro and micro pores and its natural consistency. The use of Bio-Oss® may be considered when autogenous bone is not indicated, or insufficient in quantity to fulfill the needs of the proposed surgical procedure.

INDICATIONS AND USAGE:

Bio-Oss® is recommended for:
- Augmentation or reconstructive treatment of the alveolar ridge.
- Filling of infrabony periodontal defects.
- Filling of defects after root resection, apicoectomy, and cystectomy.
- Filling of extraction sockets to enhance preservation of the alveolar ridge.
- Elevation of the maxillary sinus floor.
- Filling of periodontal defects in conjunction with products intended for Guided Tissue Regeneration (GTR) and Guided Bone Regeneration (GBR).
- Filling of peri-implant defects in conjunction with products intended for Guided Bone Regeneration (GBR).

Bio-Oss® blocks are recommended for:
- Filling of large oral and maxillofacial osseous cavities.

INSTRUCTIONS FOR USE:

- After exposure of the bony defect with mucoperiosteal flap, all granulation tissue must be carefully removed.
- Mix Bio-Oss® with autogenous bone, osseous coagulum, patients blood or sterile normal saline. If large maxillofacial defects are present, Bio-Oss® should be mixed with autogenous bone in a ratio of approximately 1:1. The further addition of microfibrillar collagen (e.g. Avitene®) allows for increased cohesiveness and moldability.
- In order to assure the formation of new bone, Bio-Oss® should only be placed in direct contact with well vascularized bone. Cortical bone should be mechanically perforated.
- Loosely pack Bio-Oss® granules into osseous defect using a sterile instrument. Use of excessive force will result in crushing of particles and loss of trabecular architecture.
- Bio-Oss® Cancellous Block may be carved to the desired size using a scalpel after moistening with sterile normal saline. The shaped block is then placed loosely into the bone cavity in direct contact with well vascularized and bleeding bone. Cortical bone should be mechanically perforated.
- Bio-Oss® Cortical Block may be carved to the desired size using a scalpel or bur after moistening with sterile normal saline. The shaped block is then placed loosely into the bone cavity in direct contact with well vascularized and bleeding bone. Cortical bone should be mechanically perforated.
- Overfilling of the defects should be avoided.
- The mucoperiosteal flaps should be sutured to achieve primary closure, if possible. A surgical dressing may be placed over the wound for one to two weeks.
- Sites grafted with Bio-Oss® should be allowed to heal approximately 6 months prior to implant placement.

CONTRAINDICATIONS:

Contraindications customary to the use of bone grafts should be observed.
Bio-Oss® should not be used in patients with:
- Osteomyelitis at the surgical site
- Metabolic diseases (diabetes, hyperparathyroidism, osteomalacia)
- Severe renal dysfunction, severe liver disease
- High dose therapy with corticosteroids
- Vascular impairment at the implant site

BIO-OSS® ≡ BIO-OSS®

PRECAUTIONS:

In order to facilitate the formation of new bone Bio-Oss® should only be implanted in direct contact with a well vascularized bony tissue (selective osteoplasty of adjacent cortical bone may be necessary).

In larger defects a mixture of autogenous bone or bone marrow may improve the formation of new bone. The implantation of titanium fixtures should not take place until about 6 months after the use of Bio-Oss® in any implant site.

ADVERSE REACTIONS:

No adverse reactions have been reported.

STABILITY:

The contents of the bottle or blister are designed for single use only. Resterilization with dry heat is not recommended. Do not use after expiration date.
Shelf-life: 3 years.

HOW SUPPLIED:

Re-Order No.	Product	Weight	Particle Size	Packaged
03-0502	Bio-Oss® cancellous granules	0.5g	0.25 - 1.0mm	Individually
03-2002	Bio-Oss® cancellous granules	2.0g	0.25 - 1.0mm	Individually
03-5002	Bio-Oss® cancellous granules	5.0g	0.25 - 1.0mm	Individually
03-0510	Bio-Oss® cancellous granules	0.5g	1.0 - 2.0mm	Individually
03-2010	Bio-Oss® cancellous granules	2.0g	1.0 - 2.0mm	Individually
03-5010	Bio-Oss® cancellous granules	5.0g	1.0 - 2.0mm	Individually
03-0202	Bio-Oss® cancellous granules	0.25g	0.25 - 1.0mm	Individually
01-0505	Bio-Oss® cortical granules	0.5g	0.5 - 1.0mm	Individually
01-2005	Bio-Oss® cortical granules	2.0g	0.5 - 1.0mm	Individually
01-5005	Bio-Oss® cortical granules	5.0g	0.5 - 1.0mm	Individually
01-0510	Bio-Oss® cortical granules	0.5g	1.0 - 2.0mm	Individually
01-2010	Bio-Oss® cortical granules	2.0g	1.0 - 2.0mm	Individually
01-5010	Bio-Oss® cortical granules	5.0g	1.0 - 2.0mm	Individually

Re-Order No.	Product	Block size (approx.)	Packaged
03-1012	Bio Oss® cancellous block	1x1x2cm	Individually
01-0712	Bio-Oss® cortical block	0.7x1x2cm	Individually

Bio-Oss® Devices:

Re-Order No.	Product	Packaged
05-1000	Bio-Oss® Funnel	Individually
05-2000	Bio-Oss® Syringe	Individually

CAUTION: Federal law restricts this device to sale by or on the order of a licensed dentist or physician.

Made in Switzerland
From U.S. source bovine bone
By
Ed Geistlich Sons
Wolhusen, Switzerland

Distributed by:
The Osteohealth Company,
Division, Luitpold Pharmaceuticals, Inc.
Shirley, New York 11967-4799
1-800-874-2334

Rev. 9/98
IN0712
MG #10401

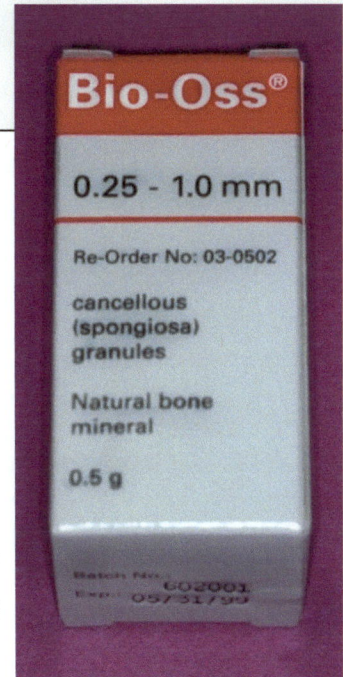

Bone graft material.
Osteohealth Company.
1-800-874-2334

The End Of The Line

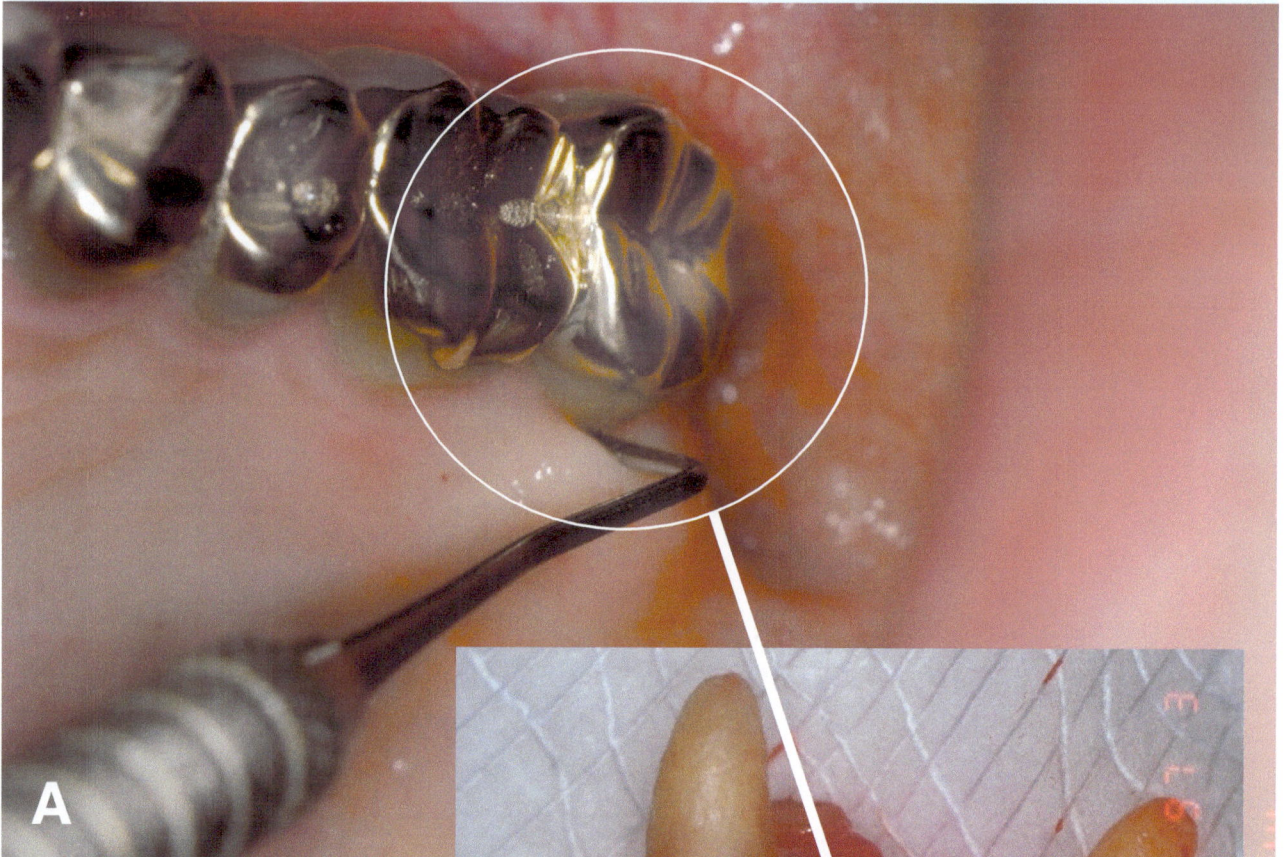

This tooth shows periodontal deterioration to the extend that 90% of its supporting bone has been destroyed. Probing indicates very deep pocketing and the tooth is loose.

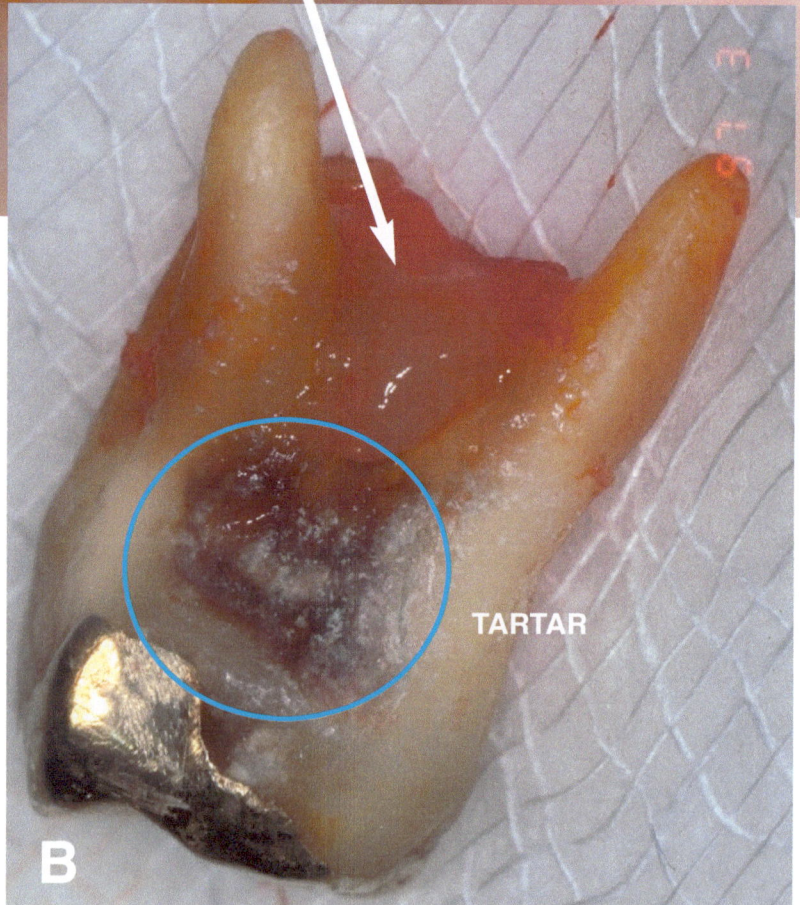

Upon extraction heavy tartar (which existed beneath the gum line) is evident.

TARTAR

Loss Of A Tooth Supporting A Bridge

(Photos A - F)

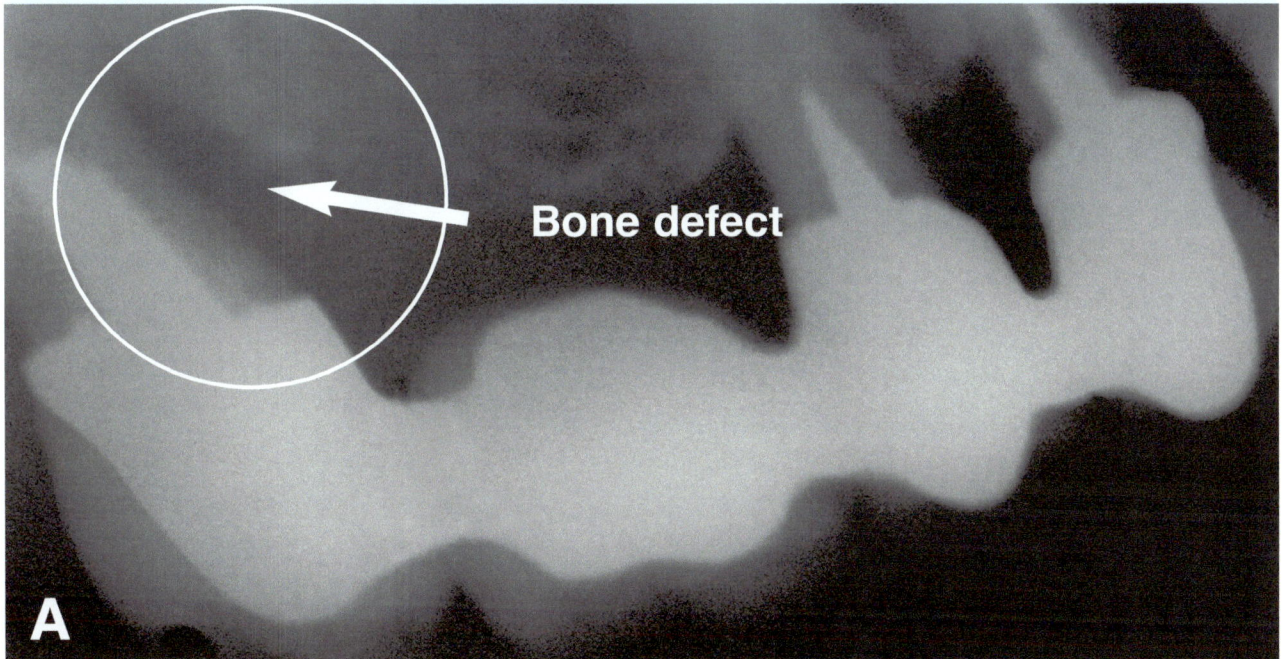

Bone defect

A

Radiographic evidence of bone destruction surrounding a critical tooth supporting a bridge.

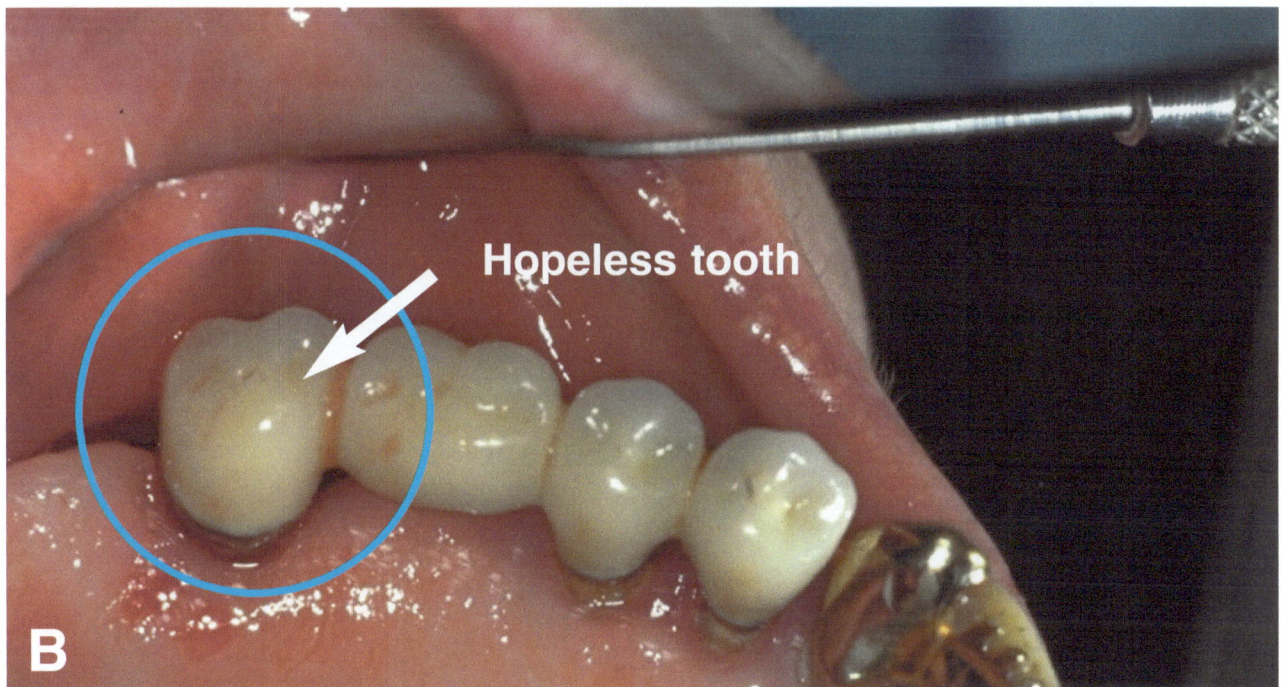

Hopeless tooth

B

Loss Of A Tooth Supporting A Bridge (Continued)

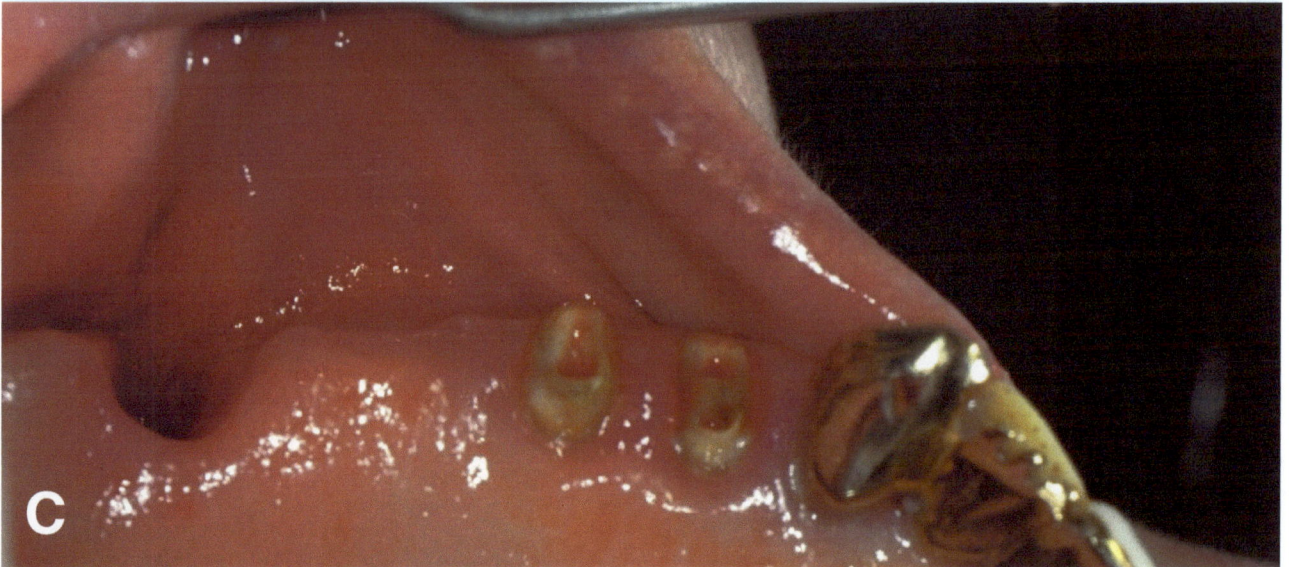

Removal of the bridge along with extraction of this hopeless tooth.

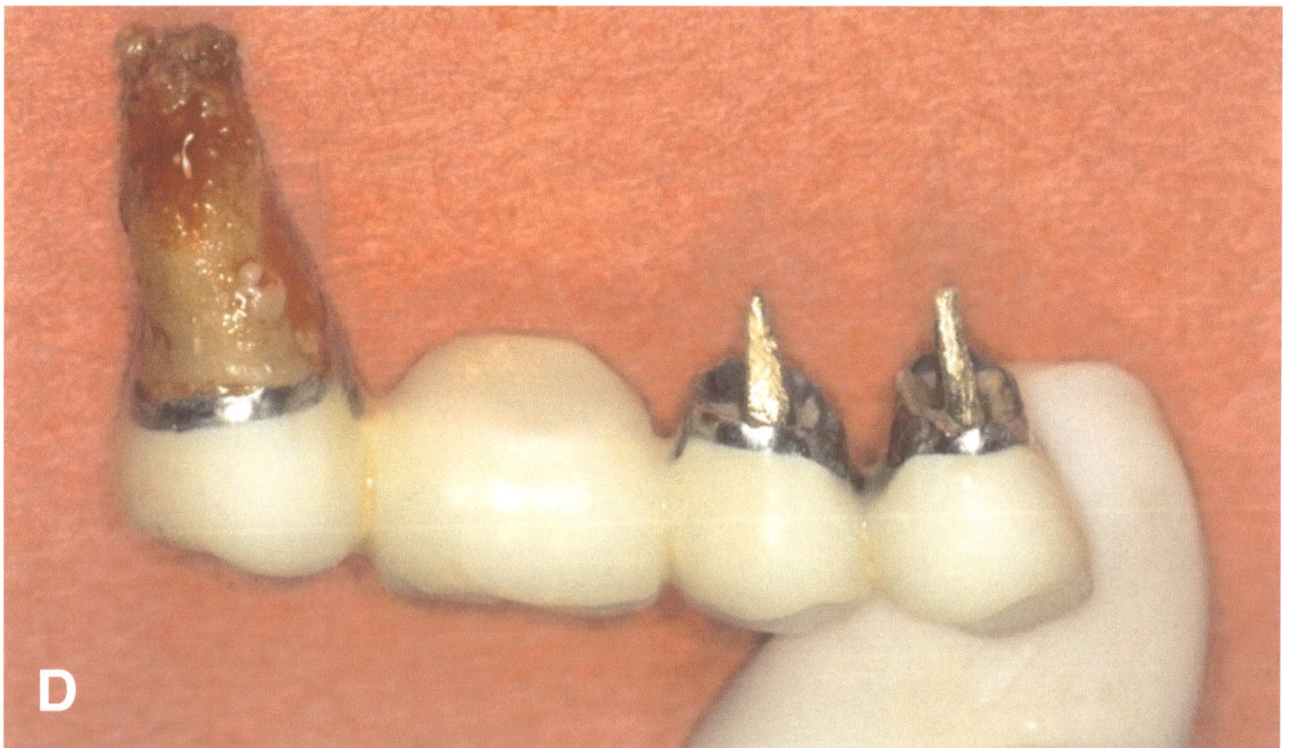

Loss Of A Tooth Supporting A Bridge   **(Continued)**

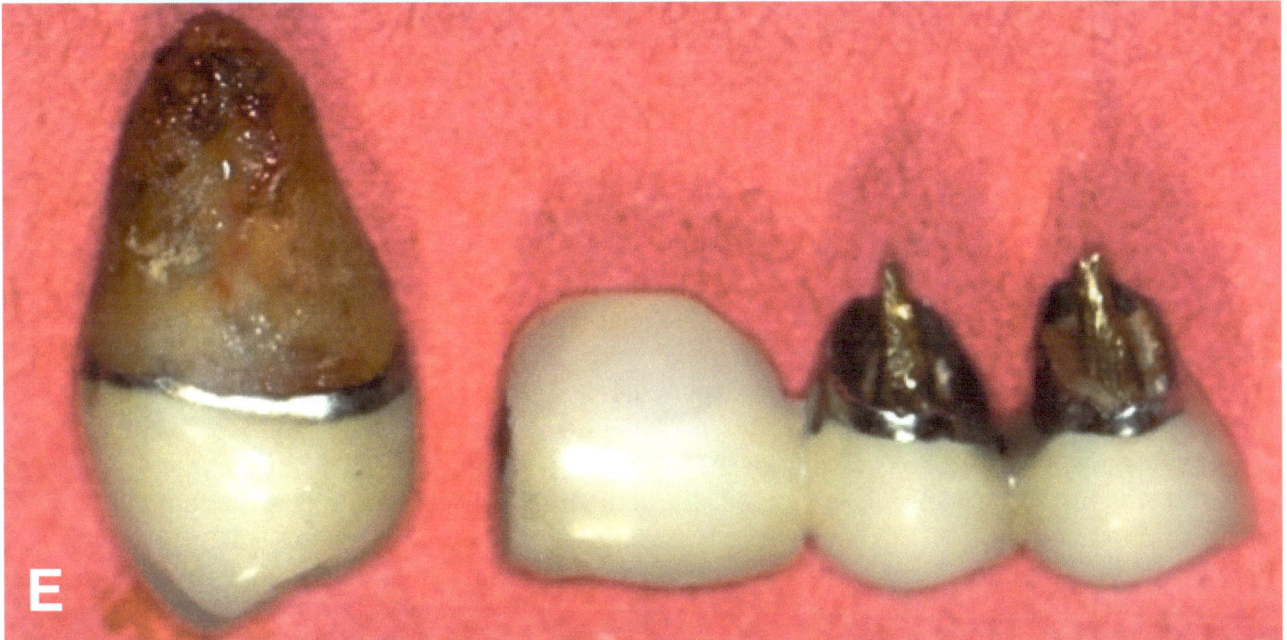

As a temporary measure, the back portion (posterior) of the bridge was cut off...

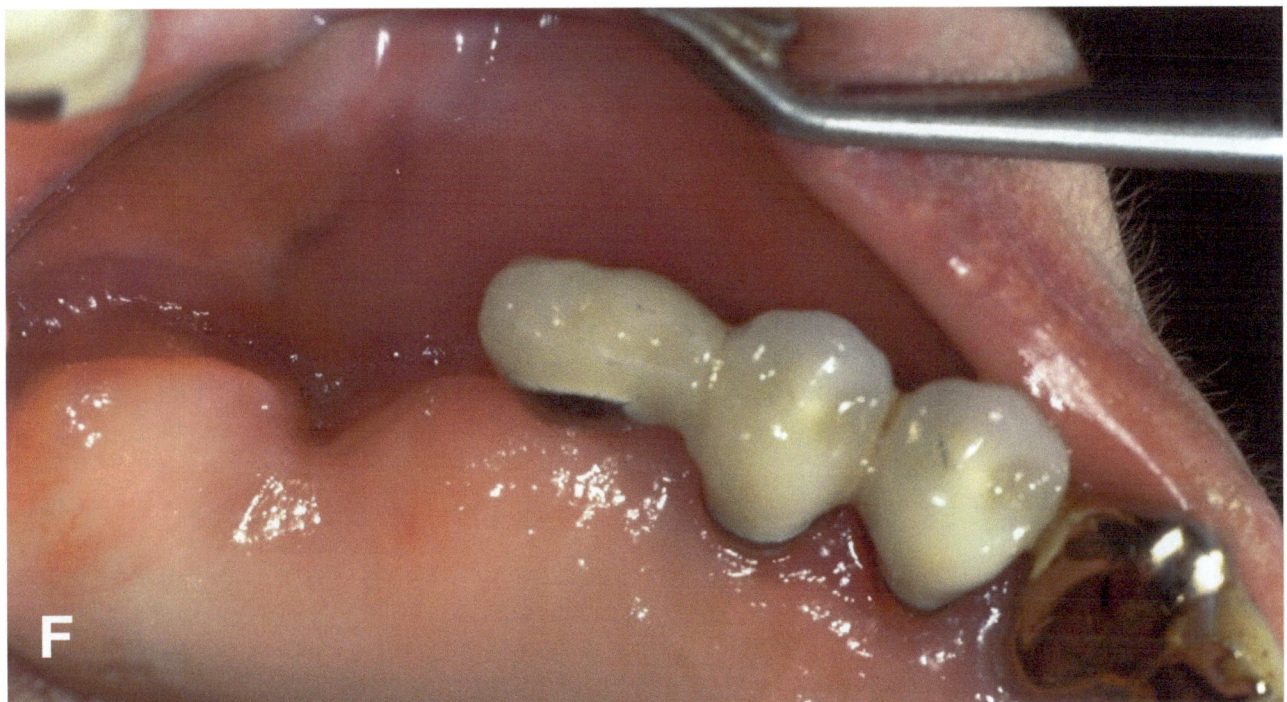

...and the front portion (anterior) was recemented.

PROSTHETICS

Prosthetics is the area of medicine that deals with artificial body part replacements. In dentistry, it is the artificial replacement of natural teeth and other adjacent structures. A natural tooth can be lost due to trauma, massive decay, or periodontal disease. (Developmental defects, whereby a tooth either does not erupt properly or fails to develop at all, is another problem.)

When a tooth is missing, the necessity for artificial replacement depends on a number of factors. Loss of a front tooth poses mostly an aesthetic dilemma, whereas loss of a back tooth creates problems with shifting teeth and decreased chewing efficiency. Since these conditions are not life threatening, the decision to replace a lost tooth is personal, depending on how intact a person wishes to be or the degree of health he or she chooses to maintain. The analogy of the brick wall is again useful. Once bricks, or teeth, are removed, the remaining bricks are subject to additional stress, which could lead to further loss and possibly a collapse of the entire structure. This analogy isn't *always* true because most people who lose teeth do not succumb to a complete oral breakdown.

The Crown

Simple or "normal" sized fillings replace lost natural tooth structure—they are durable and fulfill the requirements of a restoration. When a large filling is placed with standard filling materials, however, limits are reached in terms of adequate replacement of tooth form and function. In these situations, a more durable restoration becomes necessary—the crown.

Generally a shell form of a tooth, cemented or bonded over the remains of a natural tooth (following removal of all decay), the crown restores the proper profile, anatomy, and "biting" relationship with an opposing tooth. Crowns may be made of many different materials, but usually are constructed from porcelain fused to metal, all-reinforced porcelain or all metal. I prefer using the best materials—always— so instead of less expensive metals, I use gold. When extensive decay has destroyed natural tooth structure, a core—usually a bonded composite (reinforced plastic)—is placed to better retain a crown. When practically no tooth structure is left to build on, a post is placed within the remaining root in order to support the core (root canal therapy is necessary before a post can be placed within the canal).

Fixed vs. Removable Prosthesis

When a missing tooth needs to be replaced, the patient generally has a choice of a fixed bridge, a removable partial denture, possibly an implant-supported tooth, or a bonded-type of bridge (the Maryland Bridge). The obvious advantage of a fixed bridge over a removable denture is that it is both non-removable and more stable. In its simplest form, with one tooth missing and a natural

Utilizing A Fractured Composite Restoration As A Core

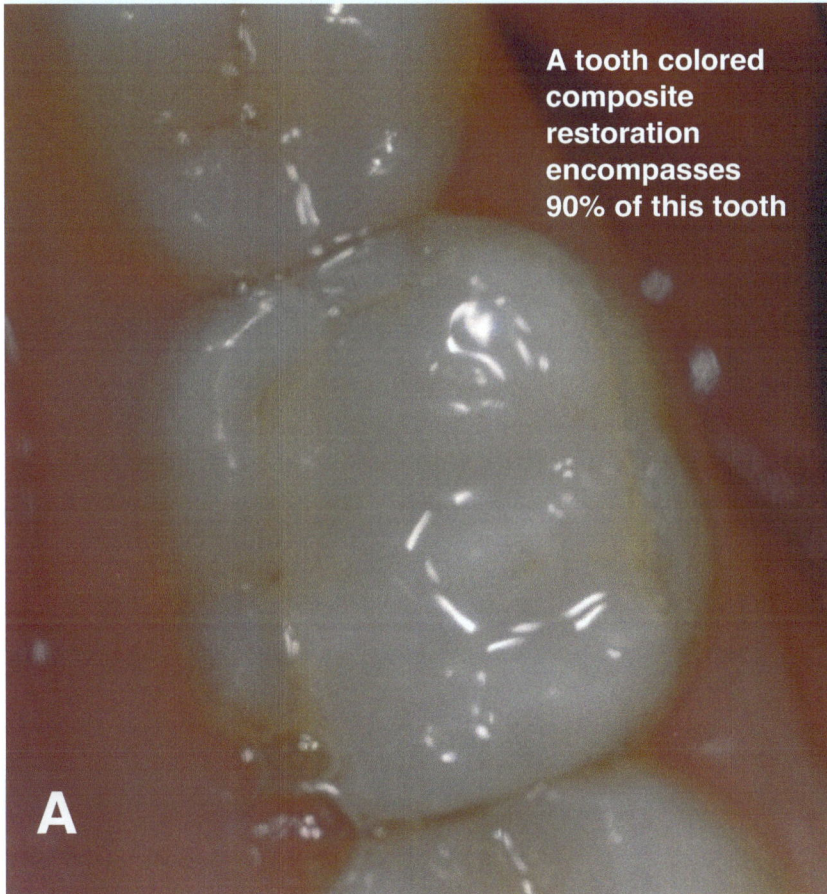

A tooth colored composite restoration encompasses 90% of this tooth

A

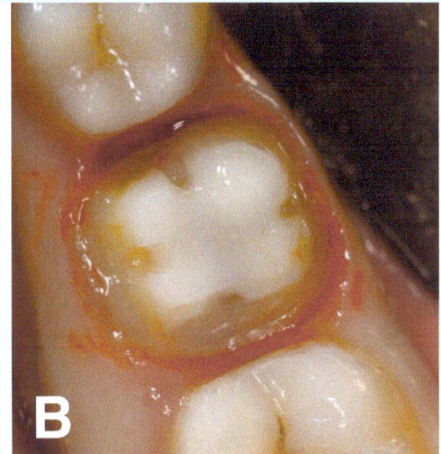

B

A - A very large composite restoration may not have the necessary durability, however it does function well as a core (B) over which an artificial crown can be cemented.

C - All gold crowns tend to be the most durable, long lasting restorations.

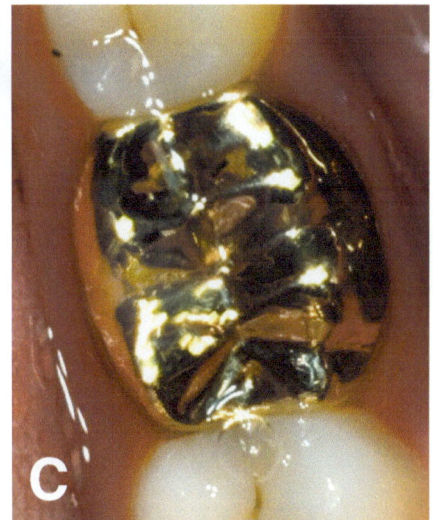

C

tooth on either side, a bridge is cemented over prepared *abutments* (abutments: the natural teeth on either side of the empty space, which have been reduced in size to accommodate the bridge). Assuming all procedures are properly performed and the bridge is correctly designed, this prosthesis can and should function for many years.

A removable prosthesis replaces a missing tooth or teeth and is retained with clasps that engage natural teeth. Though it is removable, it has advantages over the fixed bridge because it is less costly, and where adjacent teeth are otherwise healthy, it avoids the necessity of traumatizing these teeth by reducing them in size to accommodate a bridge.

Restoring Damaged Teeth With Crowns

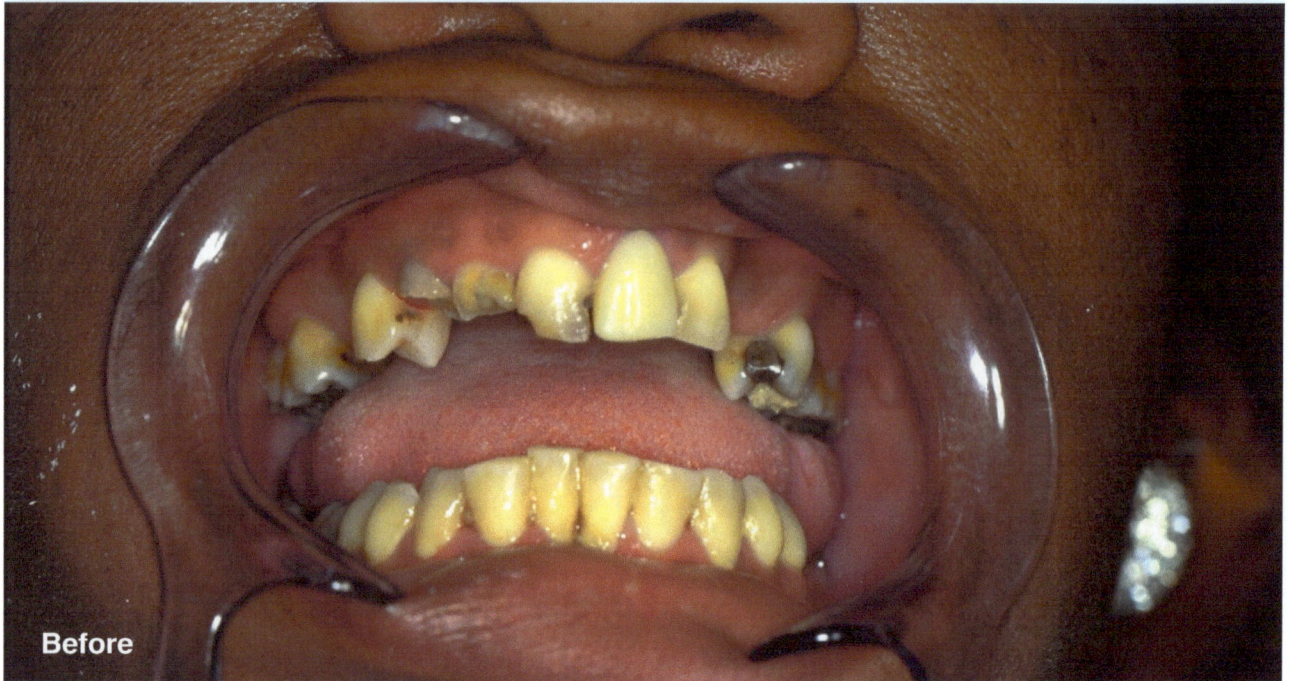

Domestic violence caused this unfortunate situation.

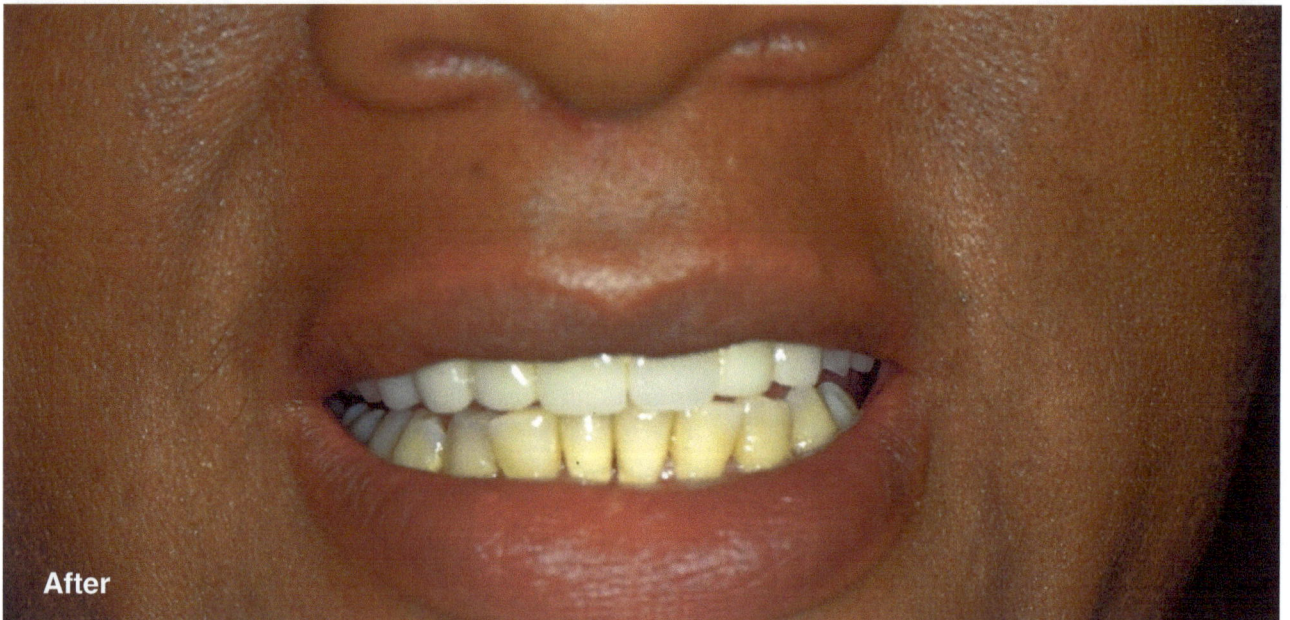

Completed reconstruction.

The Reconstructive Process

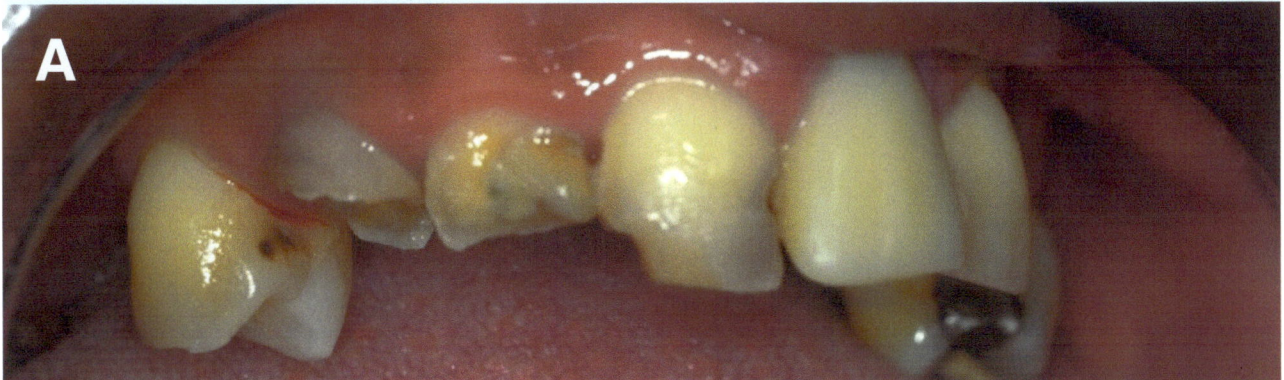

Initial appearance of fractured teeth requiring root canal therapy and placement of posts and cores.

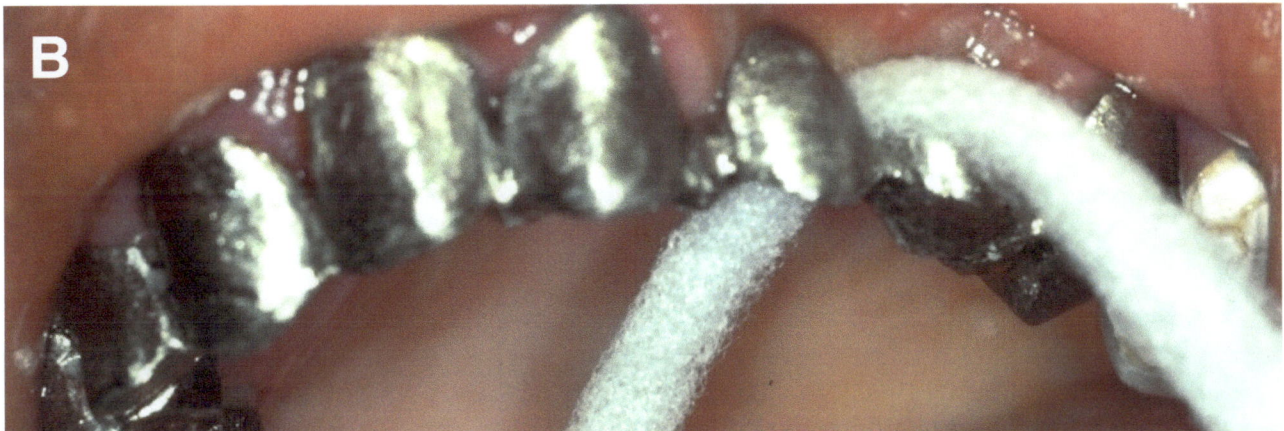

Once the teeth are built up, an impression is taken. The laboratory will then fabricate a framework (made of a gold alloy – a combination of metals that when utilized together satisfies engineering requirements). This design must allow the patient access to perform proper oral hygiene procedures. As seen here, space exists beneath the framework to allow Super Floss® to clean the area.

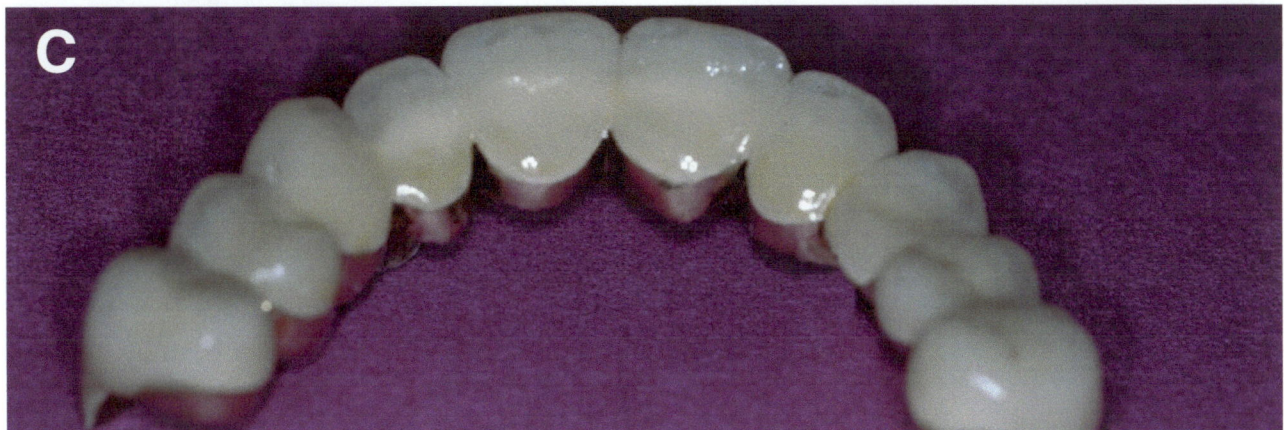

Porcelain is baked onto the framework which is then cemented onto the prepared teeth.

Fabrication of a 3-unit bridge

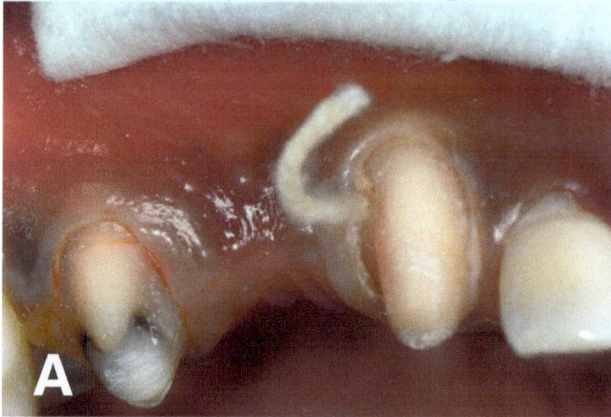

Before taking an impression for the fabrication of a bridge, retraction cord is carefully placed between the tooth and the gum. This cord is removed prior to taking the impression and allows the impression material to register the exact margin of the preparation.

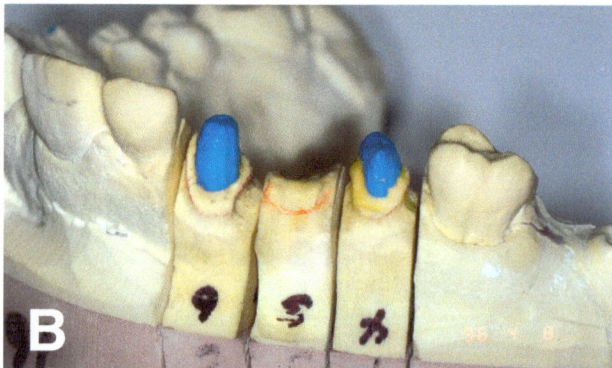

The impression is then sent to the laboratory where it is poured in stone to create a working model.

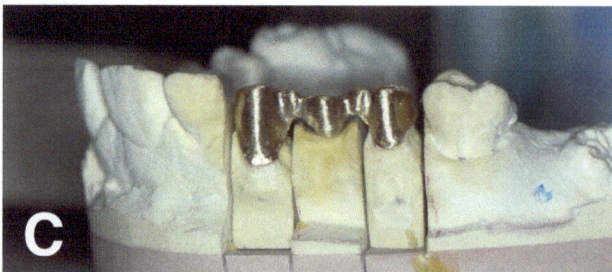

A gold framework is then fabricated.

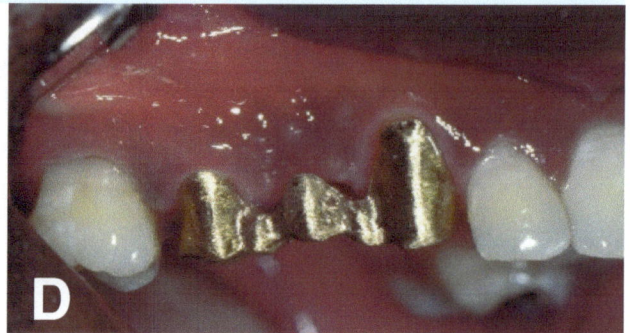

The gold framework is then tried in the mouth to assure a proper fit.

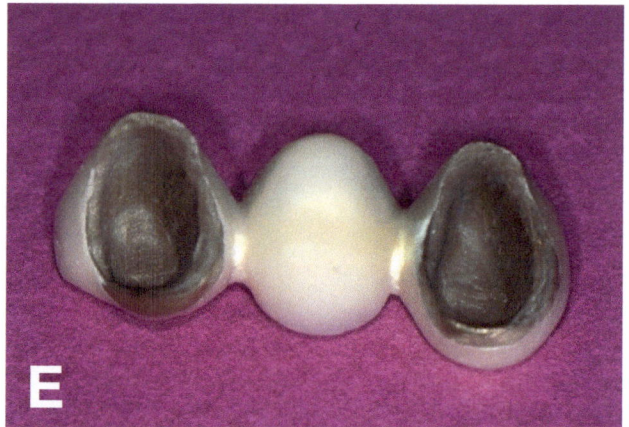

Porcelain is then baked onto the framework (underside view).

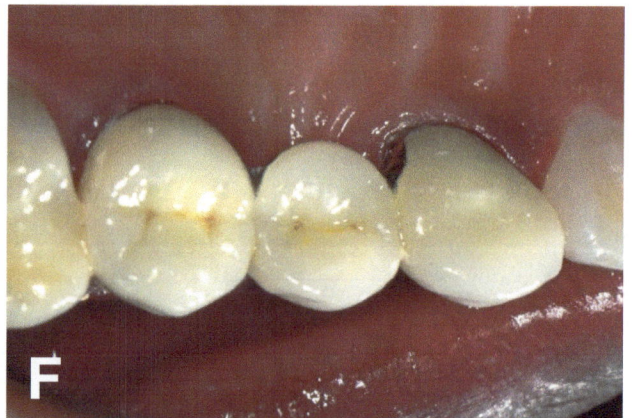

The bridge is cemented in the mouth.

Restoration Of A Root *(Photos A – G)*

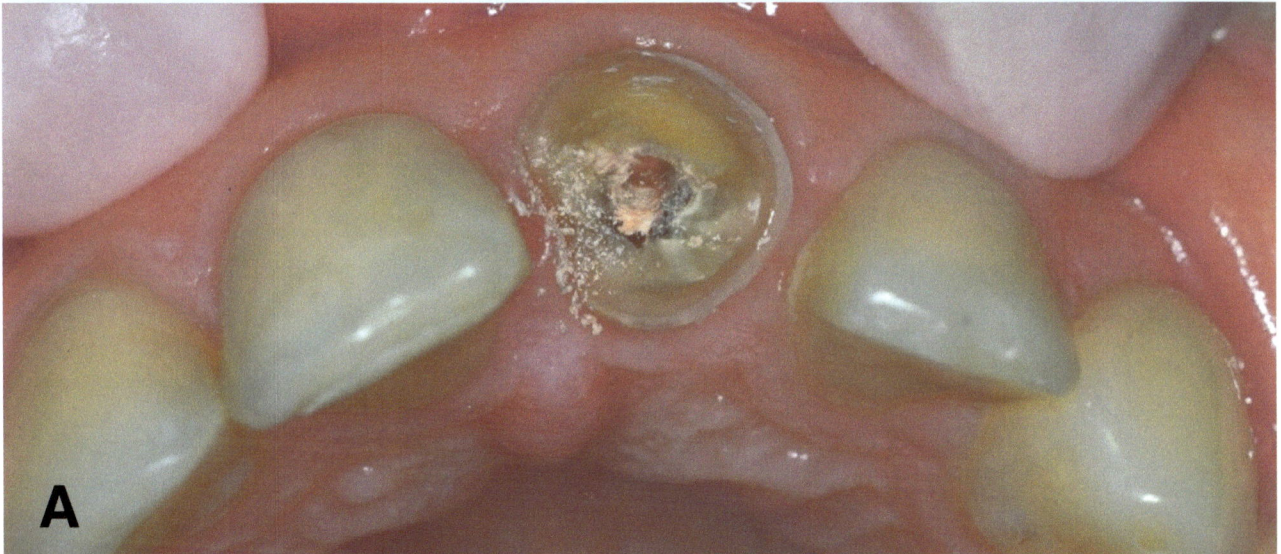

A

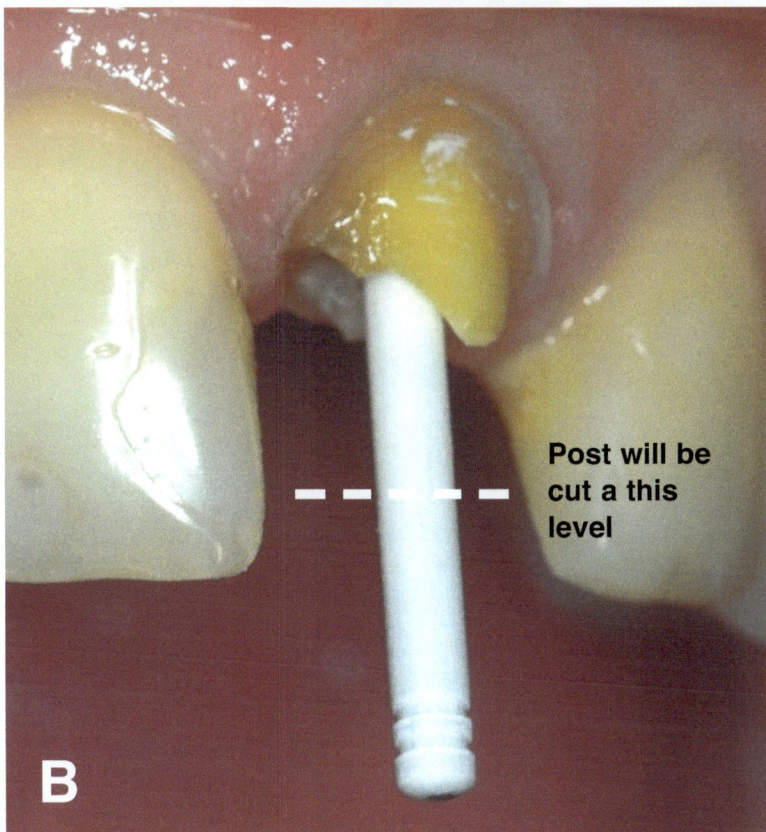

B

Post will be cut a this level

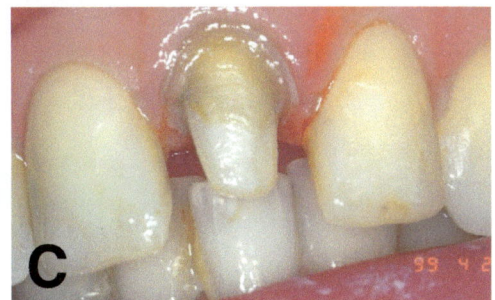

C

A - *Following root canal therapy.*
B - *A carbon fiber post is fitted, adjusted and bonded into the canal.*
C - *A core material is bonded over the remaining root and post.*

Restoration Of A Root   (Continued)

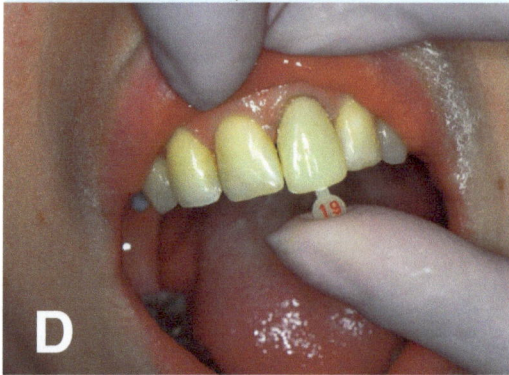

D

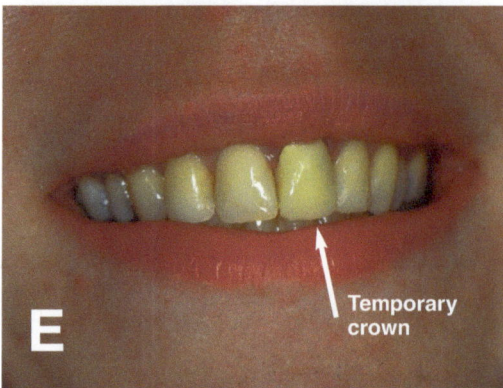

E   Temporary crown

D and E - A temporary crown should simulate the final restoration in terms of function and aesthetics.

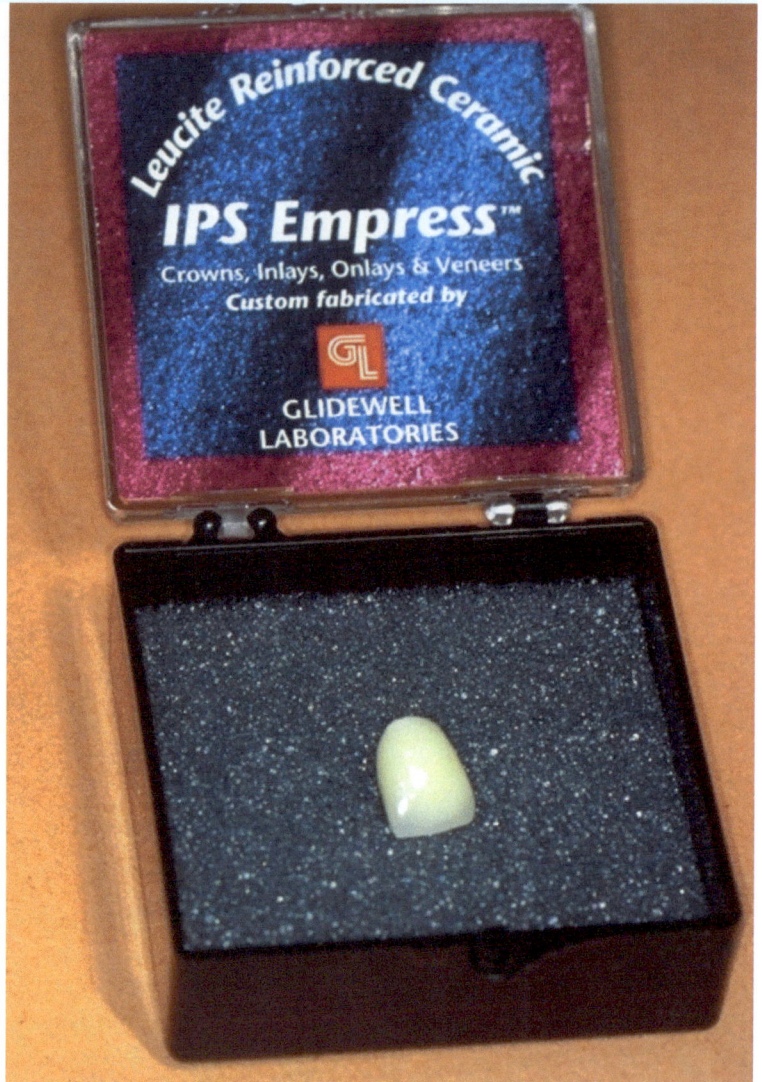

An all ceramic crown is fabricated (Advanced materials and fabrication techniques have reduced the need for metal reinforcement under porcelain crowns, therefore allowing for a more translucent and natural restoration). Glidewell Laboratories. 1-800-854-7256

Restoration Of A Root   (Continued)

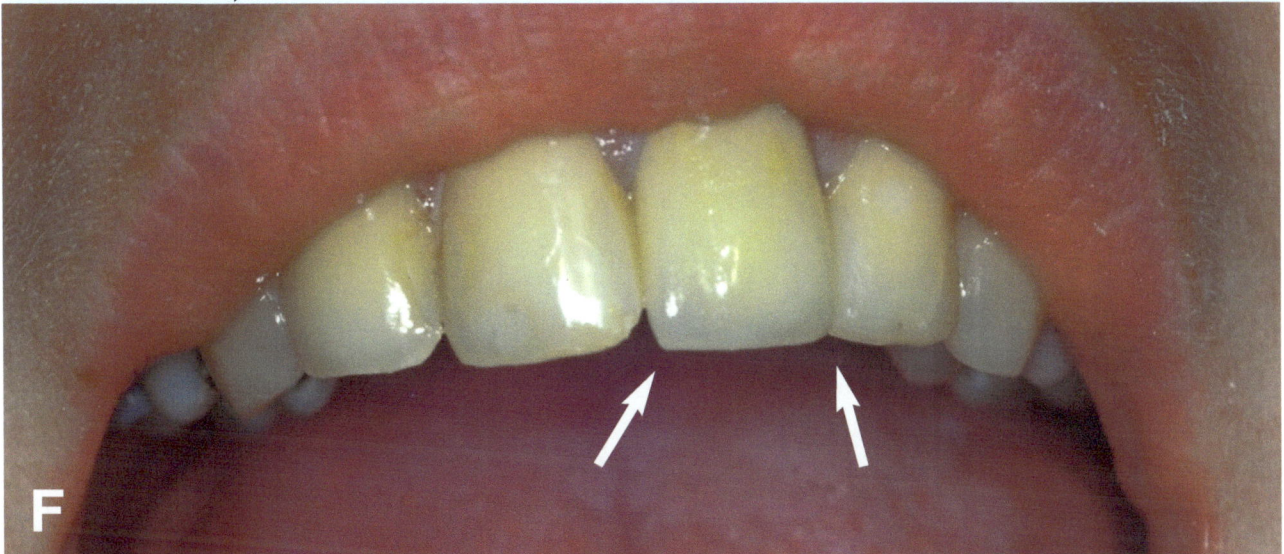

At the try in appointment the crown is checked for proper shade, fit and form.
Note that the square edges do not reflect a feminine appearance.

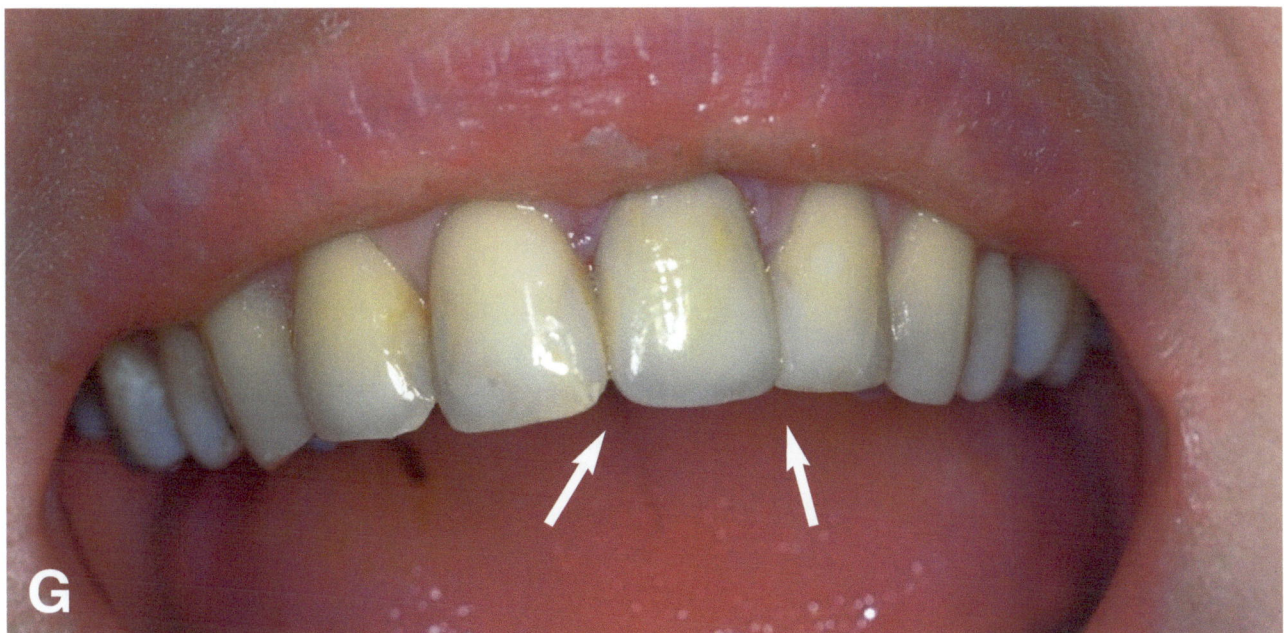

Following recontouring of the crown it is bonded to place.

Periodontal / Prosthetic Therapy　　　　　　　(Photos A – F)

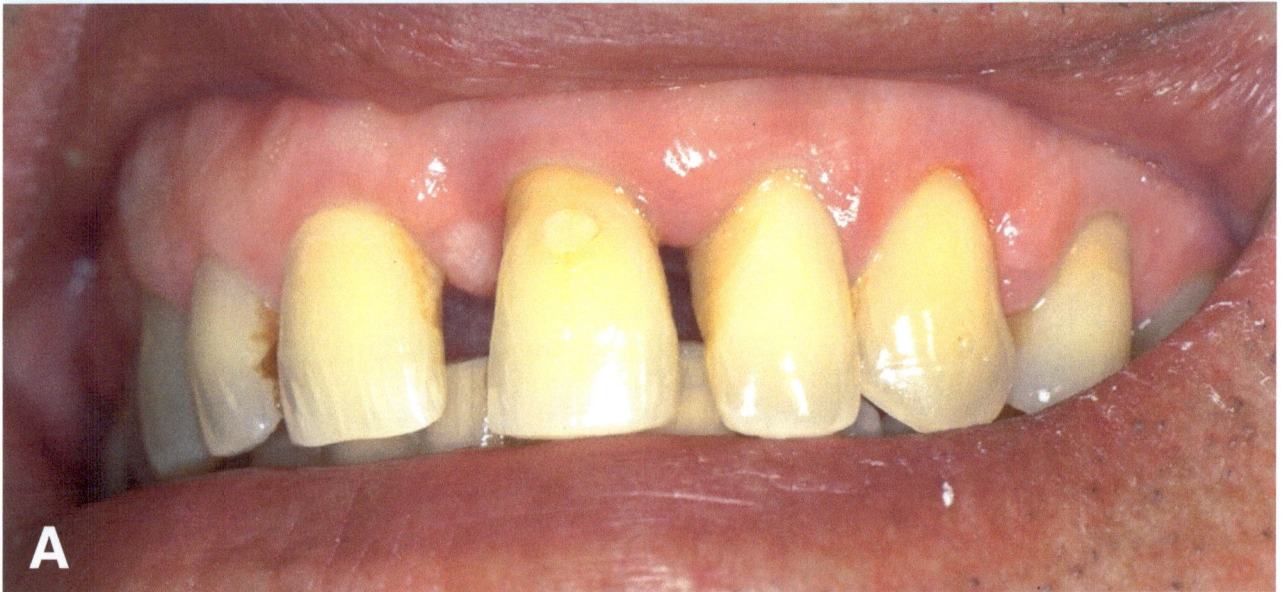

Advanced periodontal disease destroyed the bone supporting these teeth. Shifting and spacing has occurred.

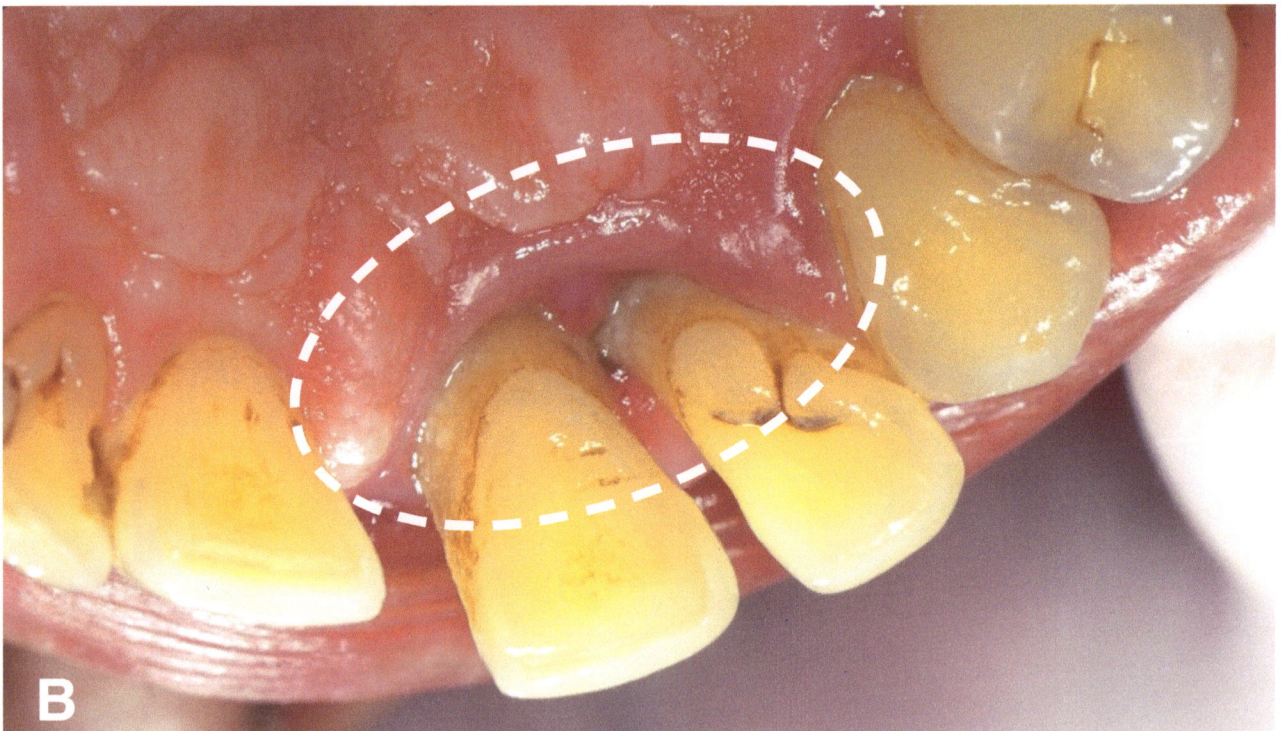

Inside view (lingual) showing separation of the gum from the teeth (periodontal pockets).

Periodontal / Prosthetic Therapy   **(Continued)**

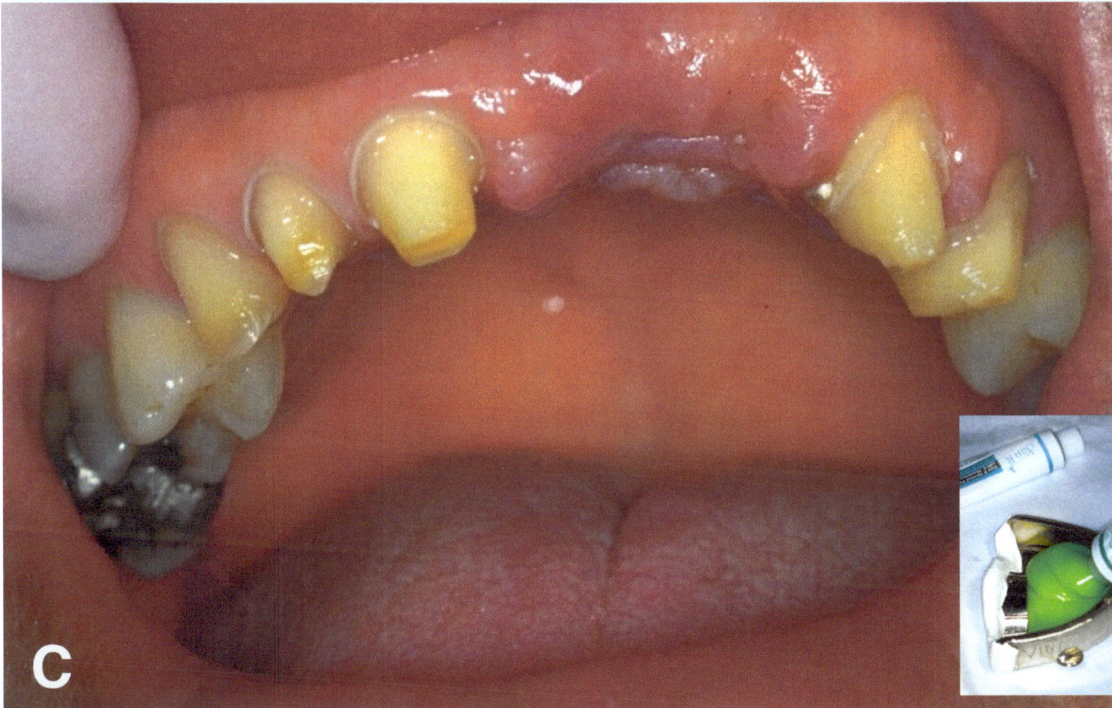

Following discussion of treatment options with the patient, it was decided that a fixed bridge would be utilized to replace the hopeless teeth. Here is the situation after extractions and adjacent tooth preparations. The patient was wearing a temporary bridge at this time (not seen here) while the tissues were healing. Many different impression materials are available. Hydrocolloid is our choice here — it is extremely accurate.

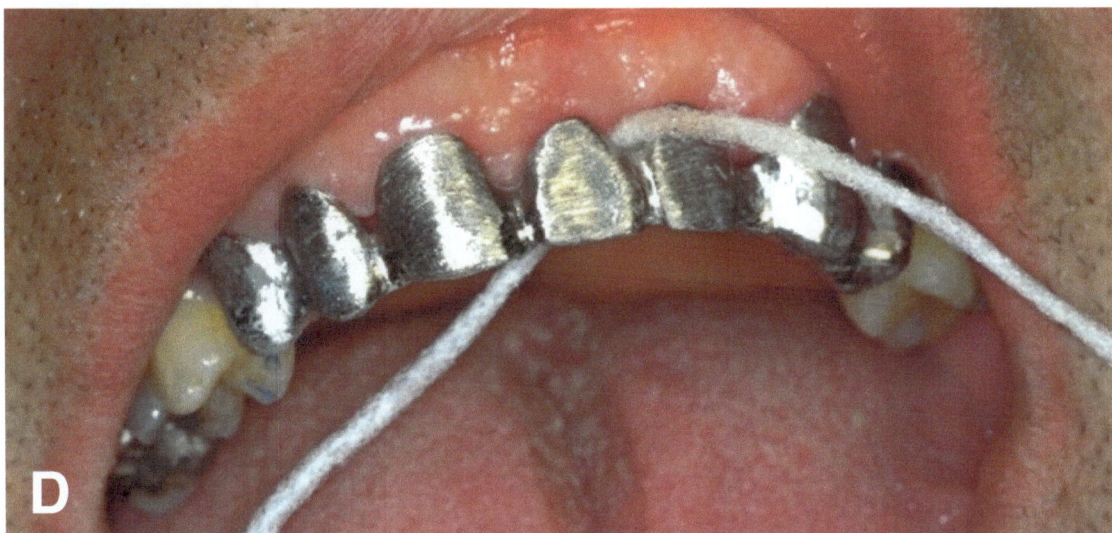

Once the impression has been taken and sent to the laboratory, a gold alloy framework is fabricated and tried in. It is designed to allow access for oral hygiene procedures (as seen here with Super Floss® – Oral-B Laboratories 1-800-446-7252).

Periodontal / Prosthetic Therapy (Continued)

E

(Before)

F

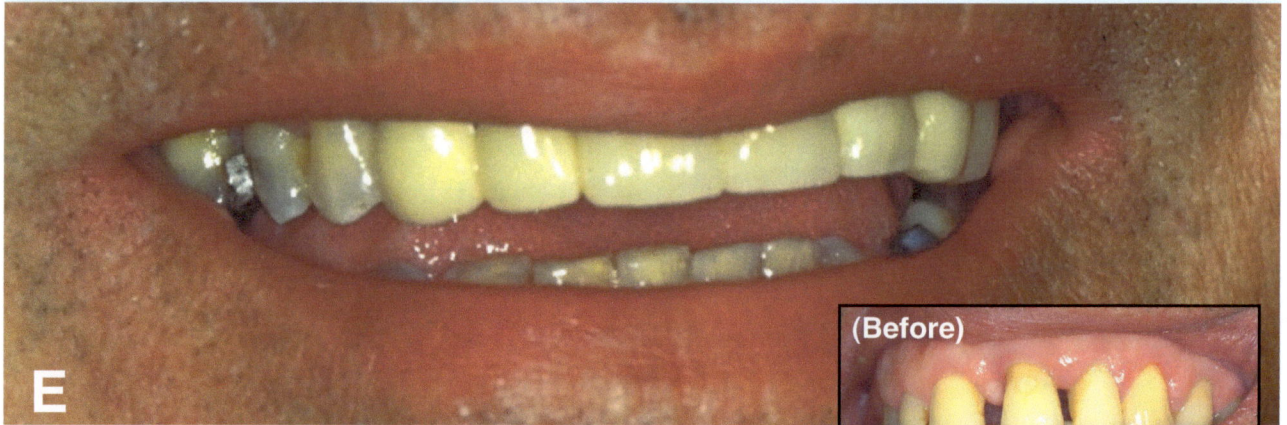

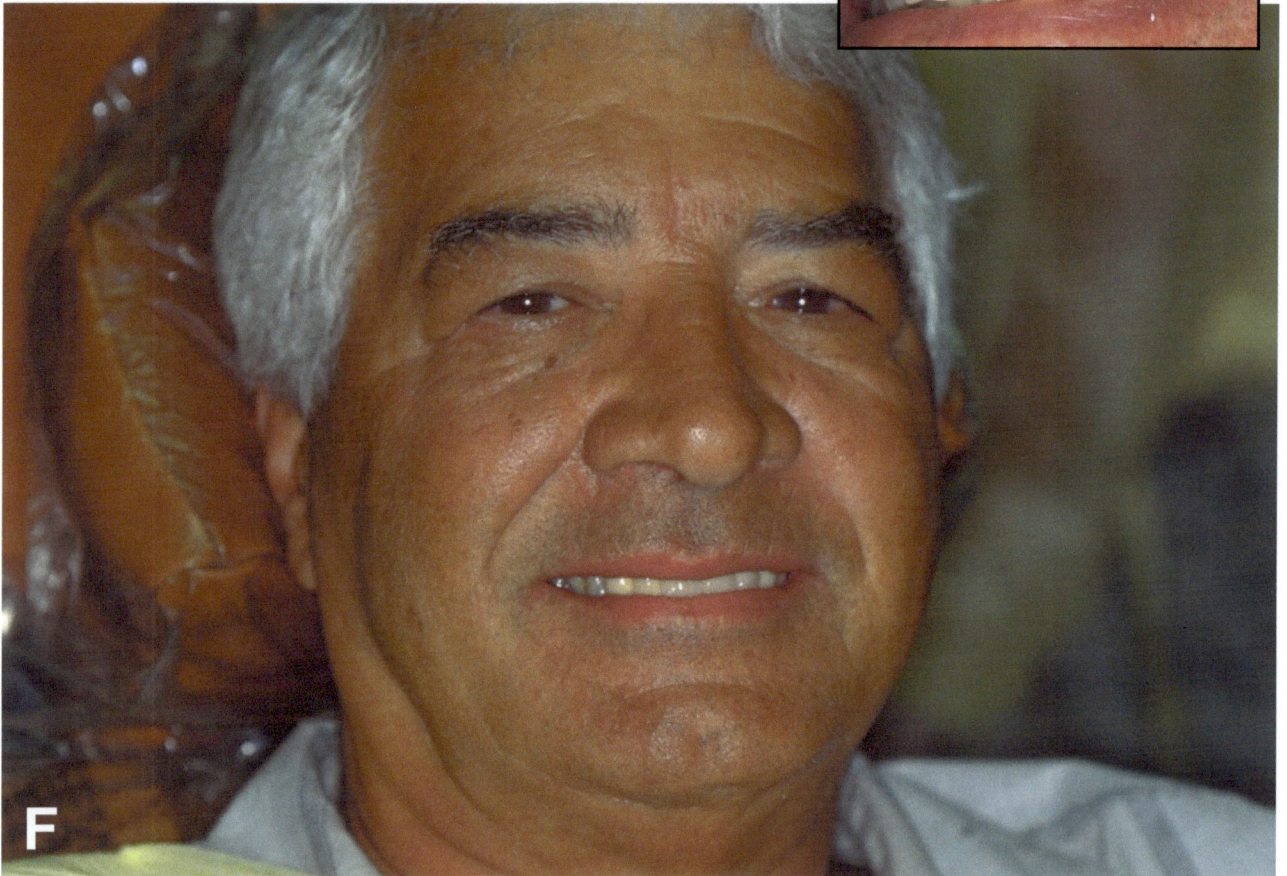

The finished prosthesis is cemented in place.

A difficult restorative case.

(Photos A – G)

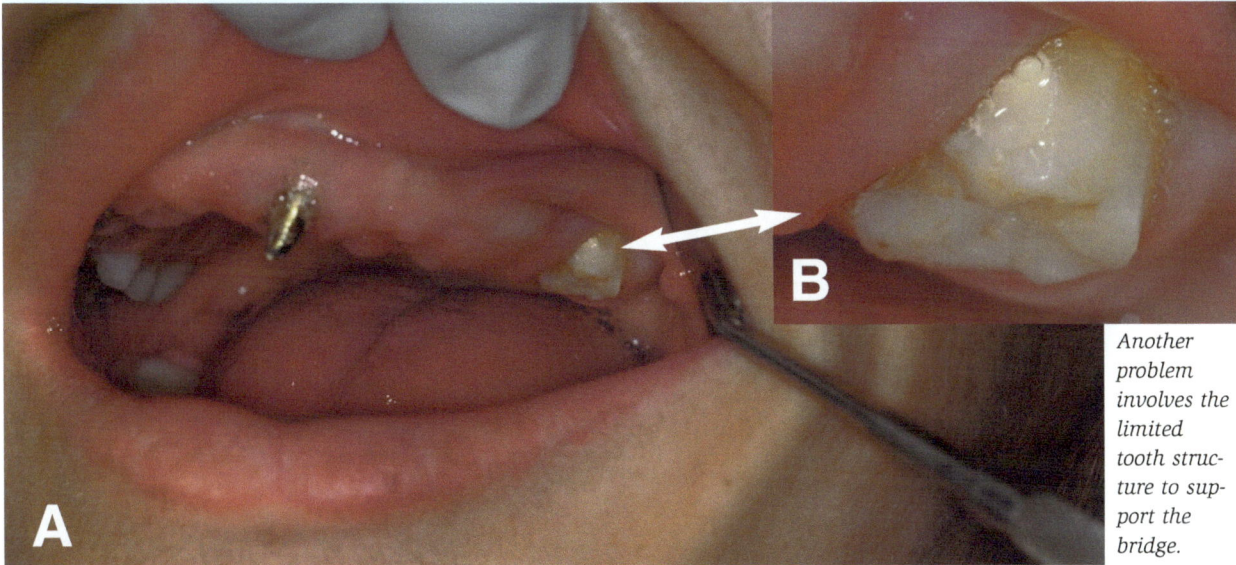

Another problem involves the limited tooth structure to support the bridge.

A young, attractive lady presented with this situation. The problem here is that there is such a long span between the supporting teeth. Treatment options to replace her missing teeth include a removable partial denture, a fixed cemented bridge or implants. It was decided to utilize a bridge.

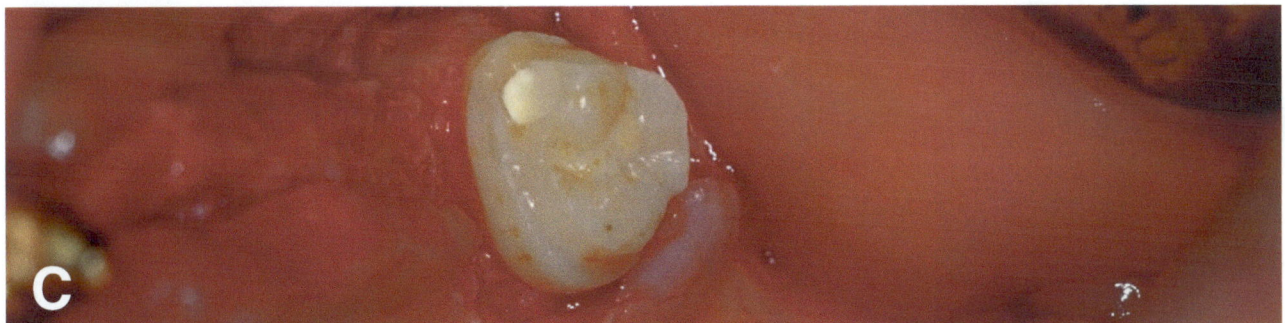

A periodontal surgical crown lengthening procedure was performed. This involves removing adjacent tissues to establish a more substantial tooth for bridge anchoring.

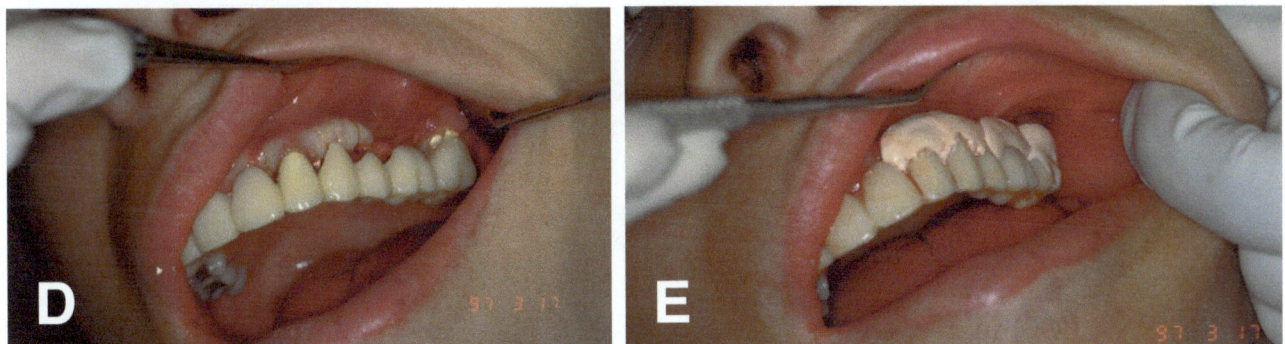

A reinforced temporary bridge is then placed along with a dressing.

A difficult restorative case.   (Continued)

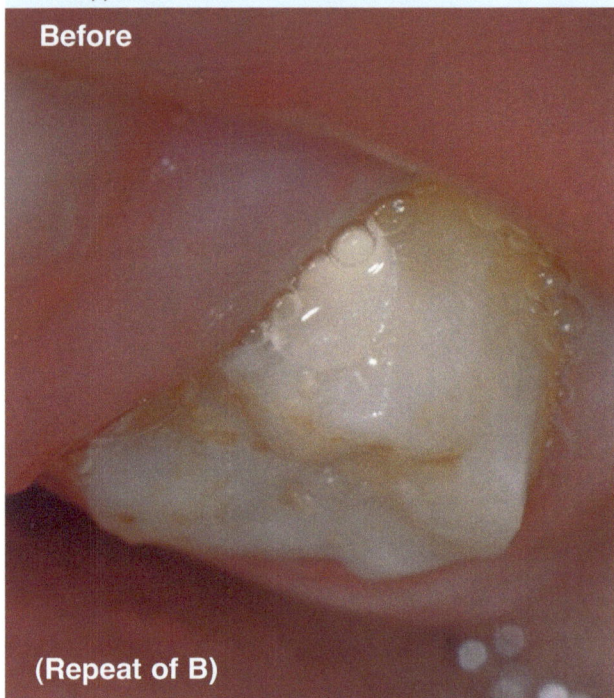

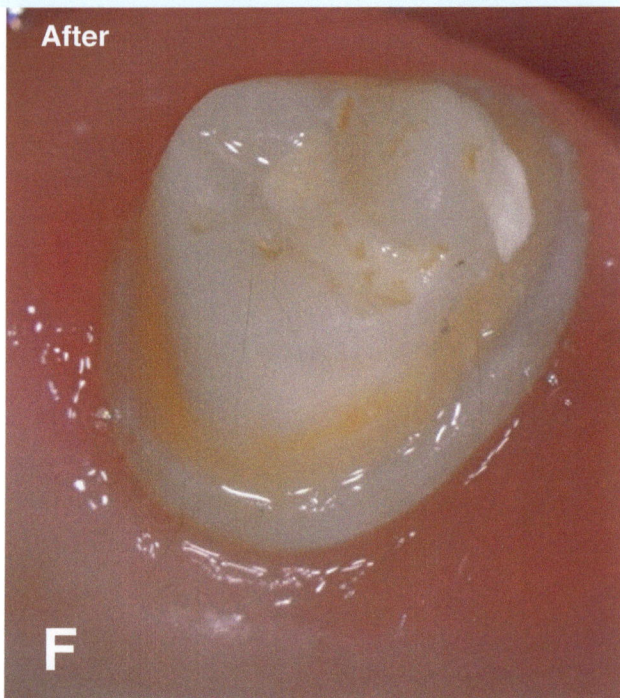

Following about four weeks of healing adequate tooth structure is now available.

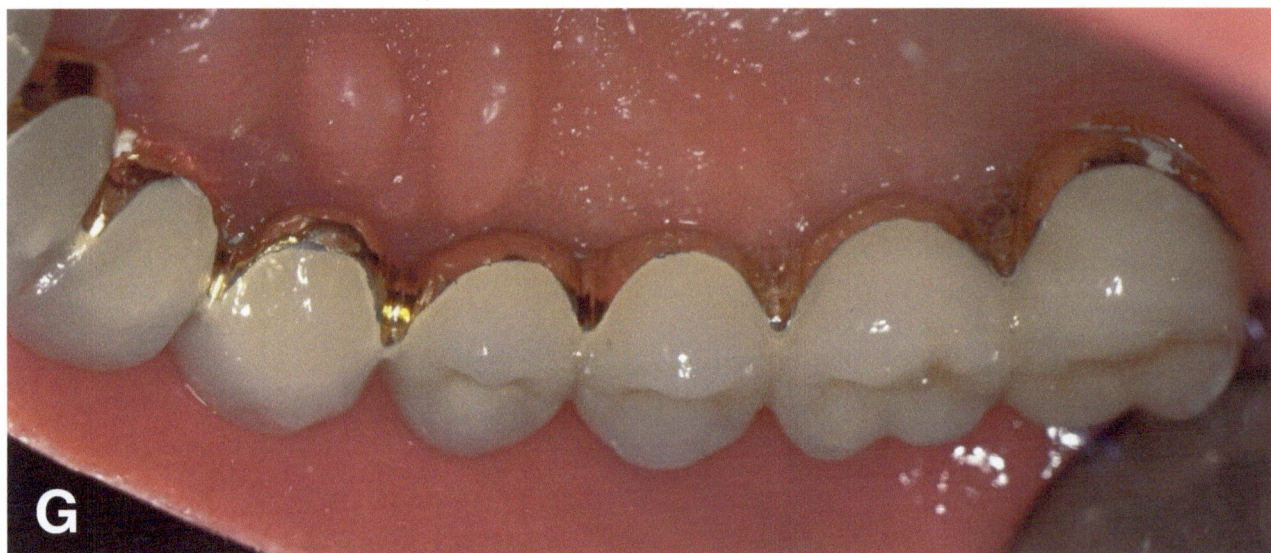

The final bridge (as seen from the palatal —inside— view). Stresses associated with this long span bridge necessitate utilizing a gold alloy (combination of metals) that is stronger than the usual metal framework.

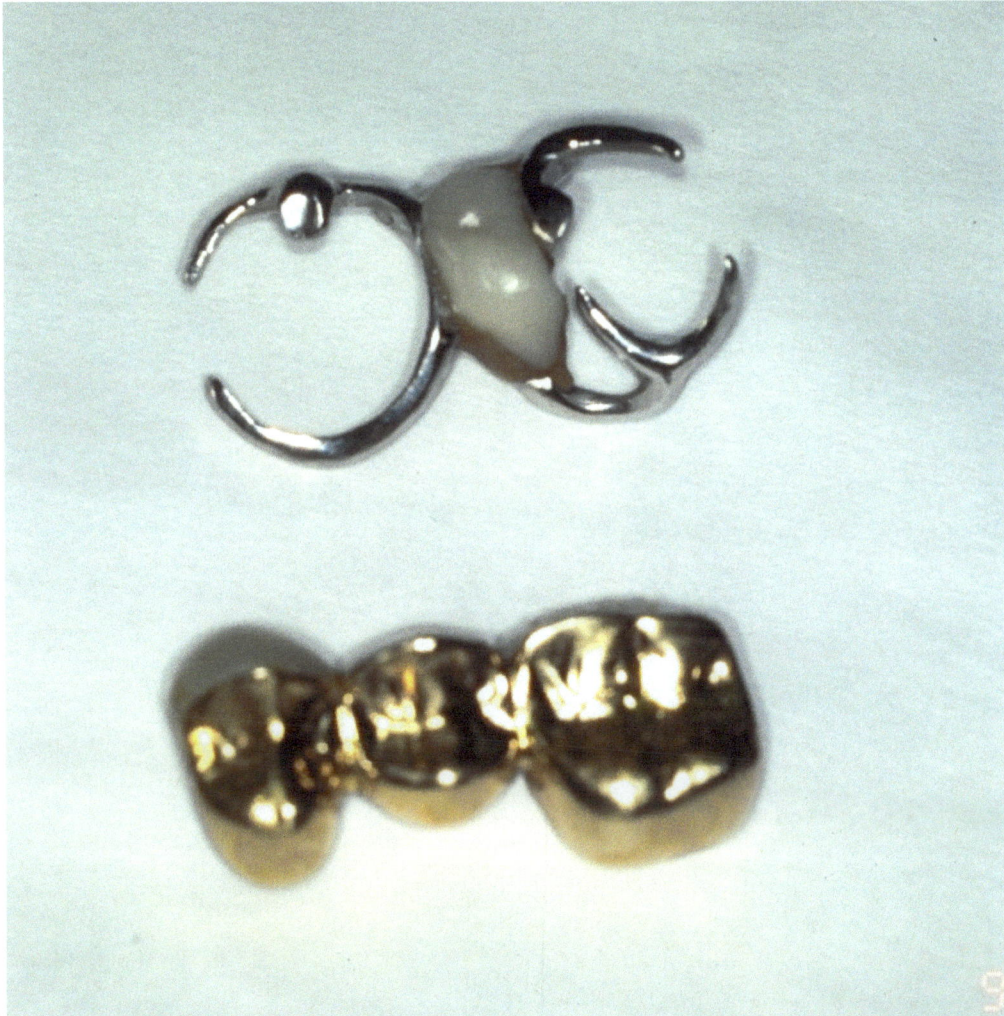

A removable one tooth replacement prosthesis and a 3-unit bridge. Both are utilized to replace one missing tooth. Though the removable device is easier to fabricate and less expensive it is unstable as compared to the fixed bridge and there is the chance that the patient could swallow it.

The Implant

An implant is an artificial root, surgically placed in bone, which supports artificial teeth. The success of an implant depends on proper planning, execution by an experienced dentist, and other factors. It is an expensive procedure, but if all goes well, it is an excellent method of replacing teeth. The "all goes well" caveat reflects my guarded opinion regarding the overall effectiveness of implant therapy to date. More will be explained on this subject in the chapter about controversies.

Single Tooth Implant

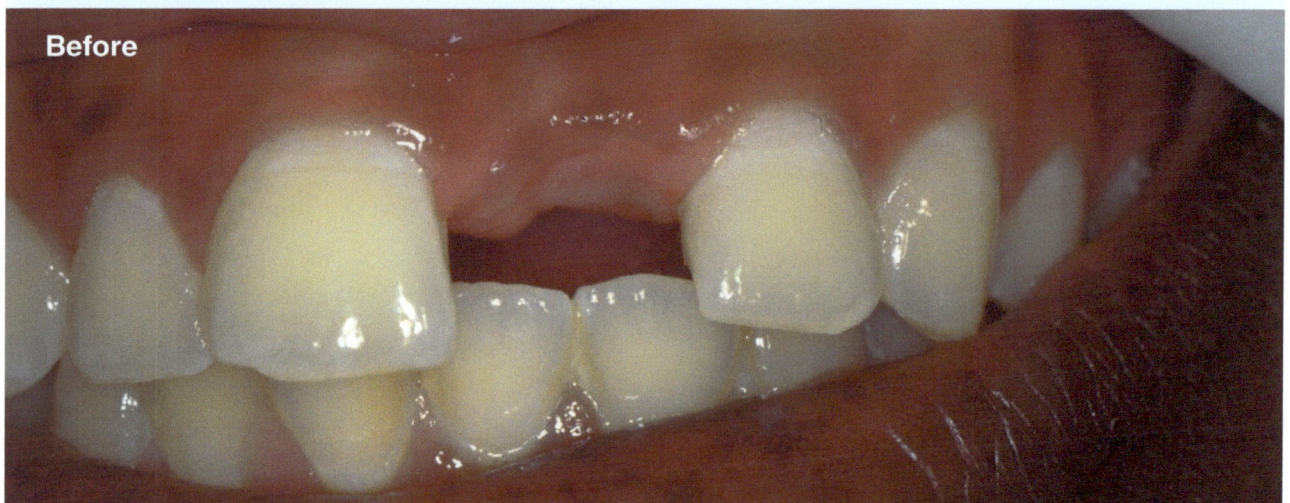
Before

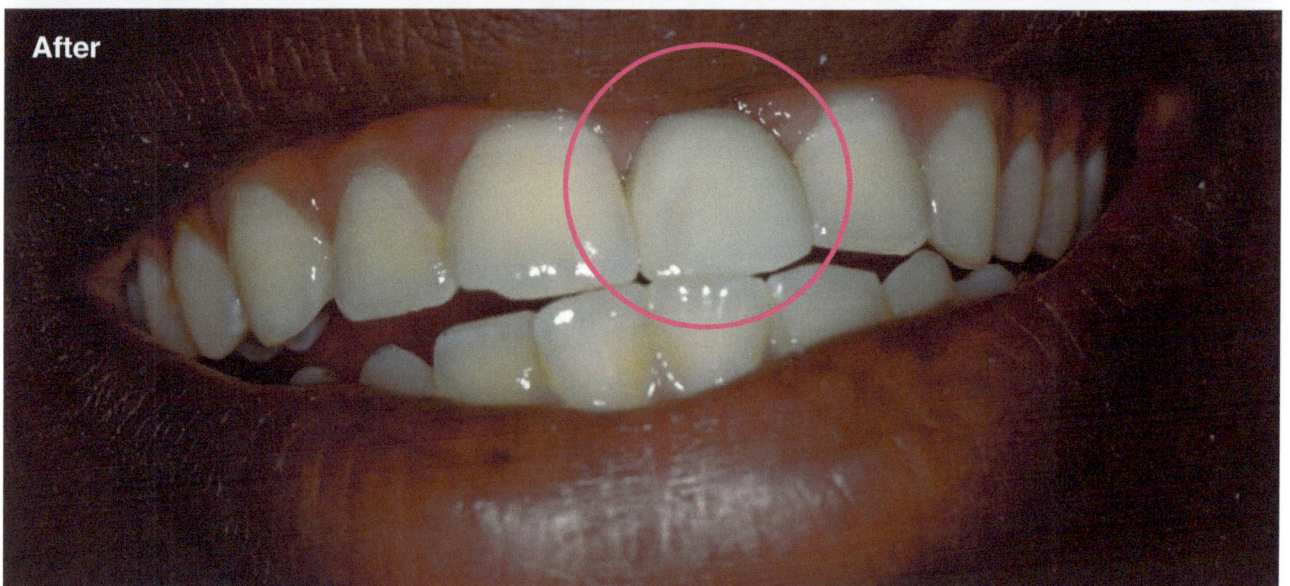
After

Single Tooth Implant

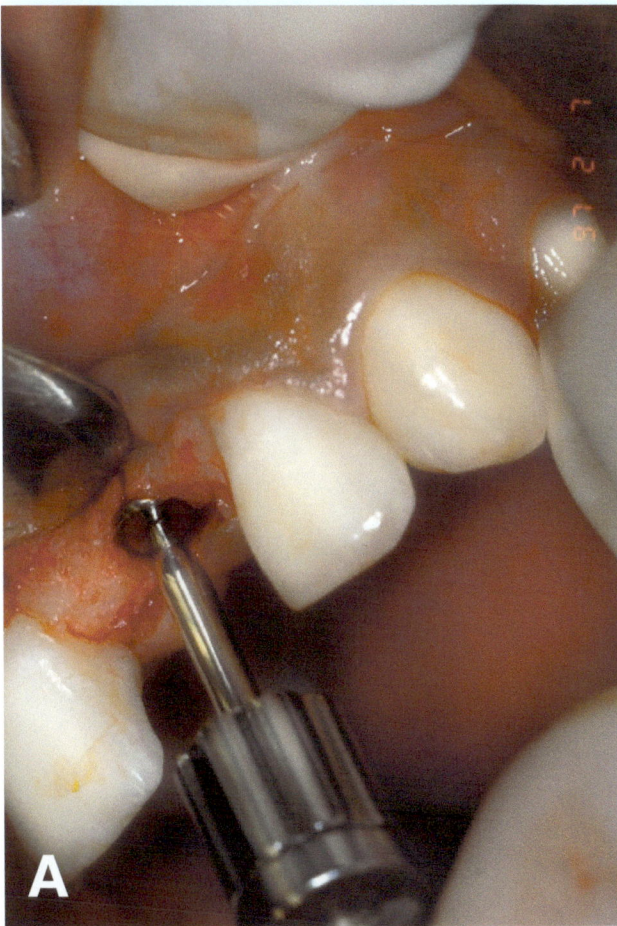

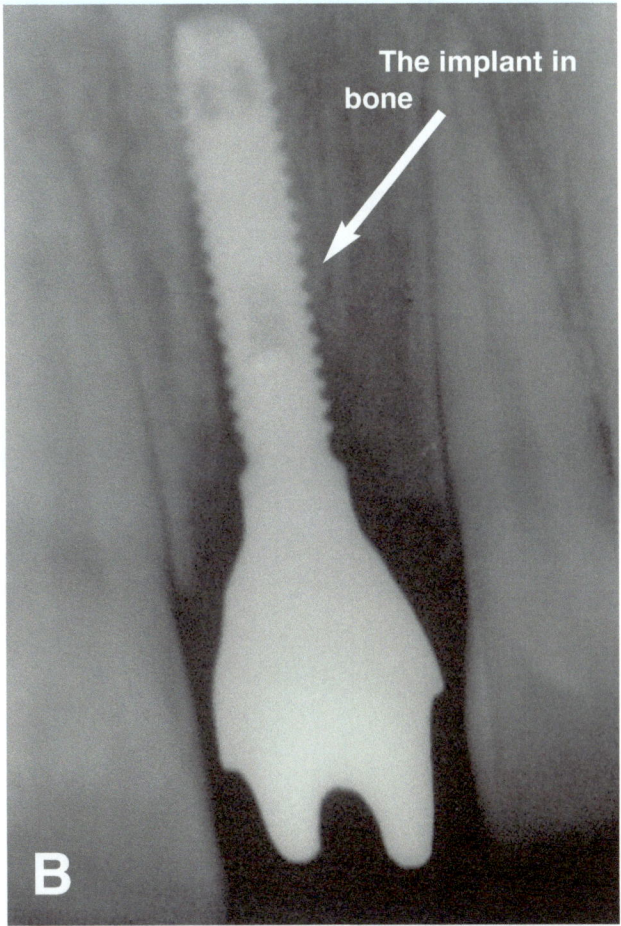

Rather than cap the teeth on either side of this empty space(A) for a bridge, or fabricate a removable partial denture, an implant was placed (B) which will support a crown.

The Implant Process

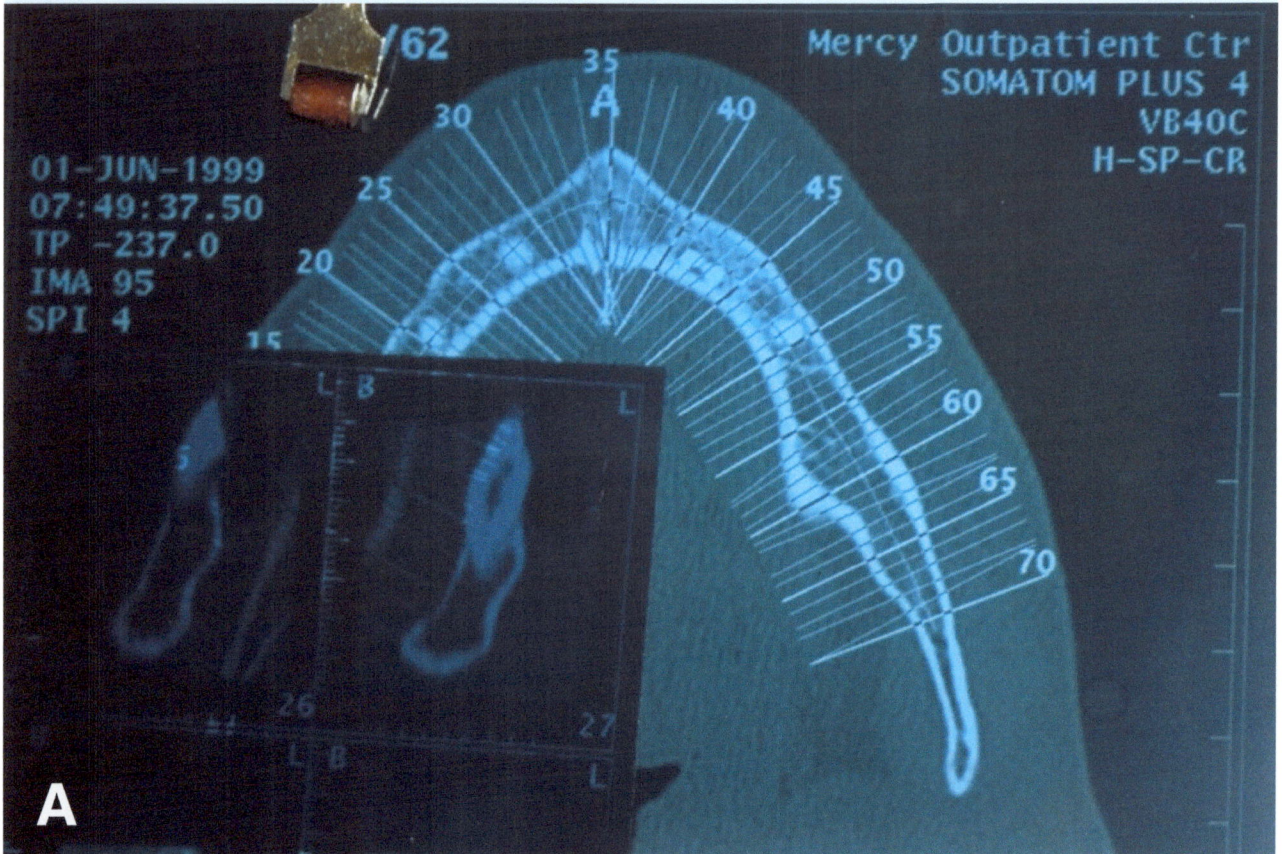

Computer enhanced radiographs are utilized to evaluate bone configuration for proper placement of implants.

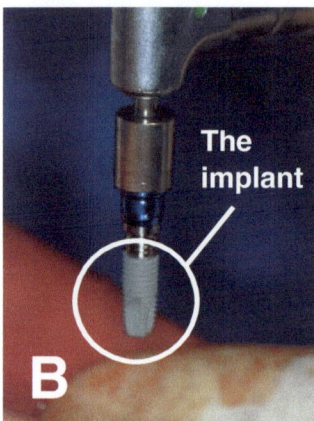

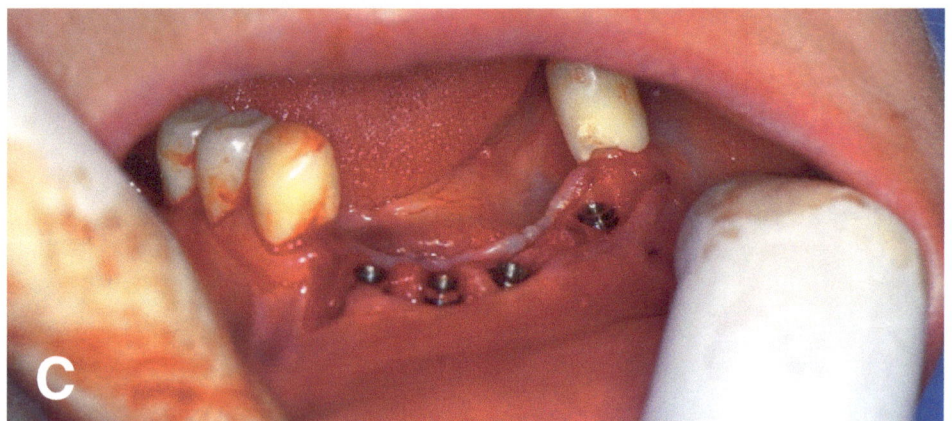

Titanium implants are placed in prepared bone "sockets".

The Implant Process   *(Continued)*

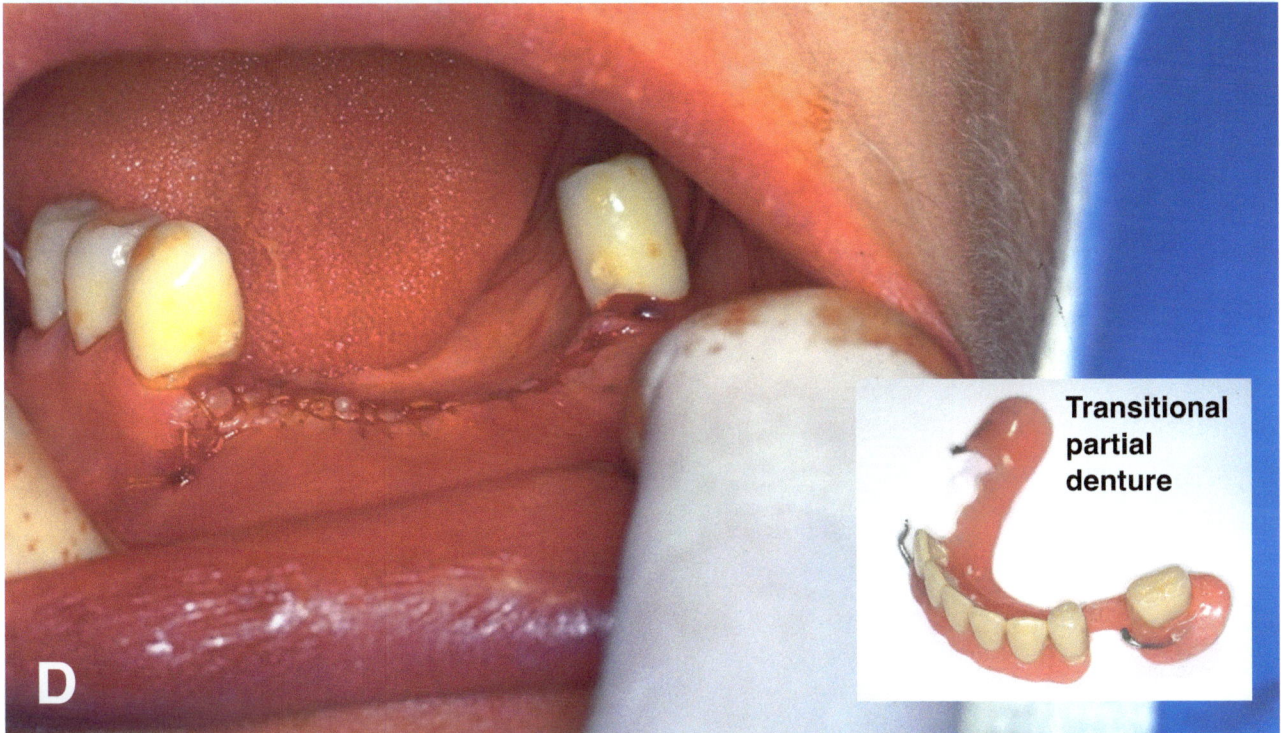

Transitional partial denture

The implants are covered and left undisturbed for four to six months during which time they fuse (osseointegrate) with the bone. The patient wears a temporary lower partial denture during this time. Advances in implant technology have reduced this waiting period. In certain circumstances, implants can be splinted and "loaded" earlier.

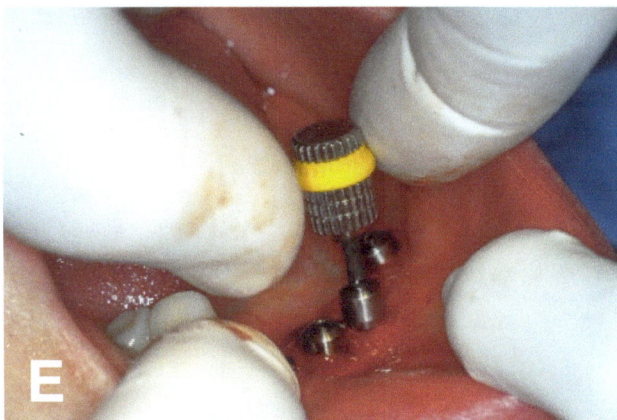

Healing caps are placed prior to impressions for the final prosthesis.

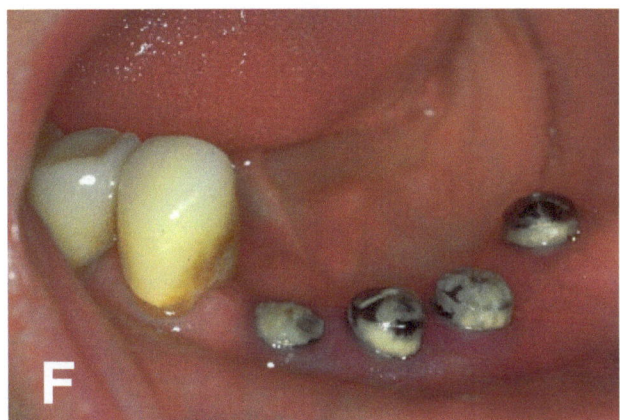

Poor oral hygiene is evident here with the accumulation of extensive plaque and tartar. This will result in failure of the case if not corrected. (The final prosthetic "artificial teeth" are not shown in this case.)

The Maryland Bridge

The Maryland Bridge is a conservative alternative to a traditional fixed bridge. With a traditional bridge, supporting teeth need to be reduced in size, necessitating the removal of natural tooth structure. The Maryland Bridge somewhat eliminates this requirement and is bonded to the supporting teeth. I like this treatment, however, problems with de-bonding do occasionally occur (and usually at the worst possible time). I feel more secure cementing a traditional fixed bridge in a patient's mouth.

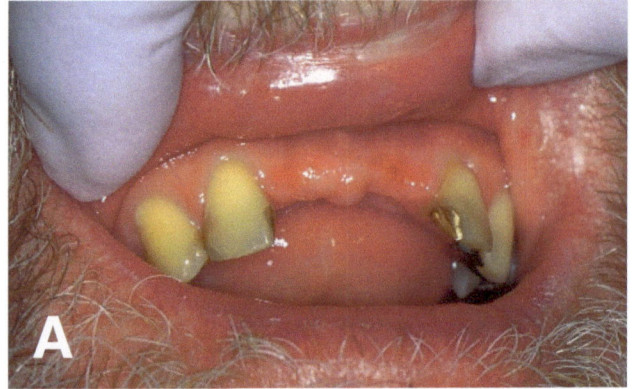

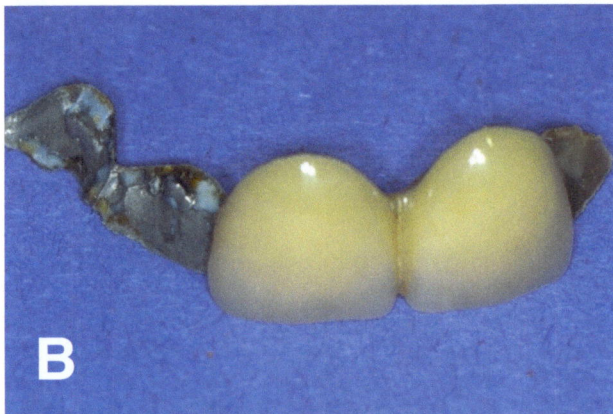

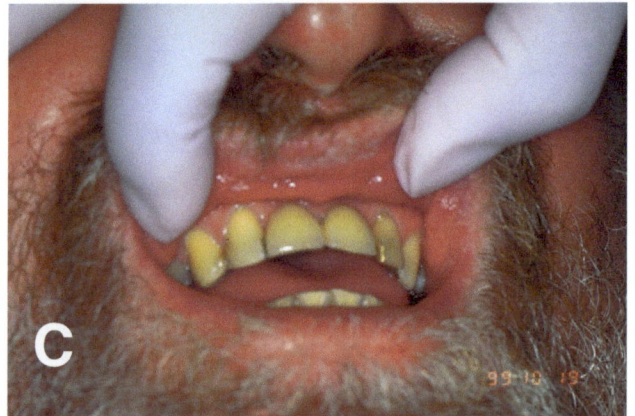

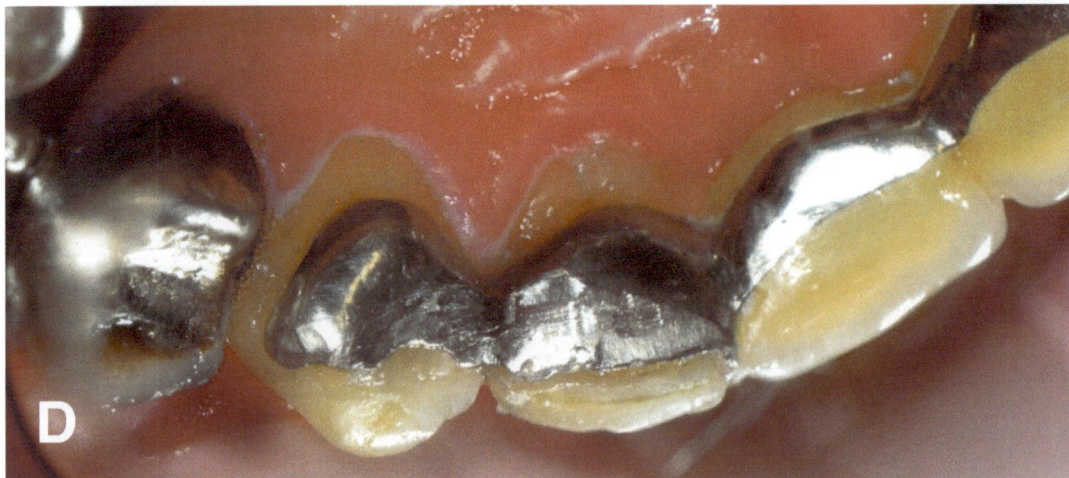

This emergency patient presented to my office with a de-bonded Maryland bridge. Improvements in materials and techniques have reduced the incidence of failures.

Utilizing The Patient's Natural Tooth Crown to Fabricate An Immediate "Maryland Bridge"   *(Photos A — E)*

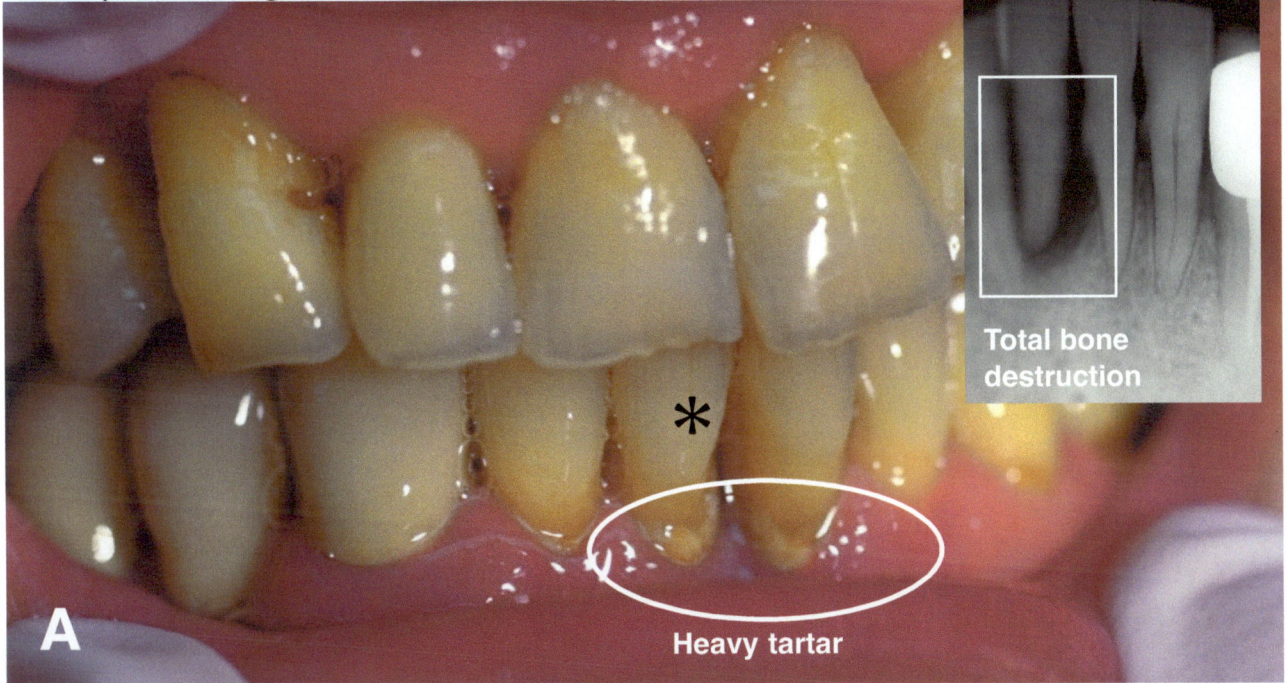

Total bone destruction

*

Heavy tartar

A

This patient has advanced periodontal disease. A lower front tooth has lost all bone support and requires extraction. In order to avoid an aesthetic deficiency (an empty space in the front of his mouth), the crown portion of the tooth(*) is bonded to the adjacent teeth before the root portion is extracted.

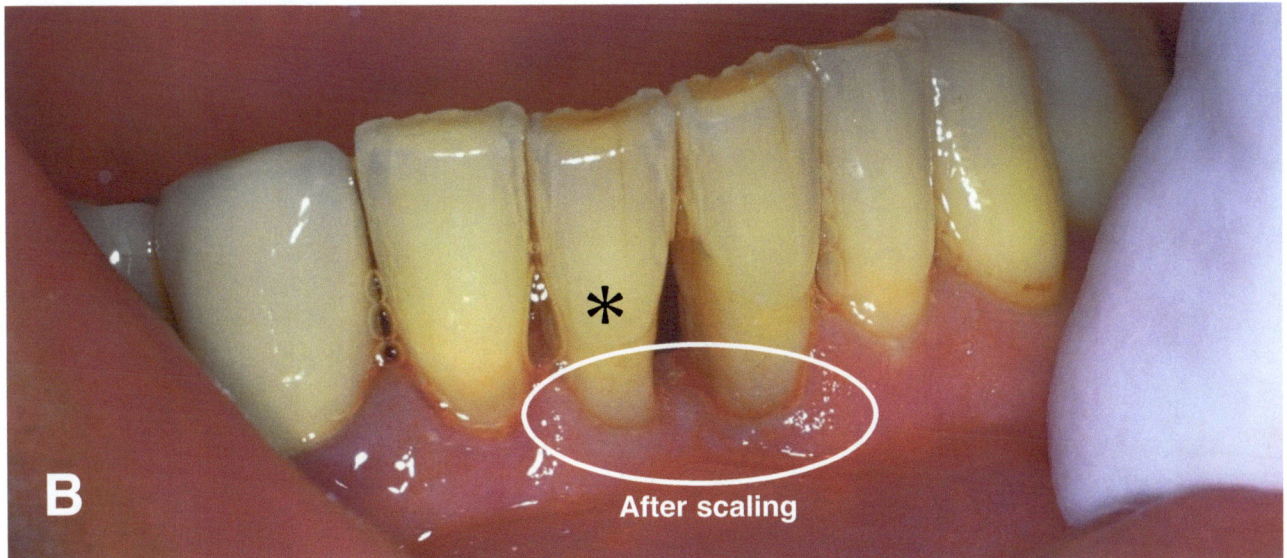

*

After scaling

B

Deep scaling and curettage has been performed.

Utilizing The Patient's Natural Tooth Crown to Fabricate An Immediate "Maryland Bridge"
(Photos A — E)

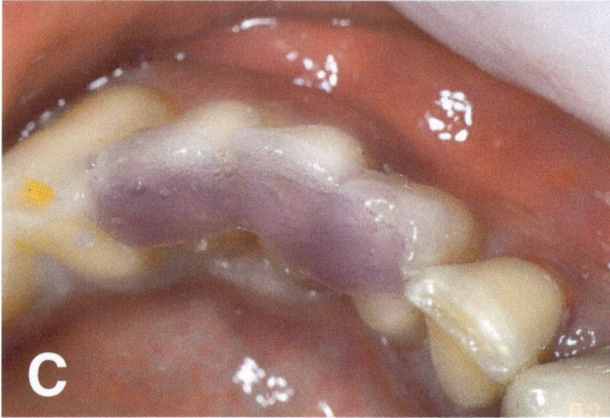

C

Treatment of the enamel surface prior to bonding.

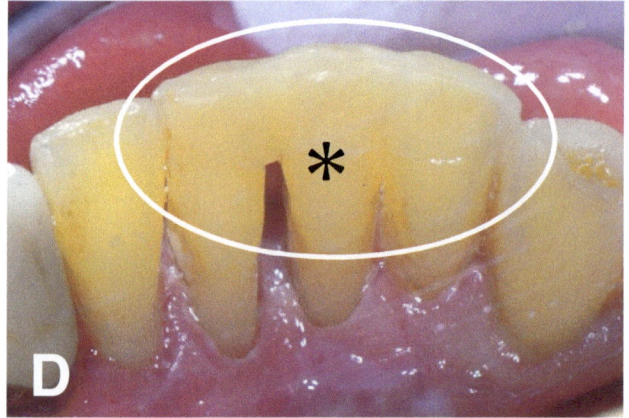

D

Composite material is utilized to bond the crown of the hopeless tooth to the adjacent teeth.

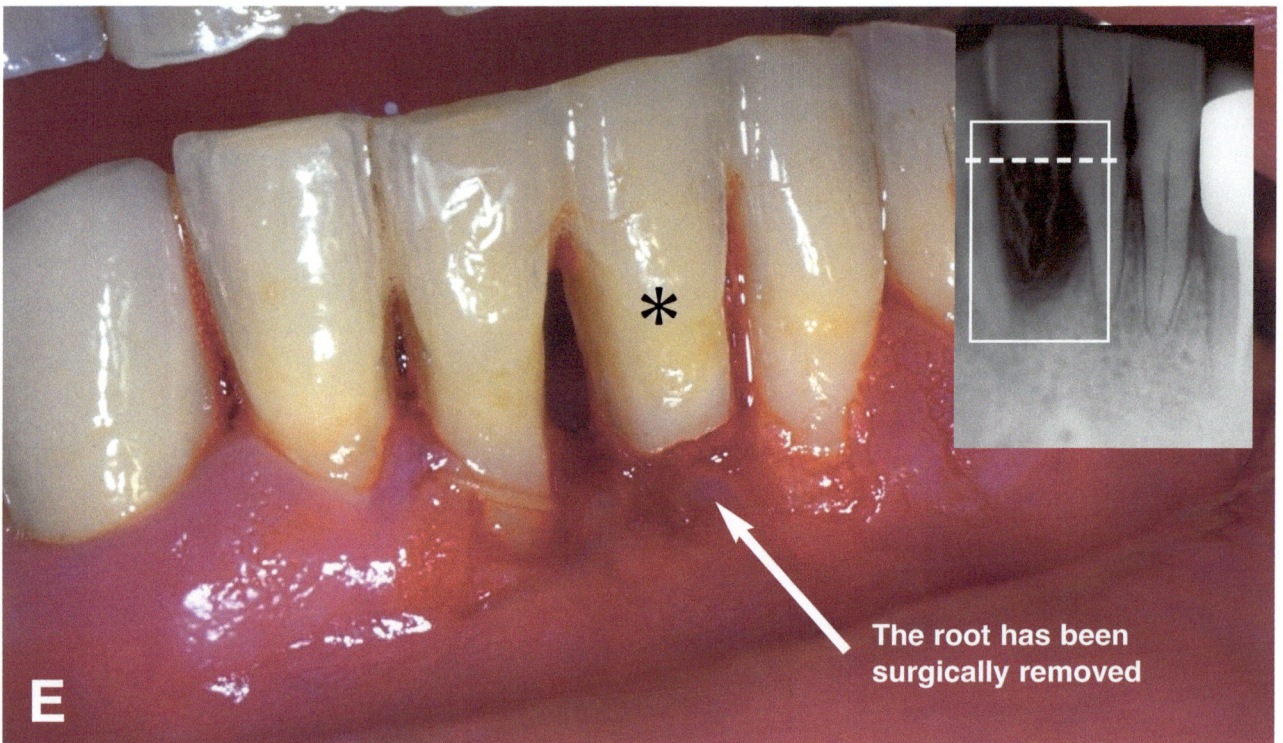

E

The root has been surgically removed

The unsupported root is cut off leaving the remaining crown bonded to the adjacent teeth. The tissues will heal in.

The Overdenture

When a tooth is lost, the surrounding bone recedes. The idea of an overdenture is to at least retain the root portion of a badly broken-down tooth (thereby preserving supporting bone) and make a denture that fits over these roots. Attachments may also be made to allow the denture to snap onto these roots for increased denture support and retention.

Prosthetic Therapy / Advanced Periodontal Disease   *(Photos A — J)*

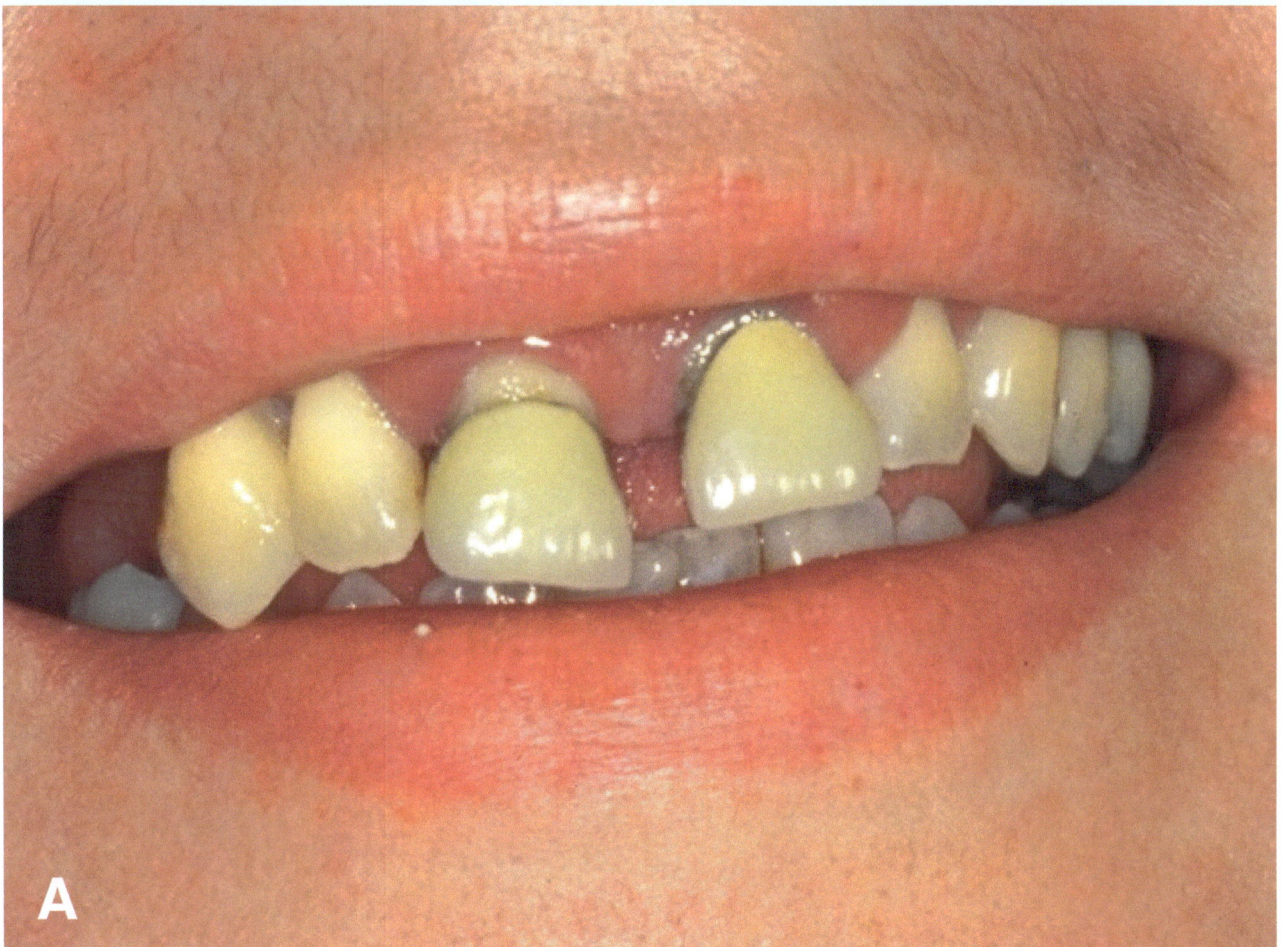

Advanced periodontal disease caused this unfortunate situation in this young lady (Shifting of her teeth due to loss of supporting bone). The exact cause of her condition was never determined. A consult and blood evaluation with her physician also failed to establish a cause (etiology).

Prosthetic Therapy / Advanced Periodontal Disease　　　(Continued)

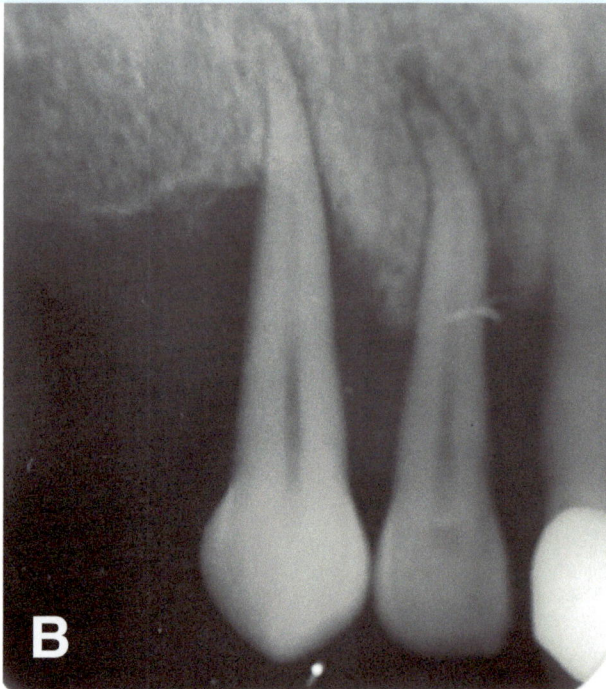

Tooth mobility and shifting of the teeth is the result of bone destruction. Shown here is 90% bone loss.

Hopeless teeth are extracted, however some roots can be salvaged and utilized to help support an overdenture. A temporary denture is then fabricated and worn as periodontal treatment and healing occurs.

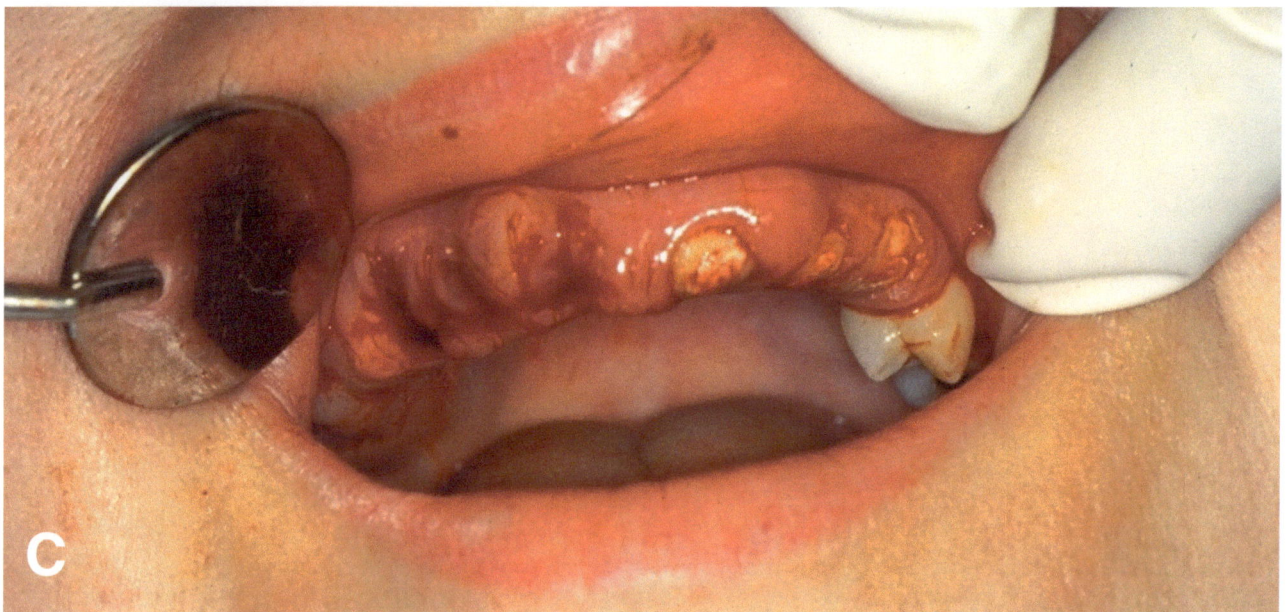

Prosthetic Therapy / Advanced Periodontal Disease   *(Continued)*

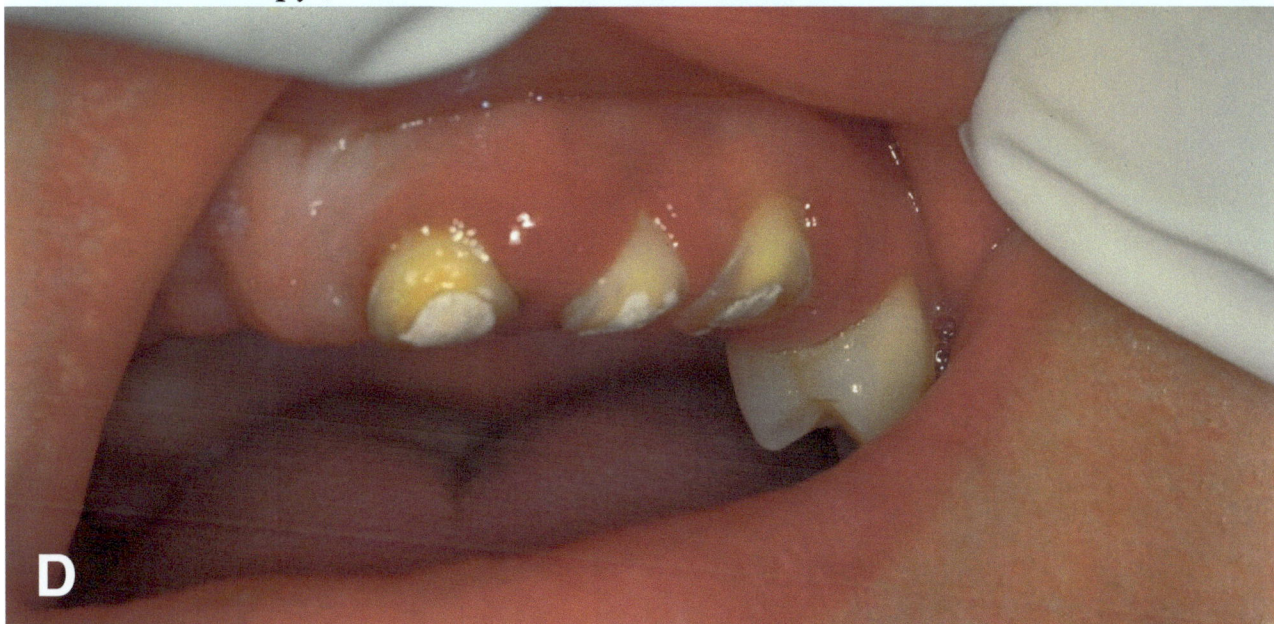

D

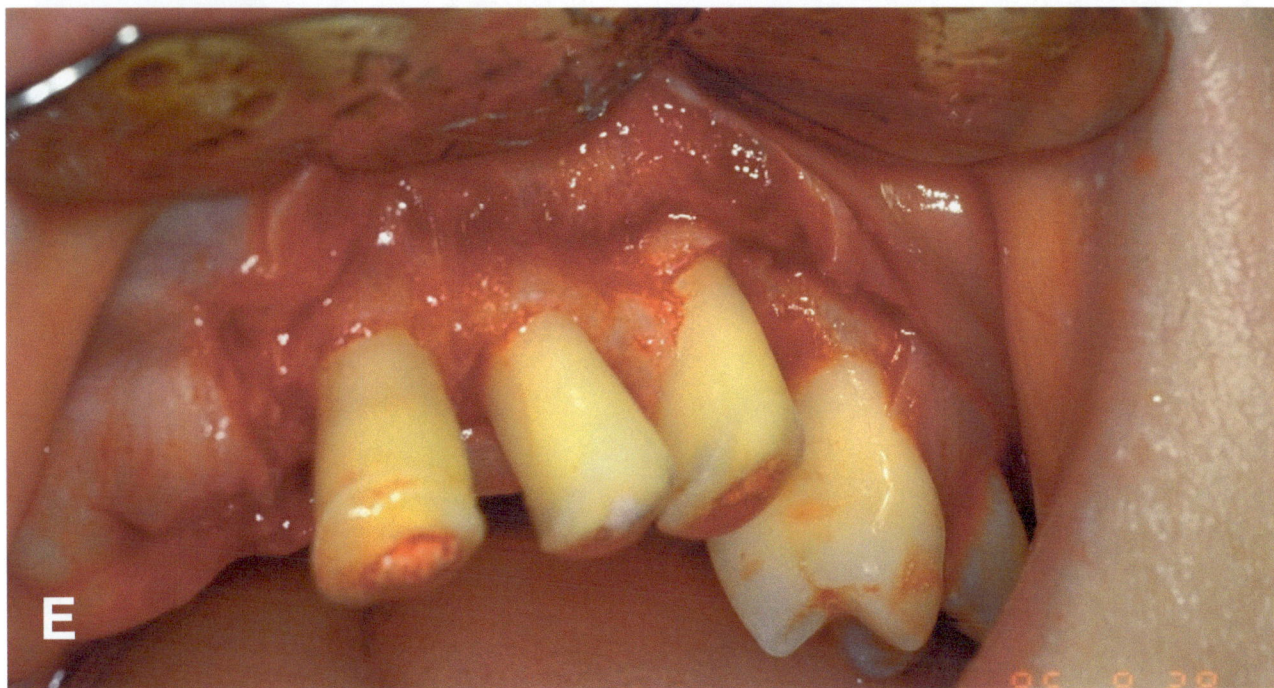

E

Periodontal surgery is performed to eliminate deep pockets and re-contour diseased bone.

Prosthetic Therapy / Advanced Periodontal Disease   (Continued)

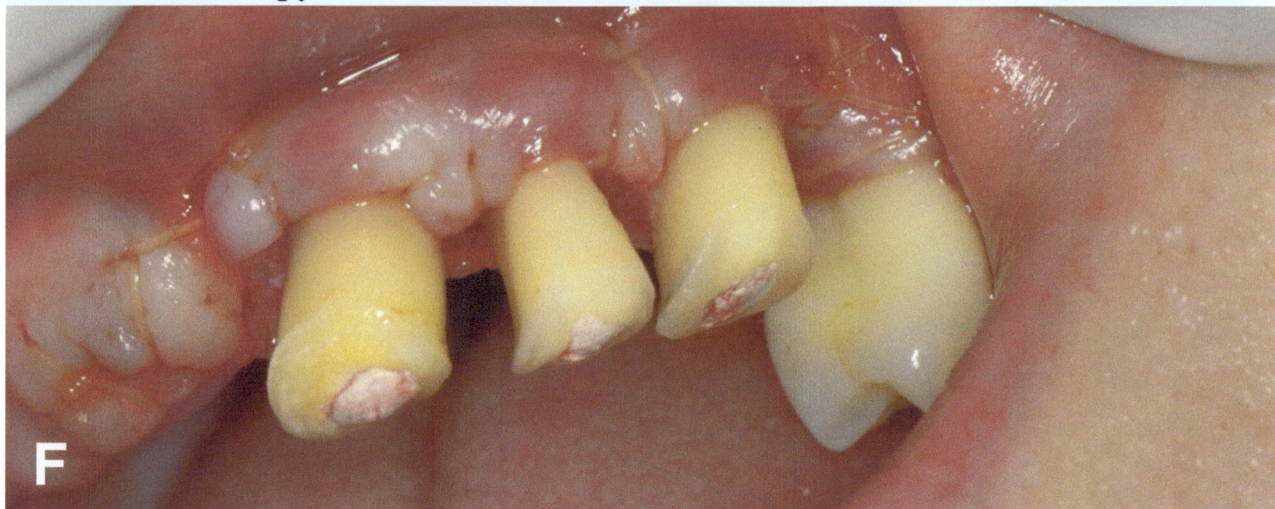

These roots are then reduced to establish a more stable foundation for the overdenture.

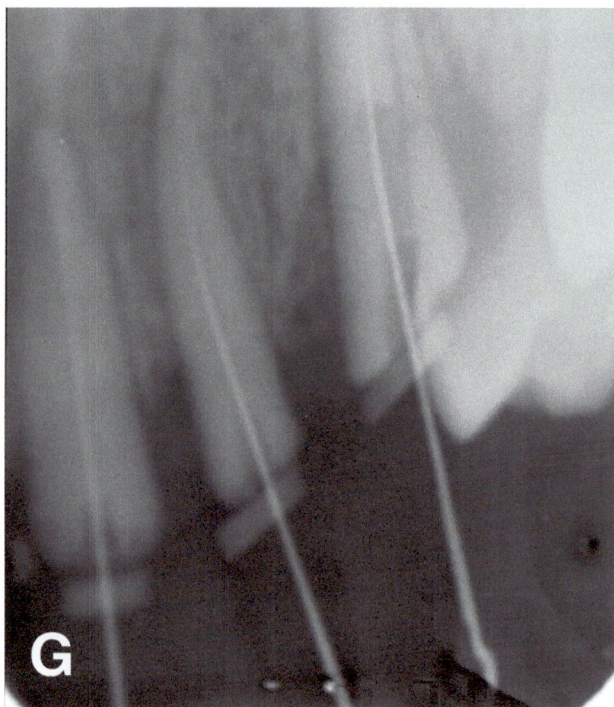

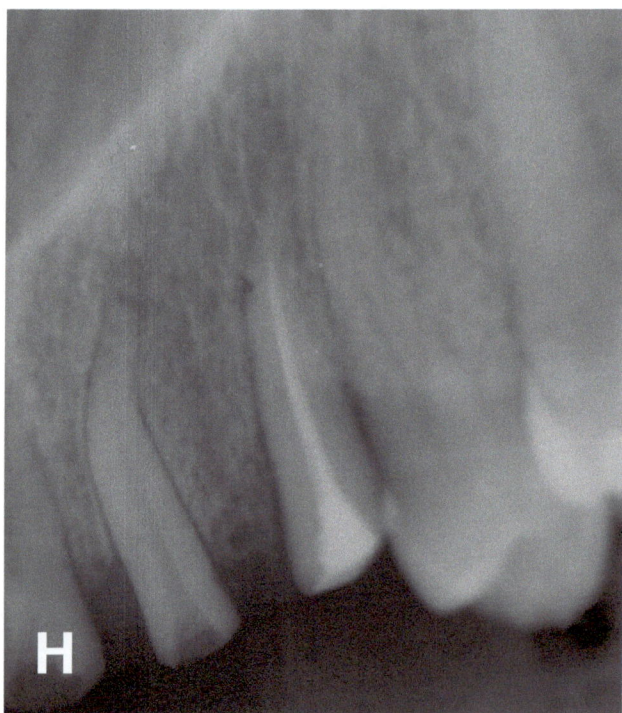

Root canal therapy is performed.

Prosthetic Therapy / Advanced Periodontal Disease   *(Continued)*

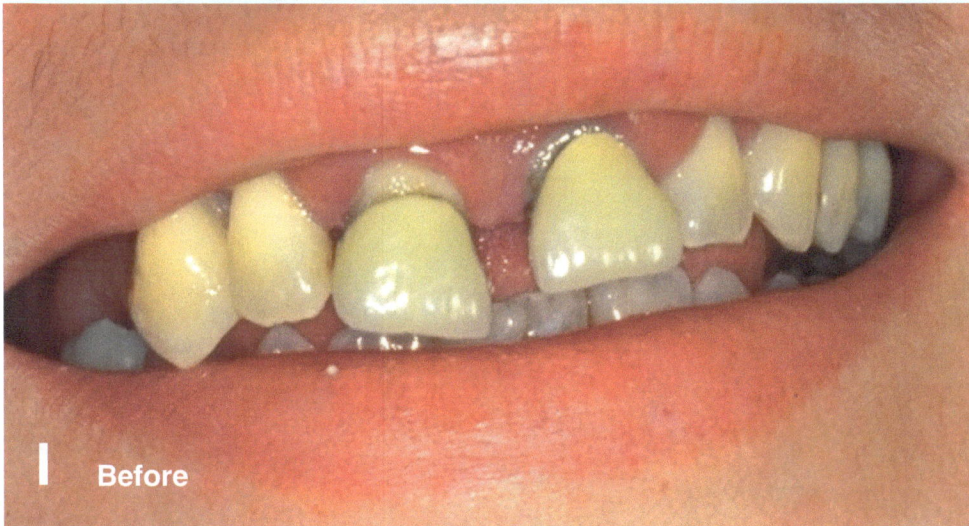

I Before

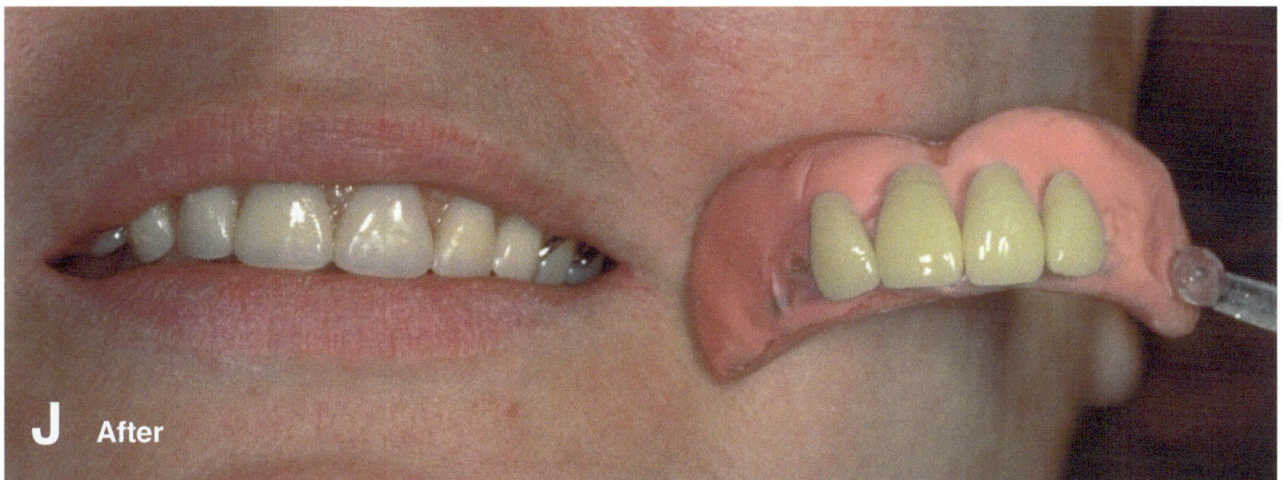

J After

Teeth are selected that match the patient's face and a final overdenture is fabricated.

Utilization of Gold Copings For Overdentures

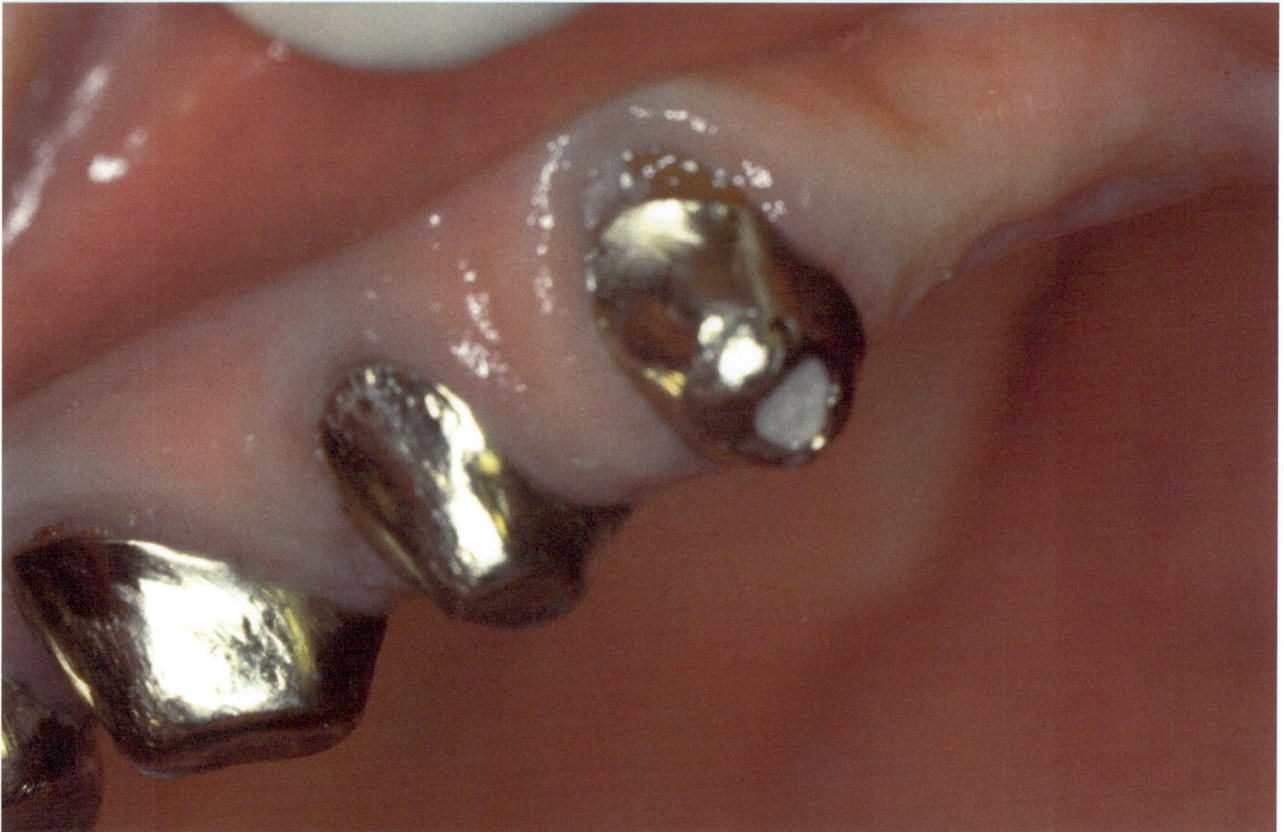

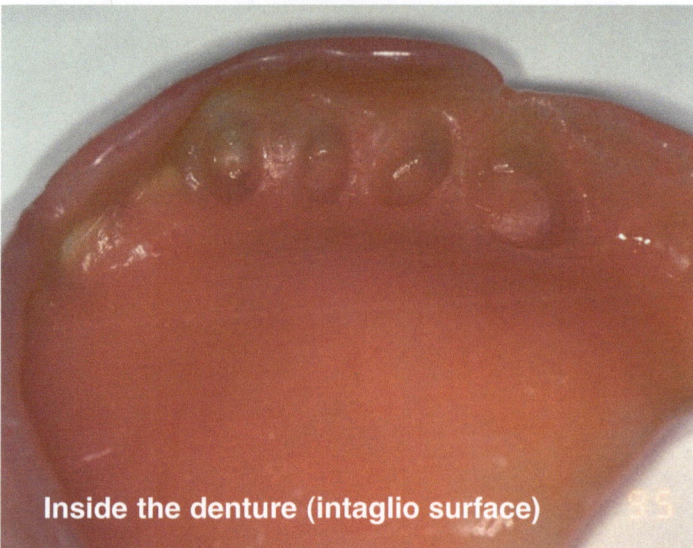

Inside the denture (intaglio surface)

These roots were saved and restored with gold "copings" to help support the overdenture. Although a more expensive therapy (then merely leaving the unrestored roots as is), preservation of the remaining roots is enhanced.

Utilization of Attachments For Overdentures

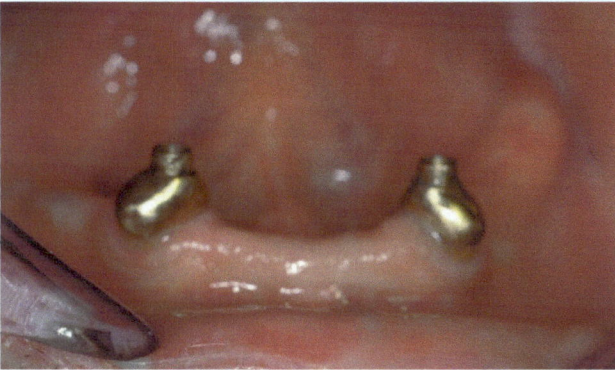

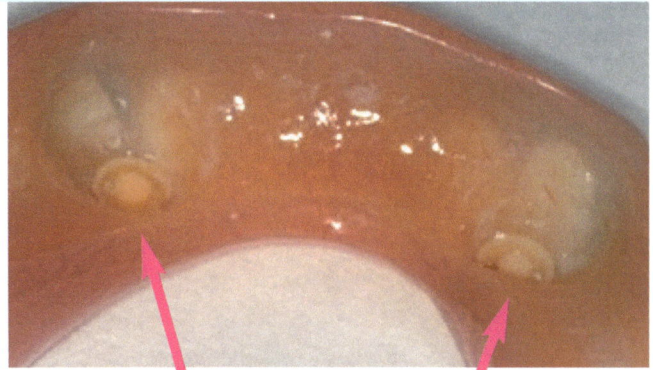

A lower arch with two gold attachments placed over remaining roots to support an overdenture. This case eventually failed resulting in extraction of the remaining roots. (The overdenture was easily converted to a full lower denture).

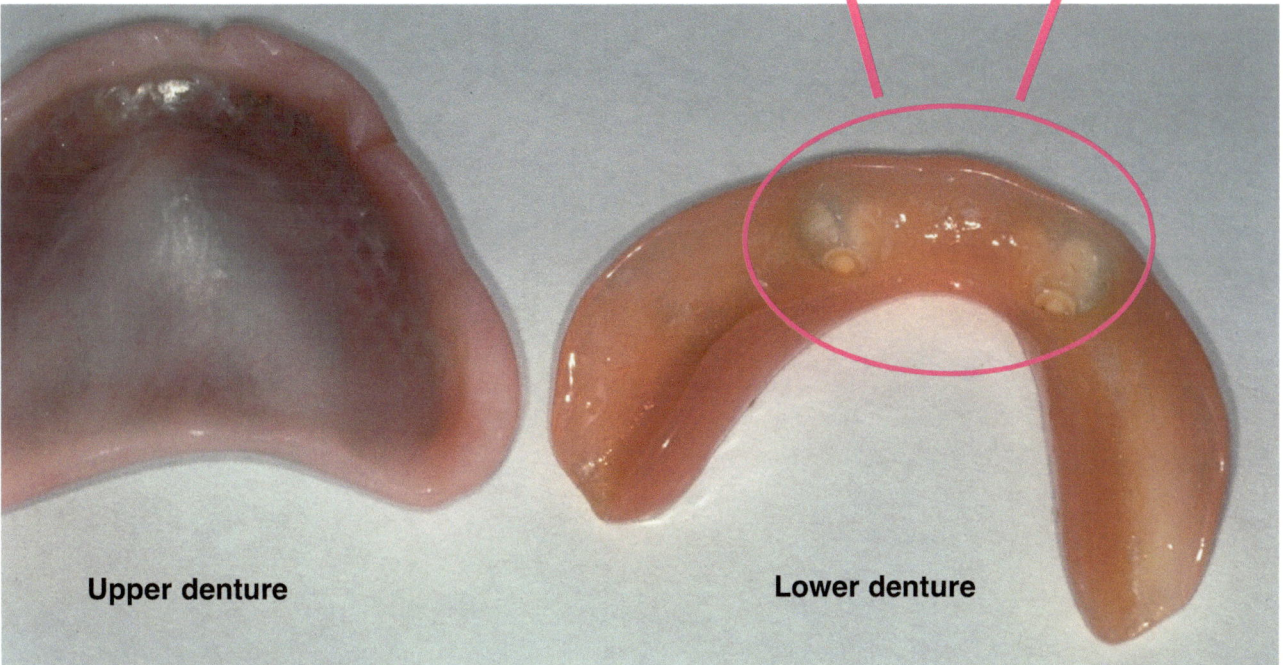

Upper denture   **Lower denture**

This patient's upper and lower dentures (tissue sides showing). Note metal reinforcement inside the upper denture and plastic snap on attachments within the lower denture.

The Full Denture

Unfortunately, many people experience a state of oral deterioration so severe that they require full dentures. If properly made and supported by an adequate amount of remaining bone, however, full dentures will satisfy most patients' aesthetic and functional needs. Implant therapy has become a valuable option in helping to support these dentures or actually eliminating the need for them.

Fabrication Technique   *(Photos A — J)*

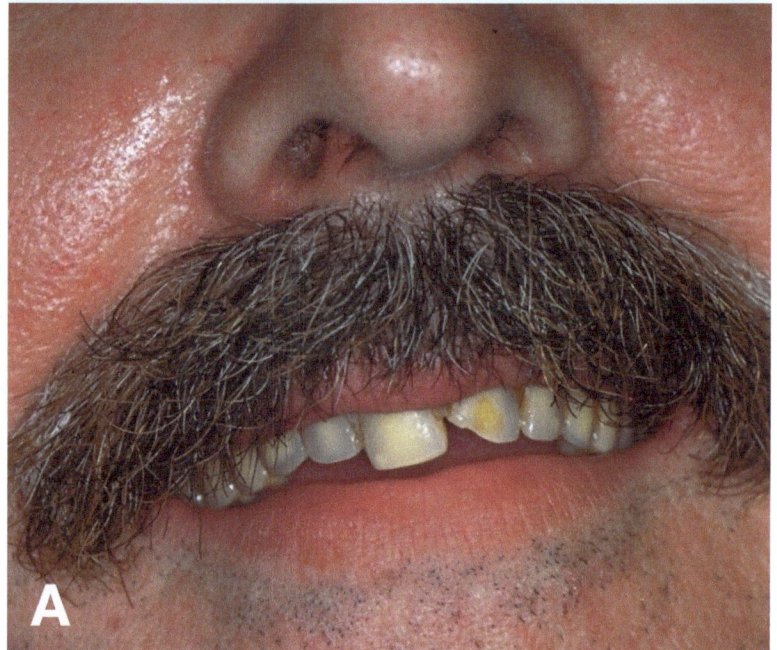

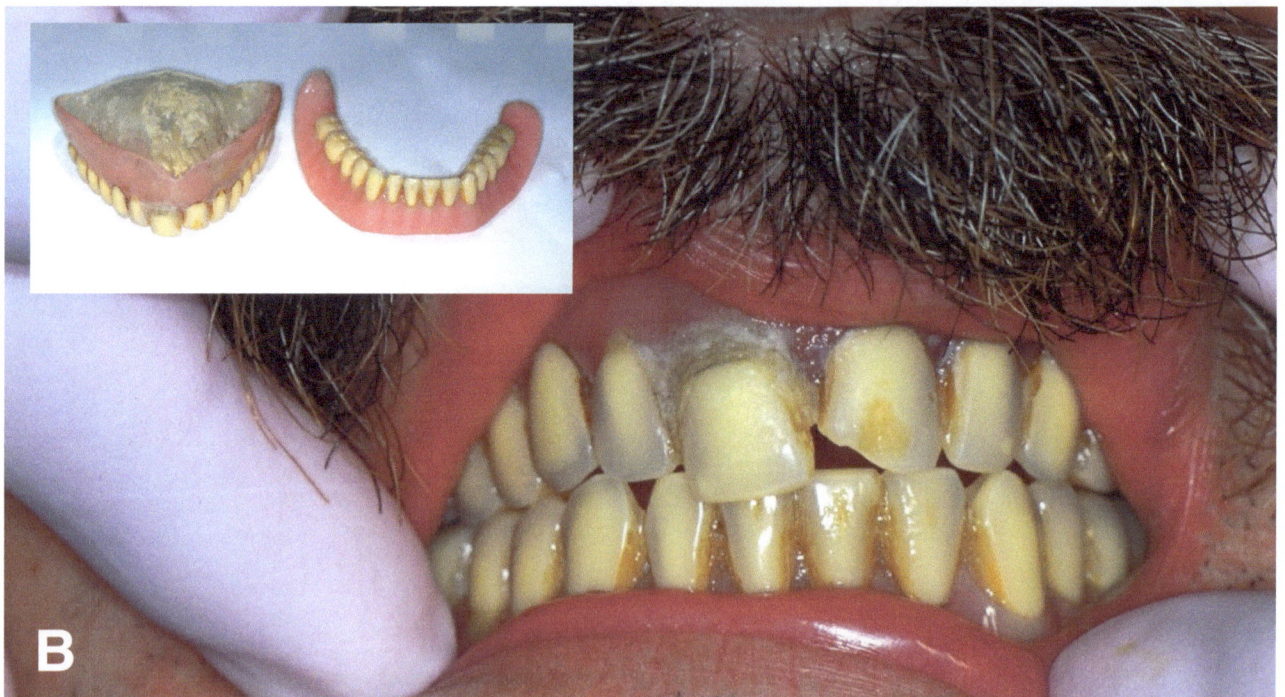

Patient presents with old, worn dentures. Notice the elongated front tooth — the patient's self-repair with crazy glue.

Full Denture Fabrication Technique   (Continued)

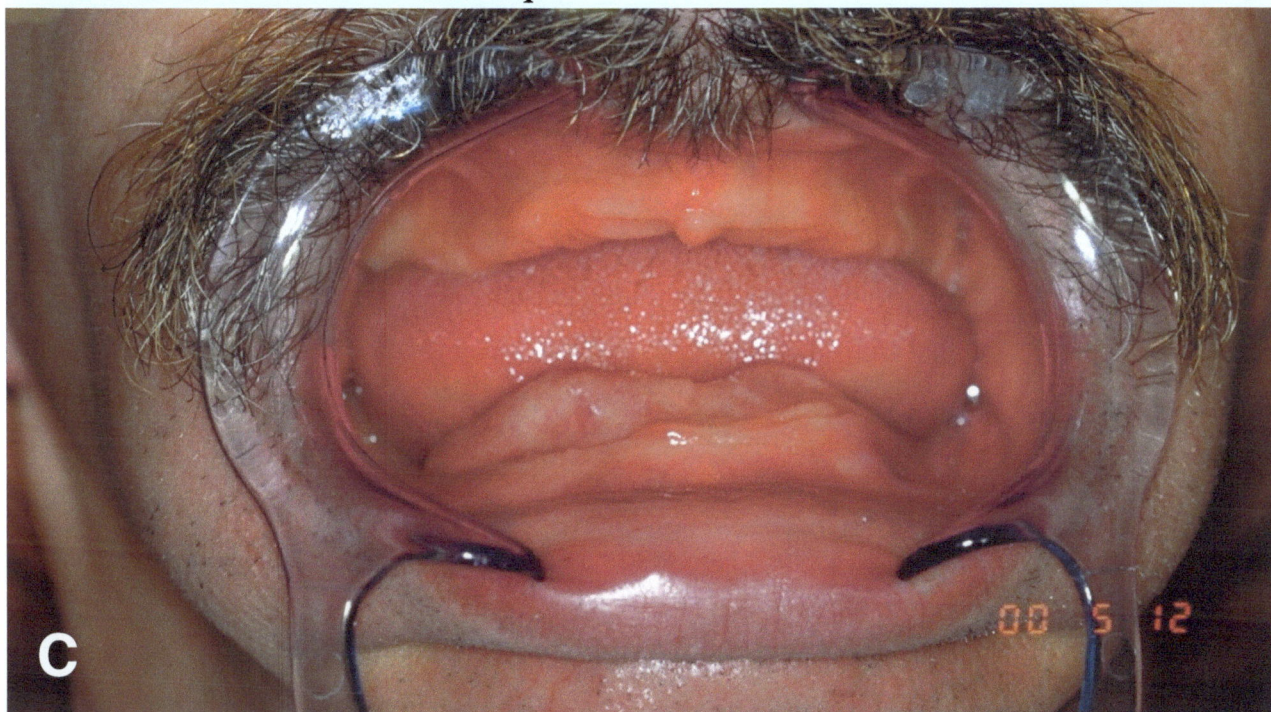

The unfortunate end result of total tooth loss.

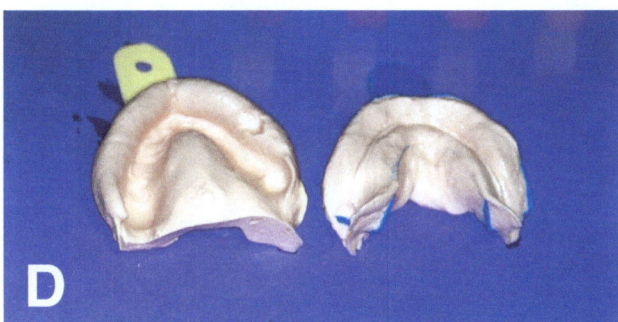

New denture fabrication begins with preliminary impressions.

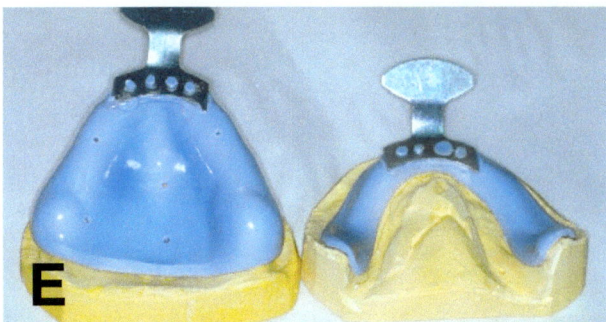

The laboratory then fabricates custom impression trays. These are utilized to record a very accurate final impression of the patient's remaining ridge form.

Full Denture Fabrication Technique

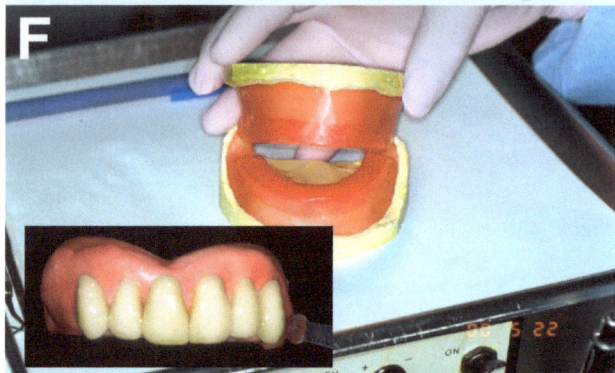

Wax bite blocks are constructed and utilized to record the upper and lower jaw relationships and also as a method of trying in the new teeth. Teeth are chosen that match the facial structure and aesthetic demands of the patient.

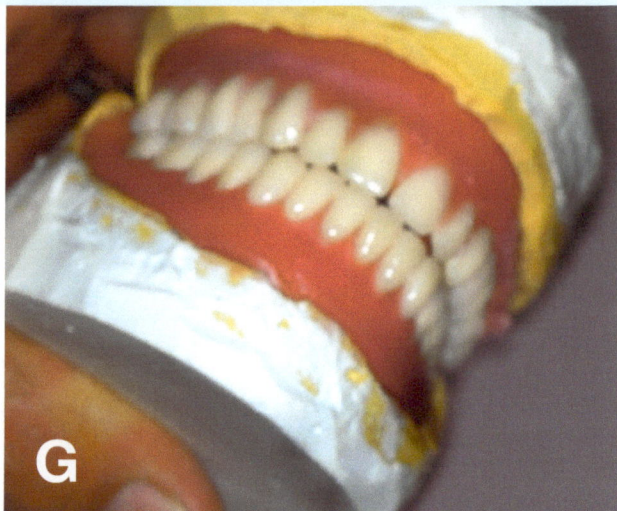

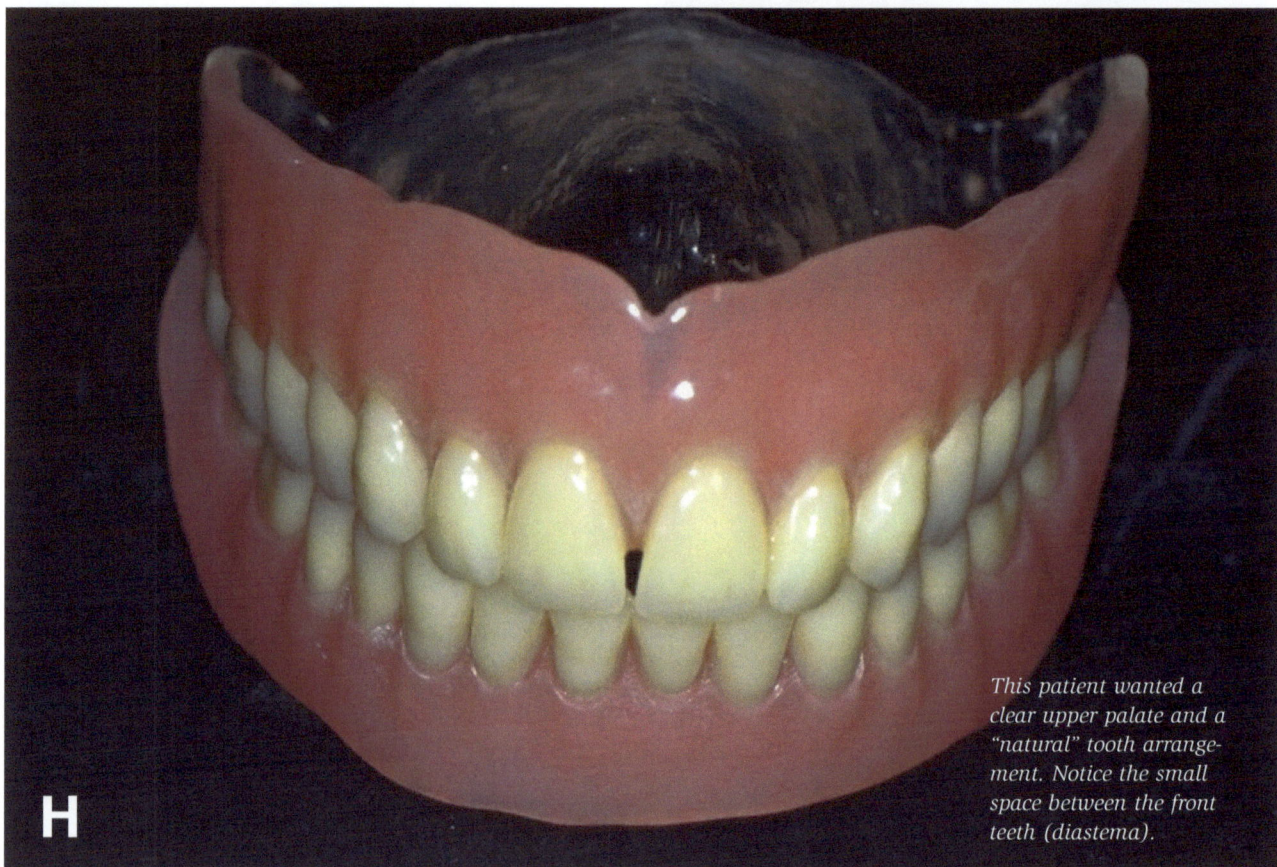

This patient wanted a clear upper palate and a "natural" tooth arrangement. Notice the small space between the front teeth (diastema).

Full Denture Fabrication Technique   *(Continued)*

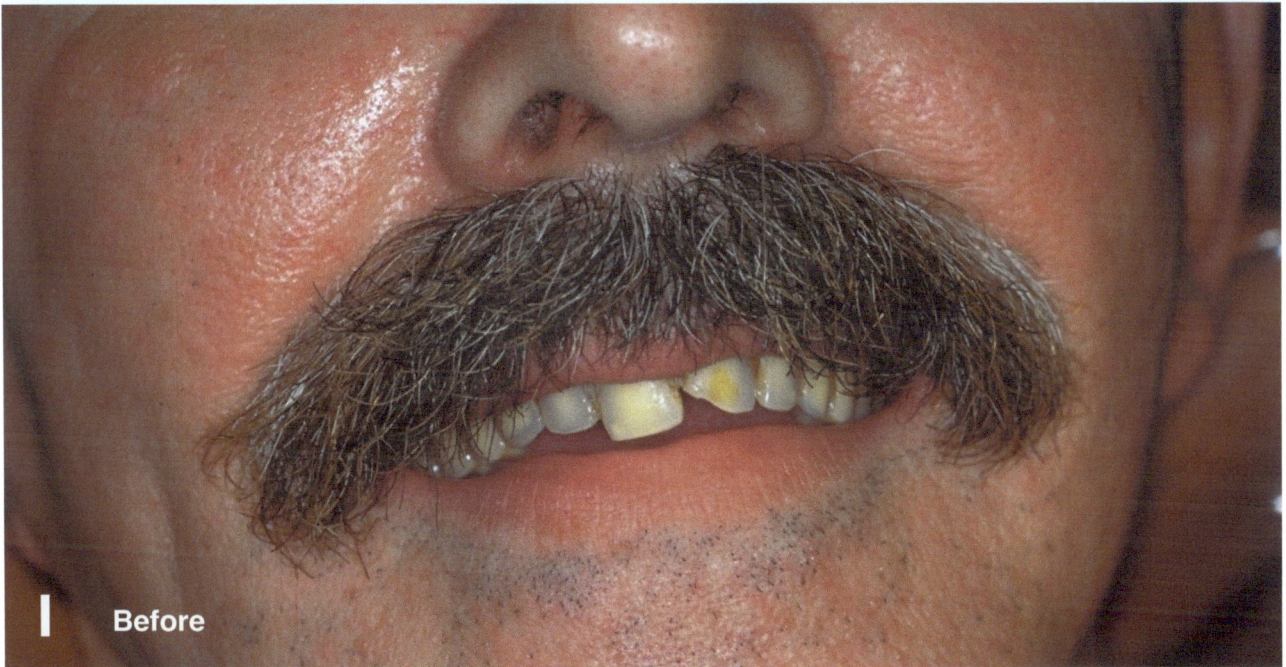

I Before

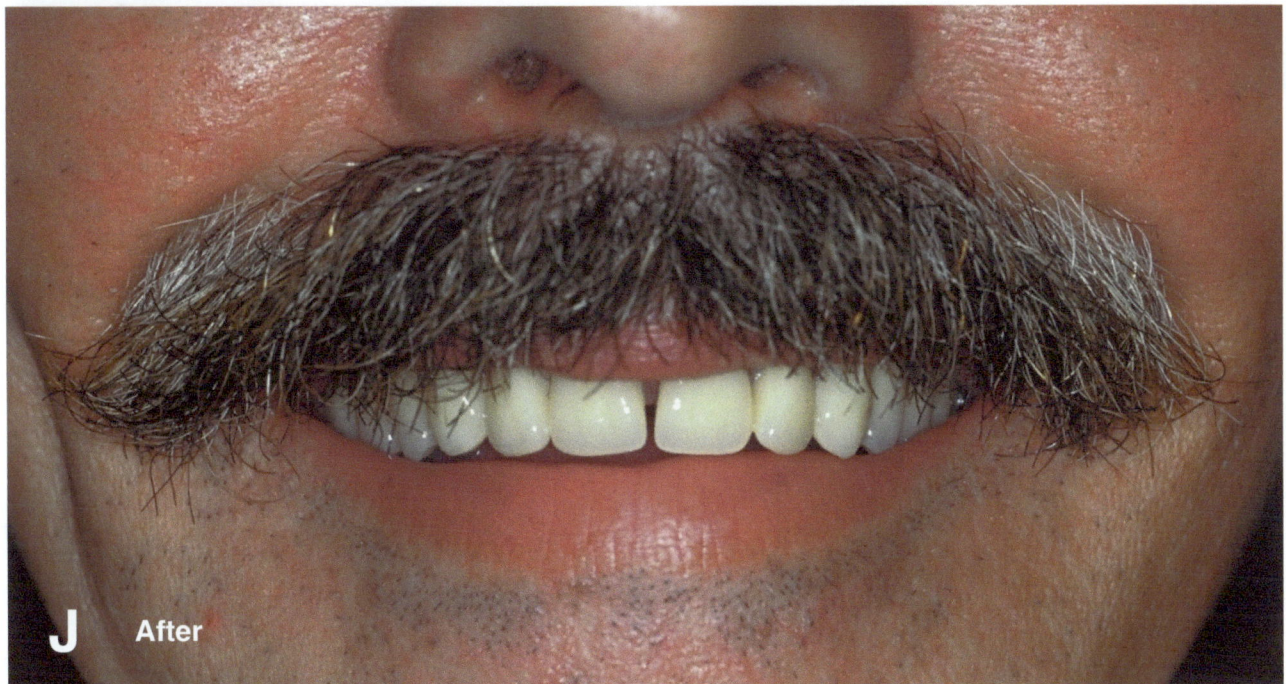

J After

Quality

Whatever prosthetic method is used, success depends on proper case planning, uncompromised choice of materials, excellent communication between the dentist and the laboratory technician, and the artistic skills of both the dentist and lab technician.

Years of experience, combined with a dedication to learning and improving, are pre-requisites to achieving success. In my earlier years, I often wished there was a simpler, faster way—a method to transfer all the knowledge from an older, more experienced dentist to myself. If that were possible, I guess we wouldn't need schools at all.[27]

The process of acquiring knowledge is never-ending. It means keeping abreast of new developments, reading professional journals, observing colleagues, and discussing cases. (Learning from failure is *also* a knowledge-producing experience). In my practice, we document all phases of treatment with intra-oral photography, which allows us to re-evaluate and critique treatment. Interested patients may also view these slides to better understand the demanding technical requirements for successful therapy.

Experience / Clinical Judgement   *(Photos A – D)*

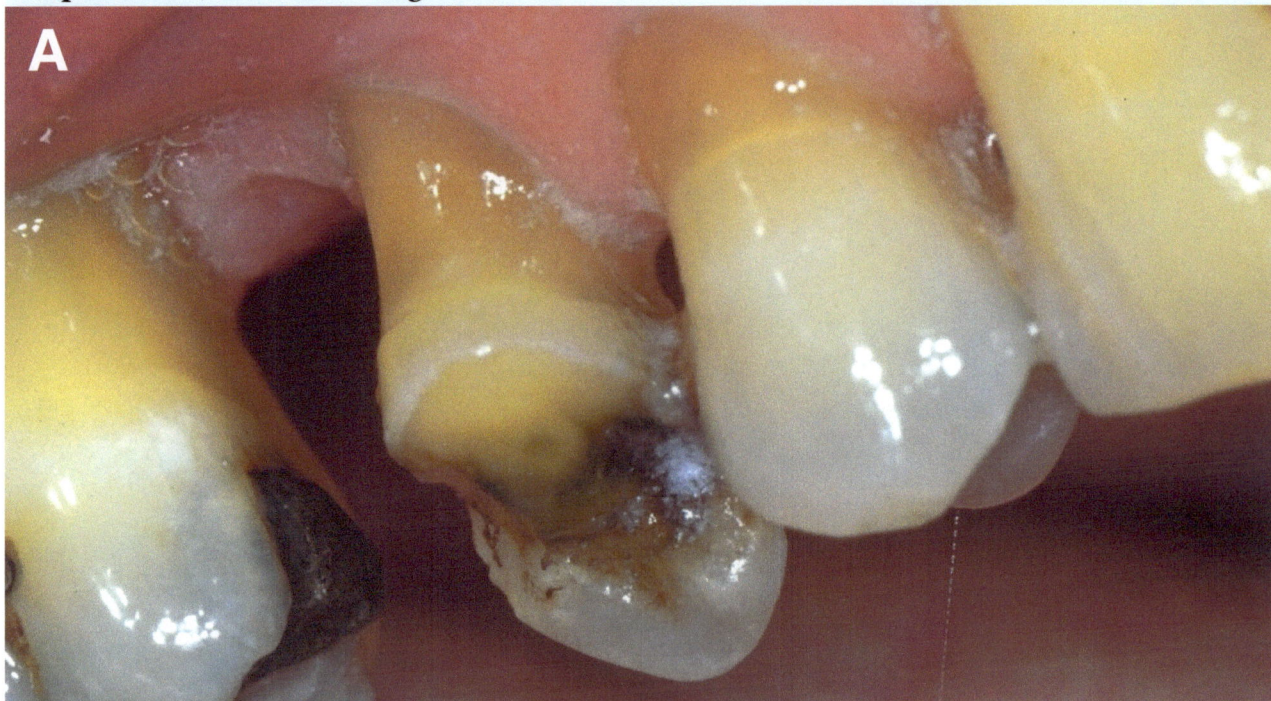

This patient presented with a silver amalgam filling that fell out. Quality in dental service is based on proper diagnosis along with an understanding of the patient's needs.

27. Obtaining superior technical knowledge without the lessons that life and time provide results in an unbalanced state of mind.

Experience / Clinical Judgement   (Continued)

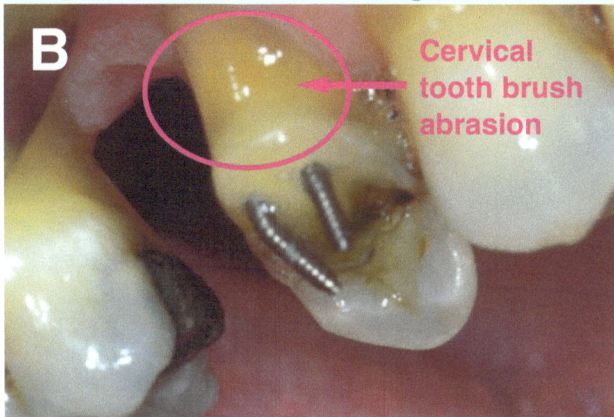

Cervical
tooth brush
abrasion

Titanium pins will help retain the bonded composite restoration.

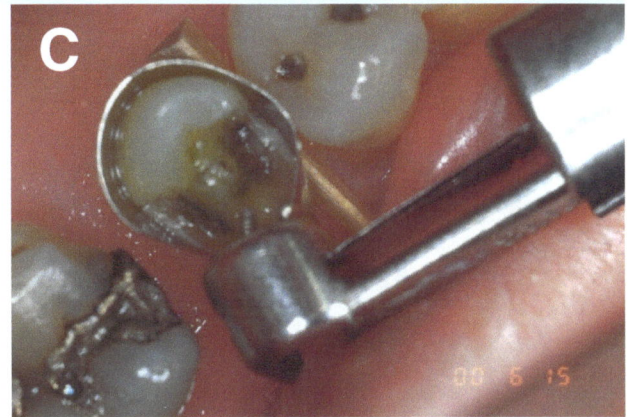

A matrix band holds the composite material and a wedge helps ensure a normal contact with the adjacent tooth.

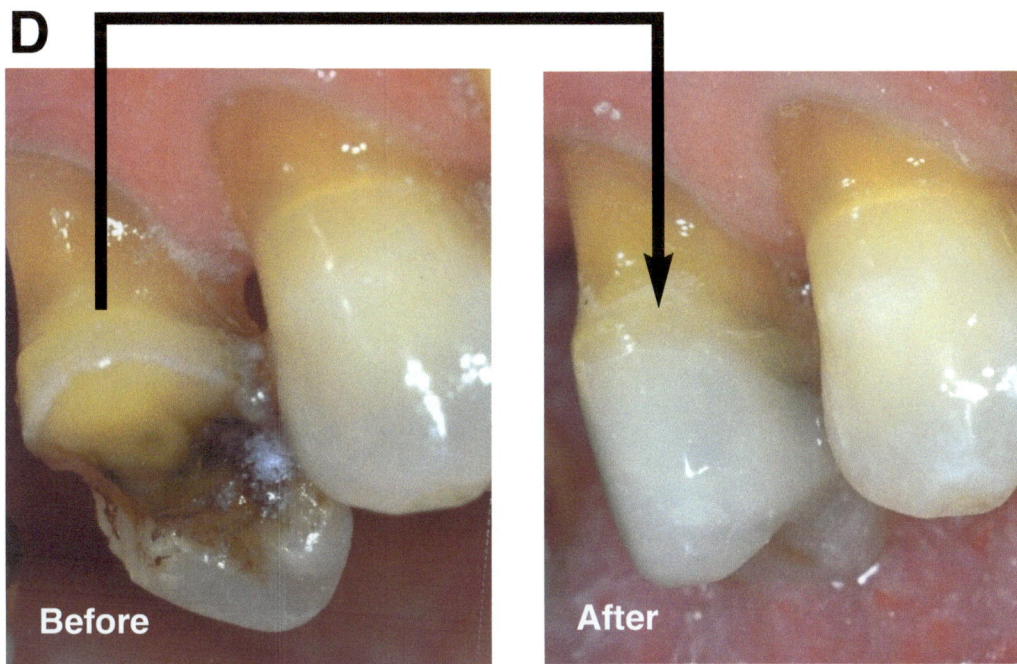

Before

After

The completed restoration. Proper shade selection along with special polishing instruments create a restoration that is indistinguishable from the natural tooth.

   A full crown might have been the restoration of choice here. However, in order to avoid the time and expense of a laboratory fabricated crown, this direct composite suited the patient's need. Also the area of *cervical abrasion* is left unrestored *(photo B)*. This area seems to be stable and placing a restoration here might create other problems later on. — This is clinical judgement.

Quality Control

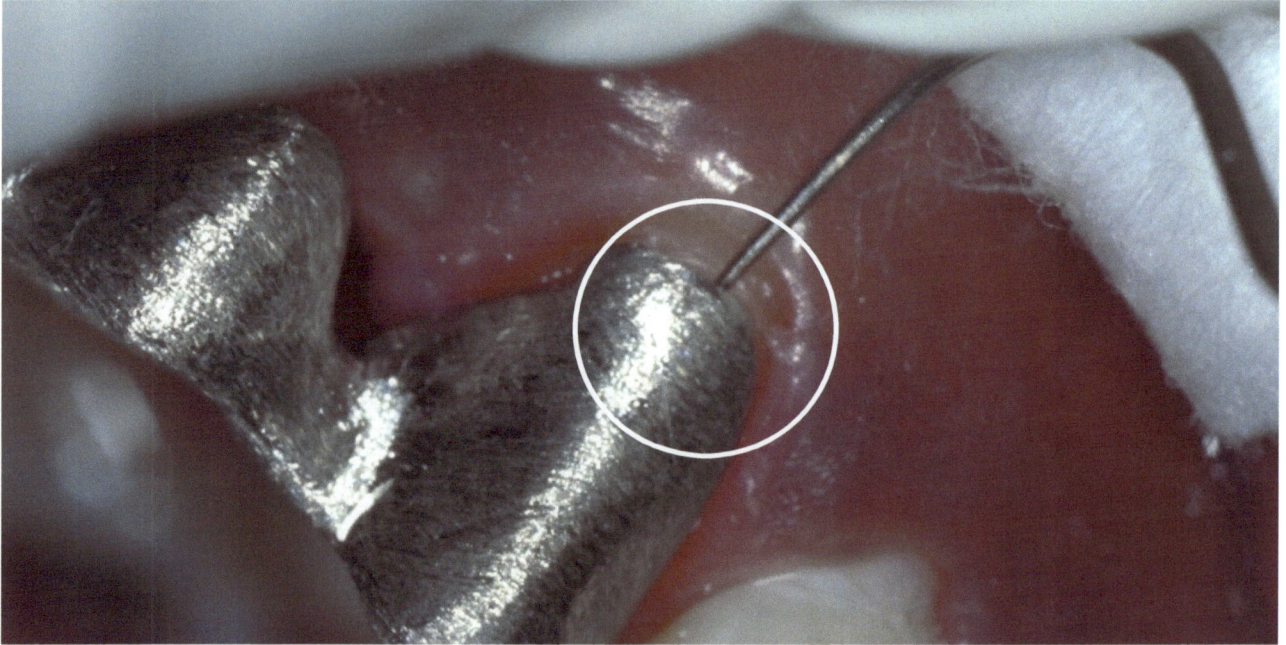

Fabrication of a bridge requires careful examination of each completed component. A metal framework is found to have an open margin during the try-in appointment. If this small opening is not detected at this stage then the final bridge could fail. (As a result of cement wash-out or ingress of bacteria and recurrent decay).

Aging

Wear and tear eventually reduces the functional capacity of any prosthetic appliance, so what happens when our patients with these appliances reach advanced years? Re-examination and subsequent treatment plans can then lead to necessary therapies. It is possible to design prosthetic appliances that outlast the patient. In that case, shouldn't we, as dentists, become more attuned to the overall aging process and coordinate care in partnership with other health care professionals? I believe so.

THE AGING PROCESS AND DENTAL NEEDS OF THE OLDER PATIENT

I was taught that the process of homeostasis (the ability of an organism or cell to maintain internal equilibrium by adjusting its physiological processes) maintains a regulatory control over our biological system, working like a feedback mechanism. For instance, when sugars are digested, certain cells within the pancreas release insulin. The insulin promotes incorporation of this food source (glucose) within the body's cells. When this is accomplished, a feedback mechanism decreases the further secretion of insulin. The body is wired and controlled by these feedback mechanisms, allowing us to maintain a healthy, functional state. For some reason, however, a slow deterioration of function eventually leads to death.

I believe the ultimate challenge in medicine is to not merely alleviate unhealthy symptoms and disease, but to cure functional deterioration and thus prevent death. What a radical concept! The idea of attempting to maintain health while gracefully dying is like a half-hearted attempt to deal with the basic problem. Naturally, I am limited in my area of expertise, but based on a sound background in the science of biology, my thinking process leads me to obvious conclusions regarding "ultimate health." The book's final chapter on the future will explore this concept in more detail. For now, let's look at the aging process regarding dental health.

I've been trying to preserve and maintain my 78-year-old mother's teeth, but so far, with only limited success. Fortunately, she has not had to deal with wearing complete dentures. I've resorted to imaginative ways of using newer composite bonding materials along with surgical procedures

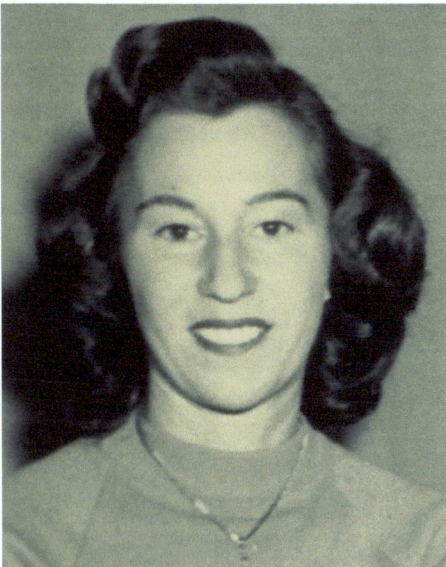

My young mother...

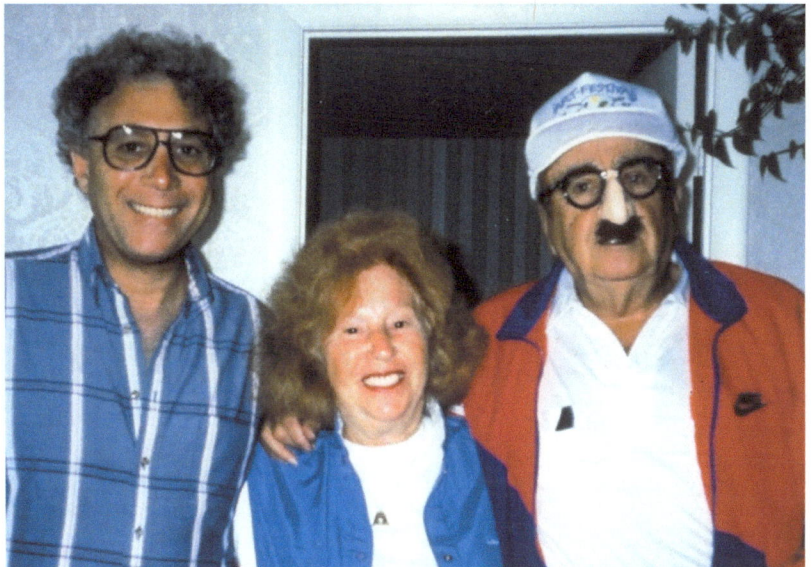

... Years later, between my father and myself.

and antimicrobial rinses. The process has been tough, but also rewarding in the sense that I am helping my mother. For patients whose children are not dentists, the situation may be more difficult. Depending on how badly you want to keep your teeth, innovative and advanced techniques are available, but they require time in the chair and added expense. It is a fact that a patient's dental health in later years of life is directly related to the quality of previous dental care. Over-aggressive "capping" of teeth and other imprudent therapies always seem to aggravate the health status later on. The less need you have had for fillings, partial dentures, bridges—the better your dental health will be as you age.

As a dentist with 29 years of experience, I have had the opportunity to get an overall picture of the problems the aging process causes within the mouth. However, like a physician who mostly sees sick patients and may not see healthy ones, my perspective is biased.[28]

The basic etiology of oral deterioration is multi-factorial—everything from "normal" wear and tear to the destructive effects of a decrease in salivary flow, which increases susceptibility to cavities. These situations are best handled by communication with a dentist and hygienist—professionals sensitive to the patient's unique requirements. Individual treatment needs are addressed and administered for the life of the patient.

The ultimate failure in dentistry is the loss of all one's teeth.[29] Properly constructed, full dentures can often fulfill the functional and aesthetic requirements from this point forward. However, changes in supporting bone do occur and can destabilize dentures. Periodic examinations are necessary, along with modifications such as "relining" the dentures or "equilibrating" the biting relationship of the teeth. The progress in implantology has allowed for improved support of these dentures, or in certain cases, complete elimination of the need for these dentures.

Premature Dental Deterioration

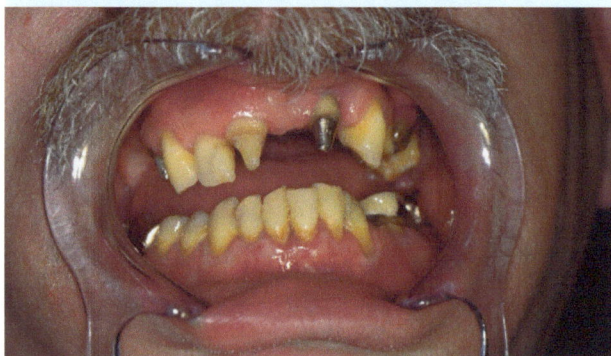

A 53 year old dentist. This is quite an unfortunate situation. Etiology (cause) — excess stress, neglect... drug abuse?

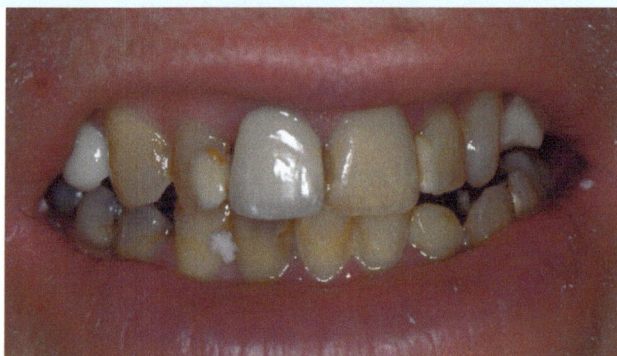

Another dentist — same age. Similar situation. This is the result of drug abuse, neglect of dental hygiene and chronic excess stress.

28. A number of years ago, I visited a private nursing home, surveyed the dental conditions of the residents, and found 95% of these patients in poor dental health. Letters relating their needs were sent to their closest relatives; the response, sadly, was negligible.

29. Many dentists enter this field rather than medicine due to this limited bottom-line consequence of failure—as compared to the physician who has to deal with death as the ultimate failure.

Restoration of a Deteriorated Oral Condition *(Photos A — G)*

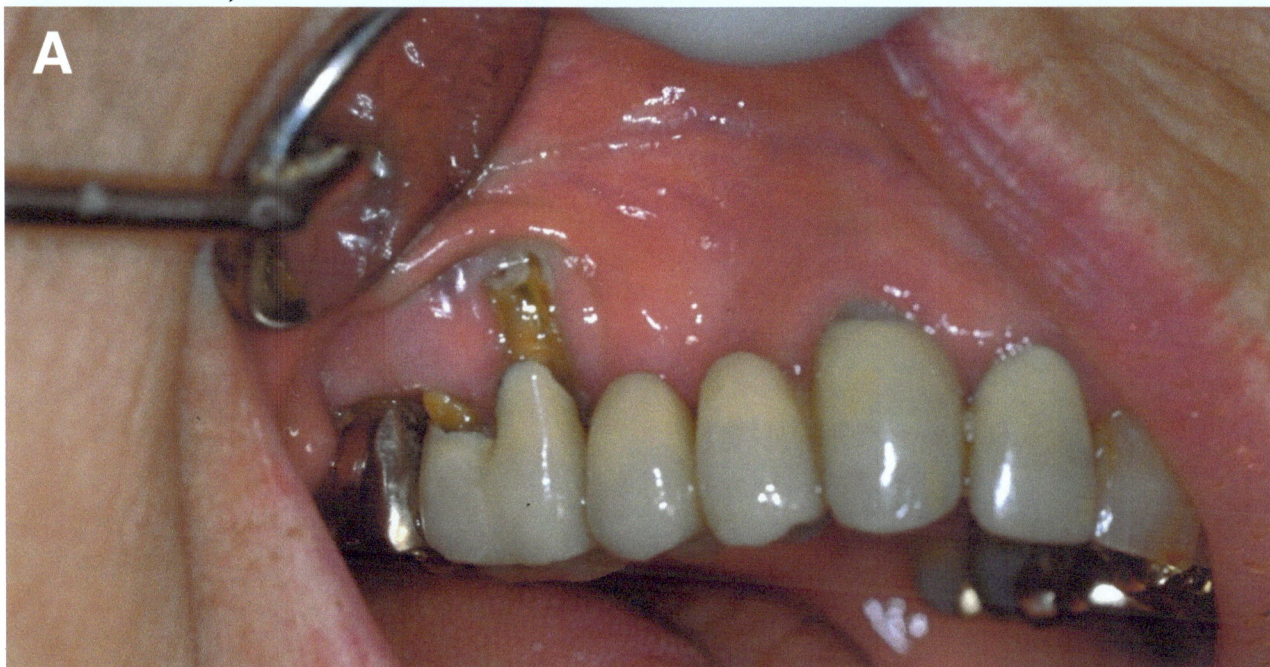

An elderly female patient presents with this deteriorating situation under an old bridge.

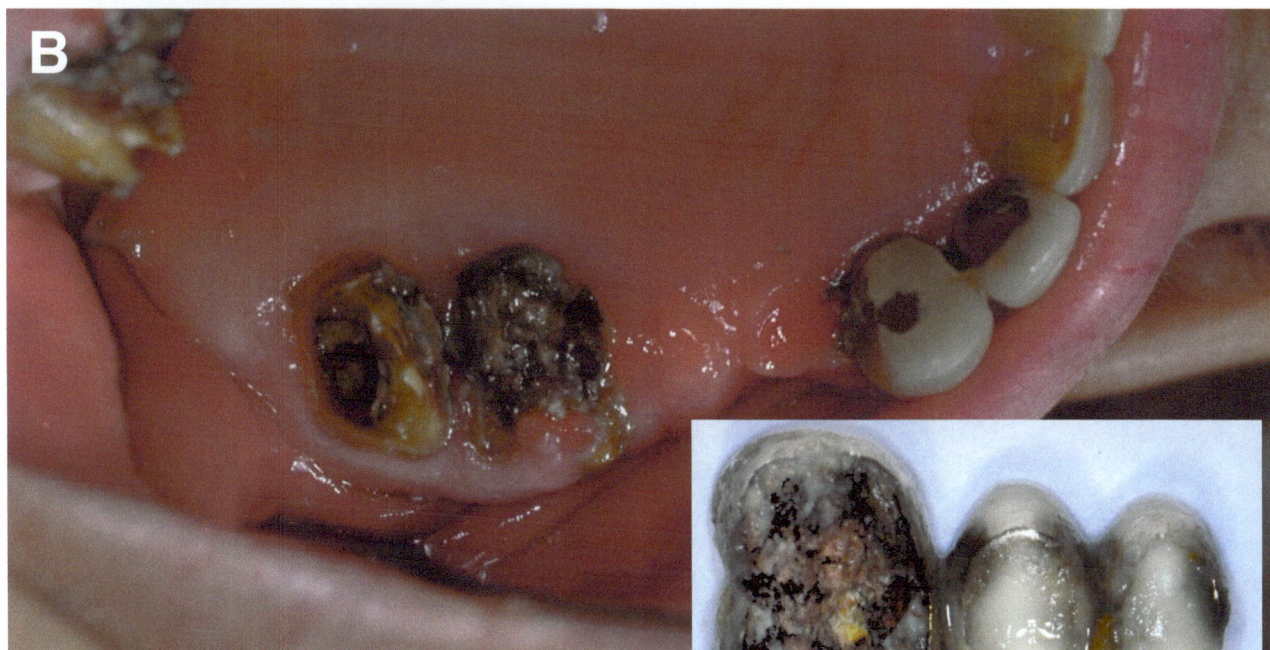

The defective bridge is removed revealing extensive tissue destruction and decay.

Restoration of a Deteriorated Oral Condition *(Continued)*

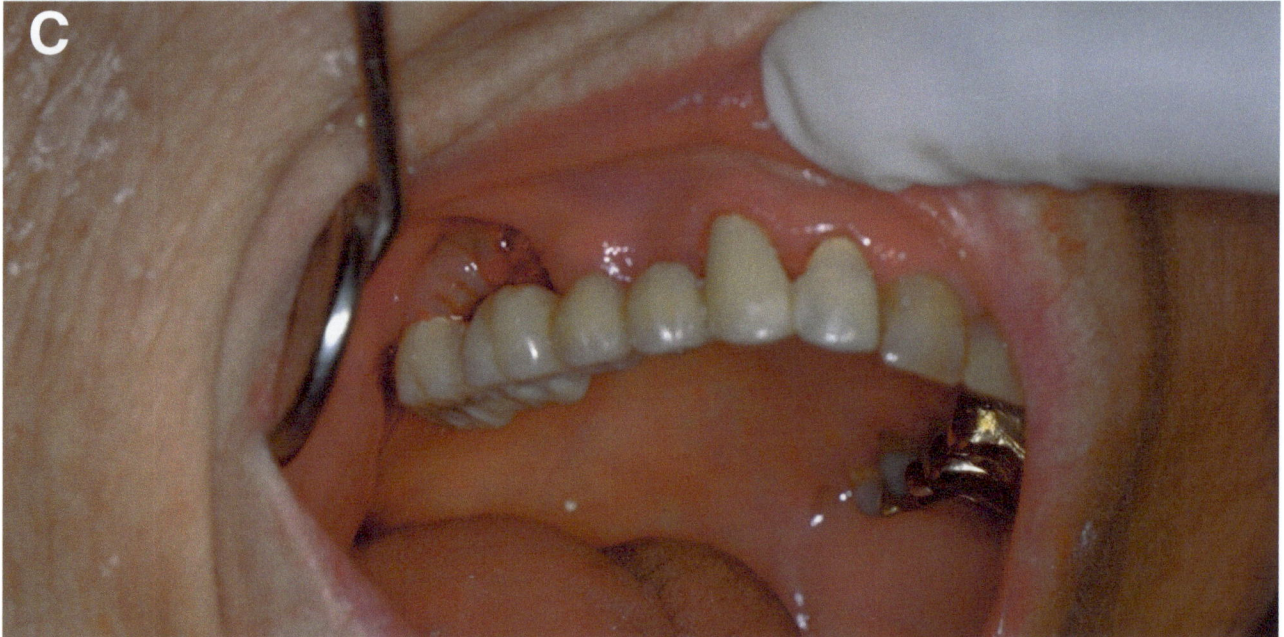

A hopeless tooth has been extracted and a temporary bridge inserted. Once total healing occurs, a final bridge will be fabricated.

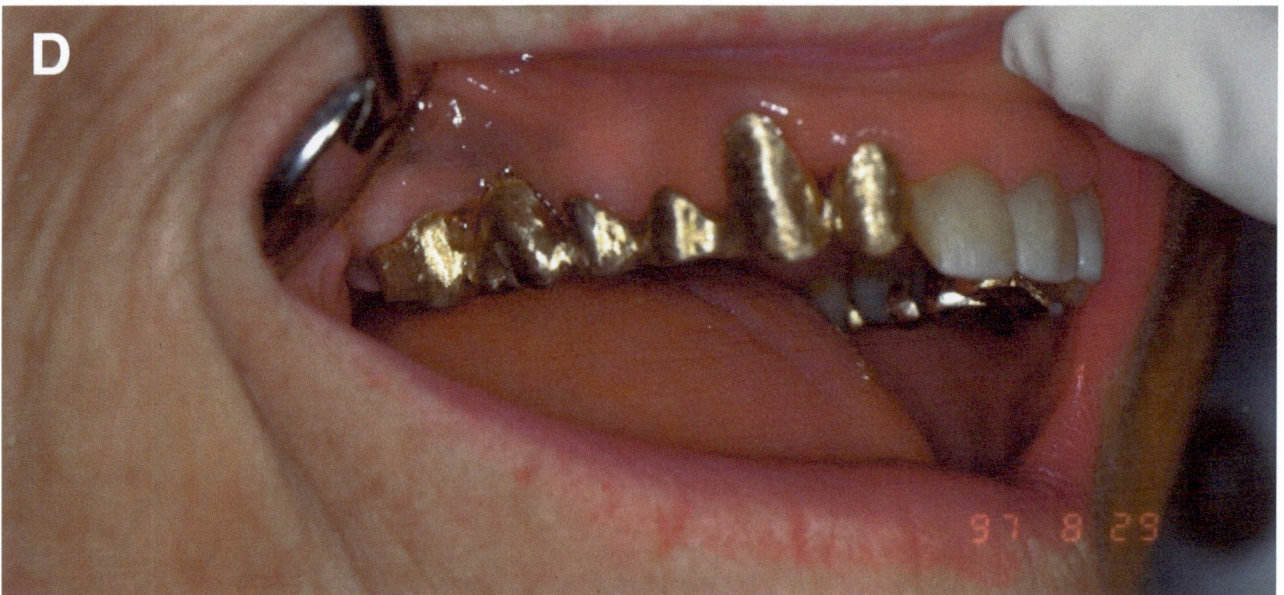

A gold frame work is tried in.

Restoration of a Deteriorated Oral Condition (Continued)

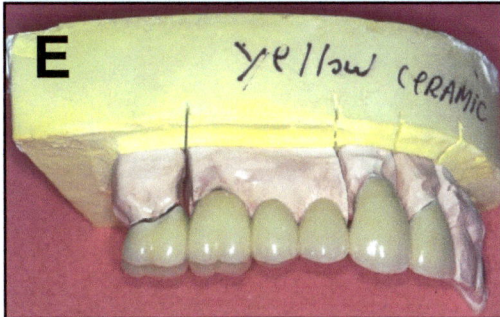

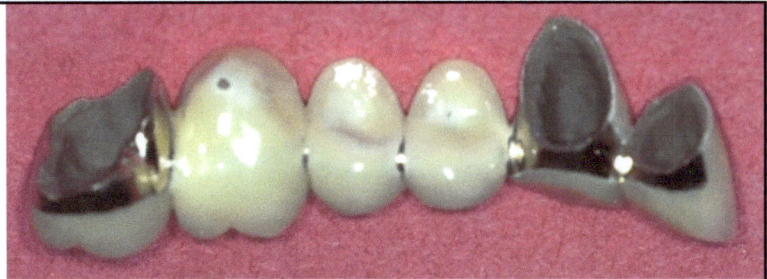

Porcelain is baked onto the framework.

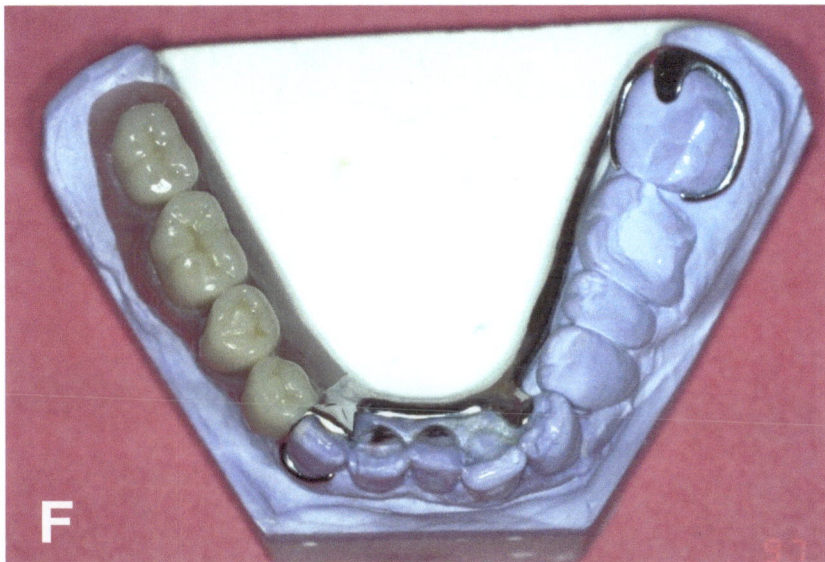

A lower partial denture is also fabricated.

The bridge and partial denture in place. — The clasp will be hidden when the lower lip is in a natural position.

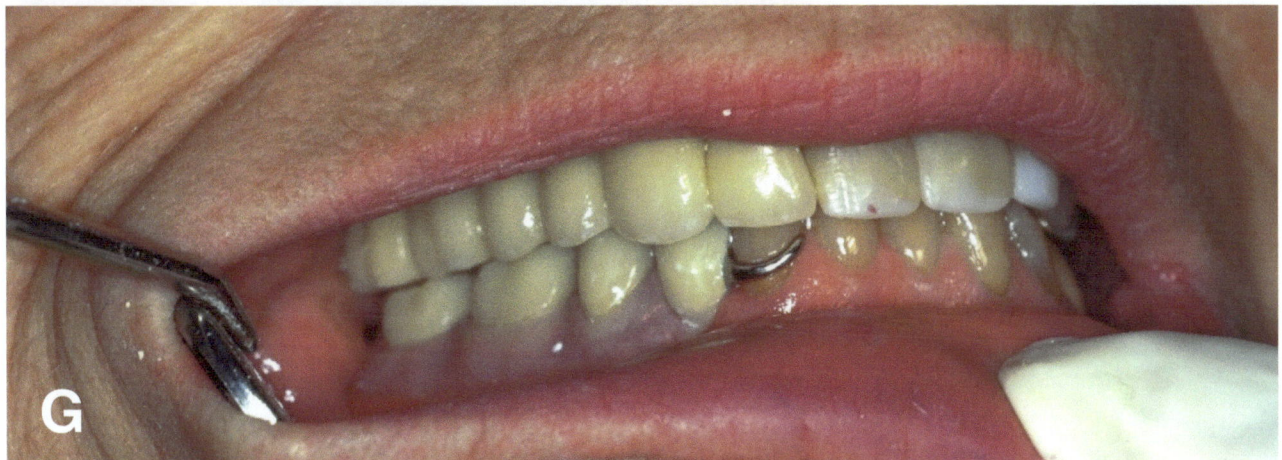

The Problem Of Recurrent Decay

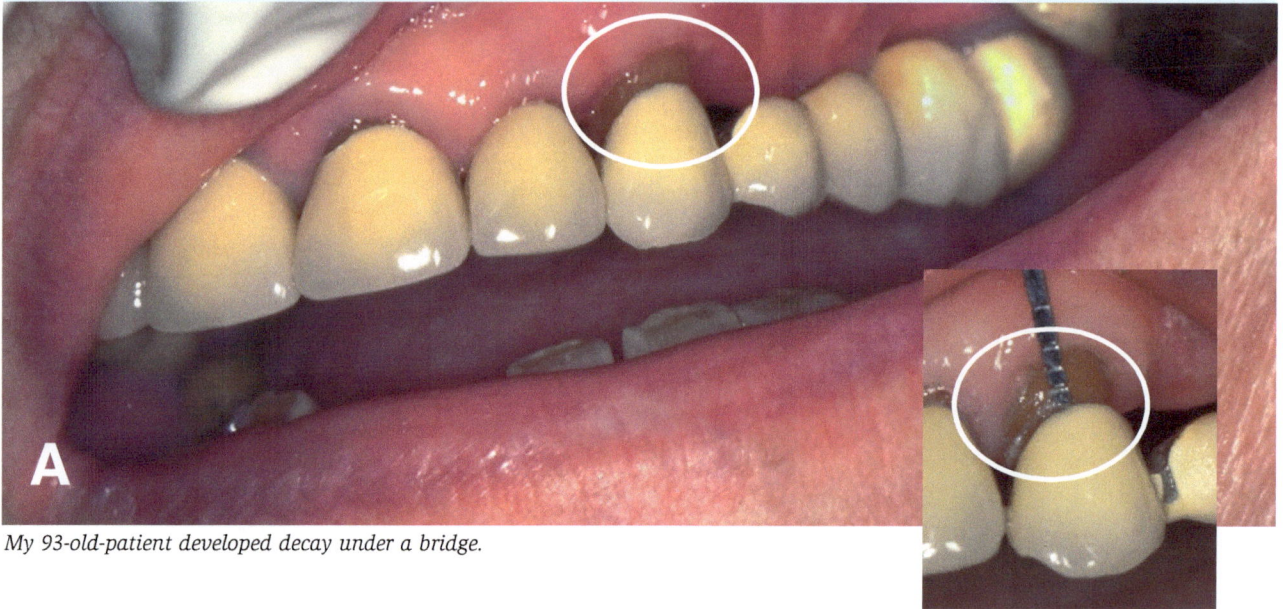

My 93-old-patient developed decay under a bridge.

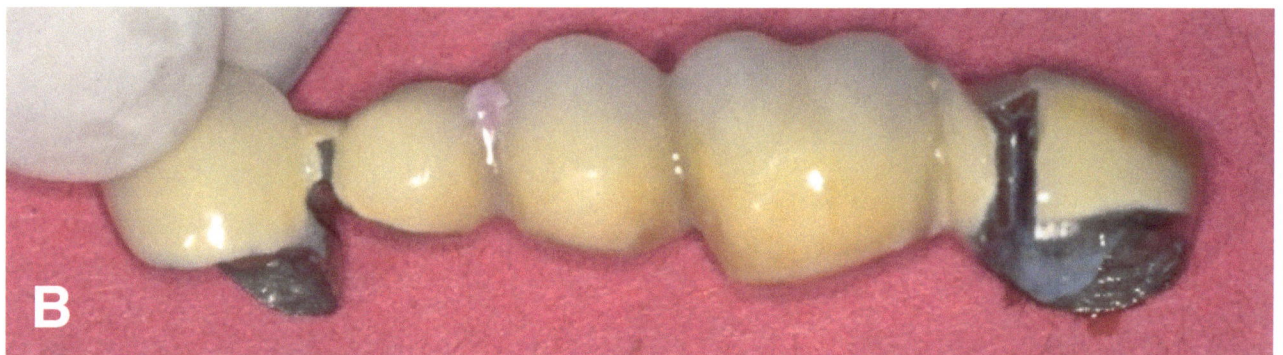

The bridge is removed. Rather than subject this patient to the time and cost of remaking a bridge, bonding composite materials were utilized to readapt her existing bridge.

Is there confusion regarding proper medical care of the elderly?

The most likely etiology for this patient's recurrence of dental decay is reduced salivary flow (*xerostomia* or *dry mouth*) as a result of medications that she is taking. This is a widespread problem, especially among the elderly.

Upon upgrading this patient's medical history it was determined that she is being treated by a *primary physician*, a *neurologist*, a *gastroenterologist* and an *ophthalmologist*.

The patient is currently taking the following medications:

1. *Pepcid*: antacid

2. *Mestinon*: for treatment of myasthenia gravis, a muscular-neurologic disease

3. *Nitro-Dur Patch*: designed to provide continuous, controlled release of nitroglycerine through the intact skin; indicated for the prevention of angina pectoris due to coronary artery disease.

4. *Remeron*: an anti-depressant

5. *Xanax*: anti-anxiety medication

6. *Buspar*: anti-anxiety medication

7. *Flonace Nasal Spray*: for management of allergic rhinitis (rhinitis: inflammation of the nasal mucous membranes)

8: *Allegra*: for relief of symptoms associated with seasonal allergic rhinitis

9. *Prozac*: for depression

10. An eye lubricant

11. A nasal spray

12. *Centrum Silver*: a multi-vitamin

13. B-complex vitamin

14. Calcium citrate

Is this really a coordinated and well thought out treatment plan? **When I asked this very intelligent and alert 93 year old patient about this degree of medication, she said that it was "keeping me out of the hospital".**

Aging / Deterioration

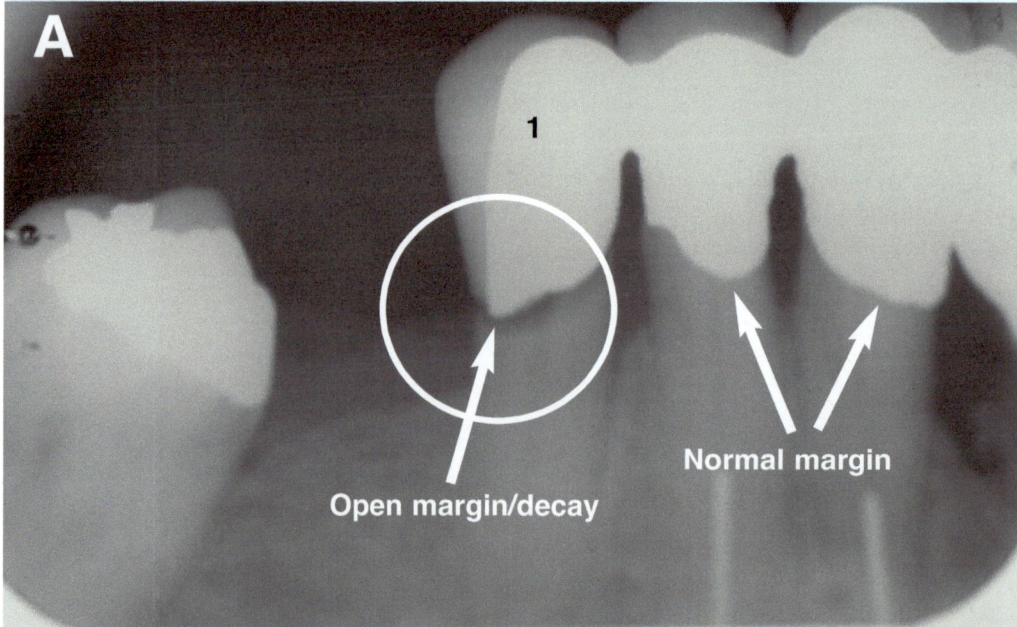

A

1

Open margin/decay

Normal margin

Radiographic appearance of decay under a bridge — unknown etiology.

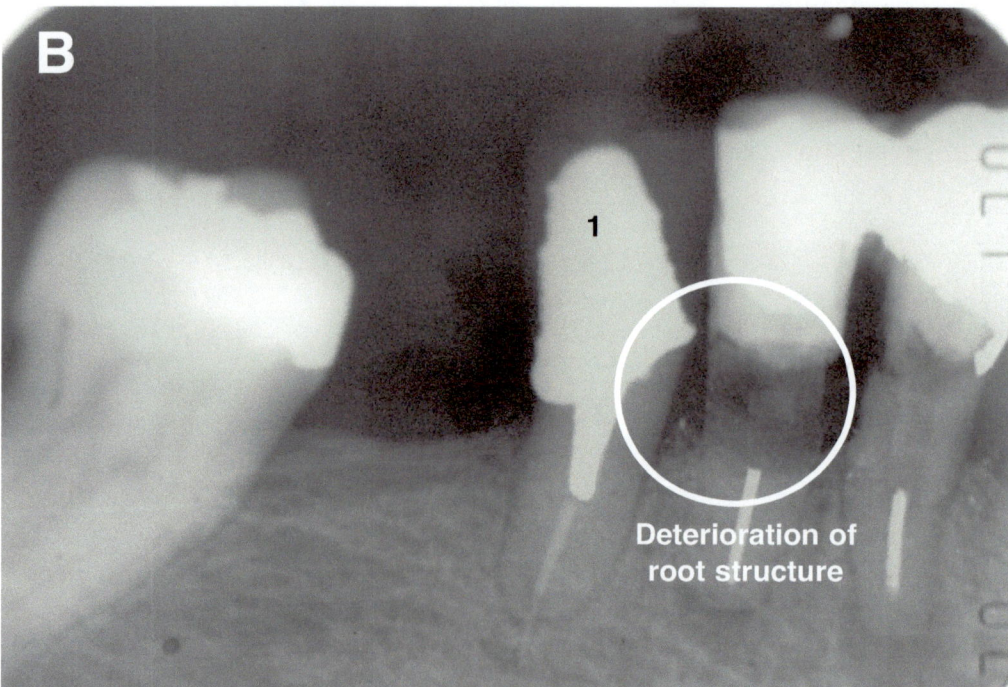

B

1

Deterioration of root structure

Same patient after restoration of tooth (#1) about a year later. This relatively healthy 73-year-old woman experienced this continued rapid deterioration on another tooth. She was not taking any medications, her diet had not changed and her medical history gave no indication of etiology (cause).

Replacing Failing Prosthetics   (Photos A — R)

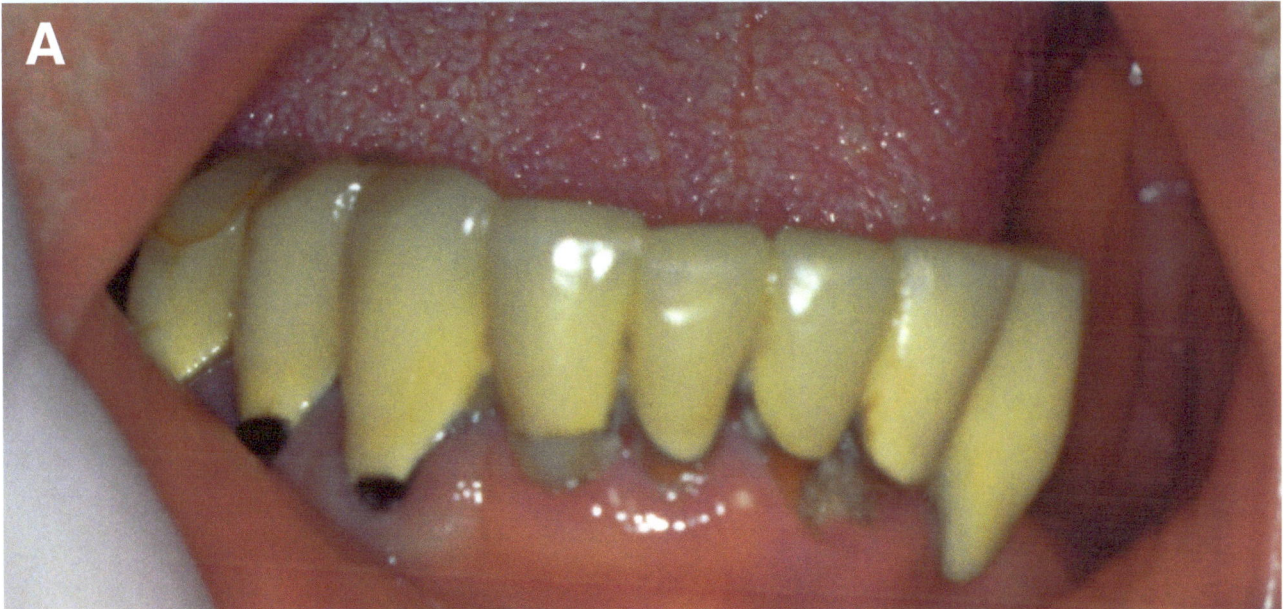

This very nice 80-year-old young at heart lady presented with a very deteriorated oral condition.

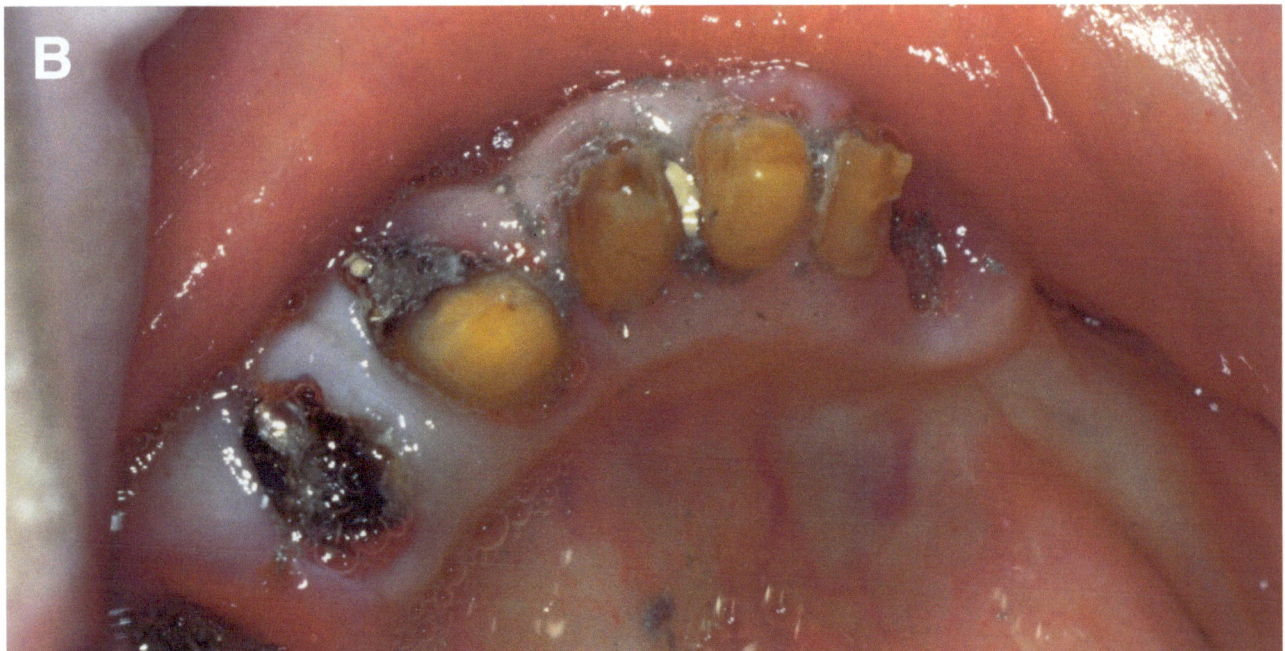

Upon removal of her lower porcelain/metal splint, deterioration is apparent. It was decided to attempt to save as many lower teeth as possible.

Replacing Failing Prosthetics   *(Continued)*

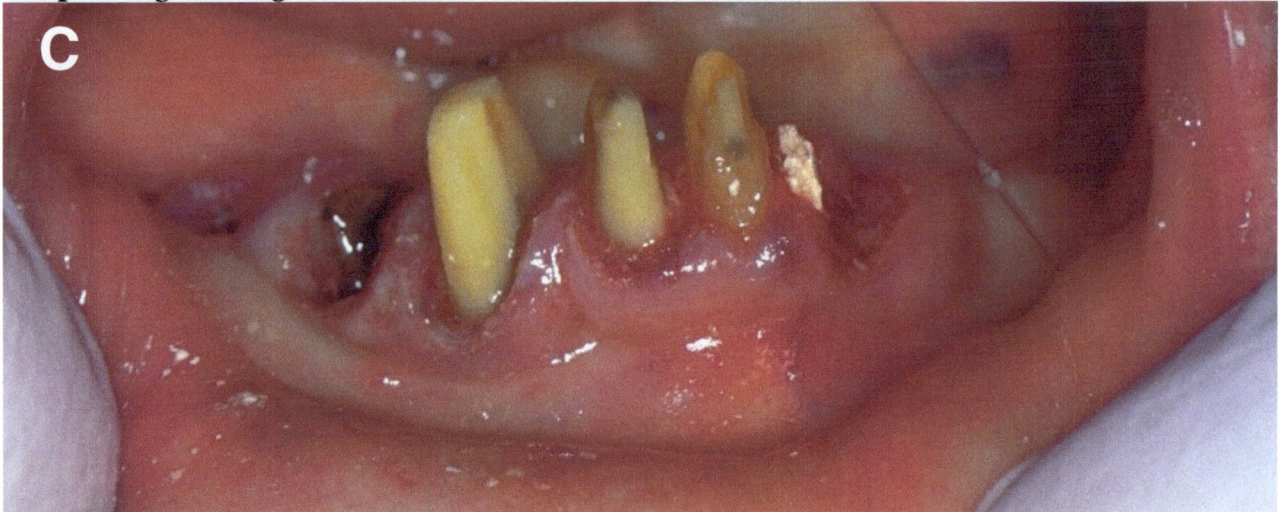

Decay was removed and composite restorative material was bonded initially.

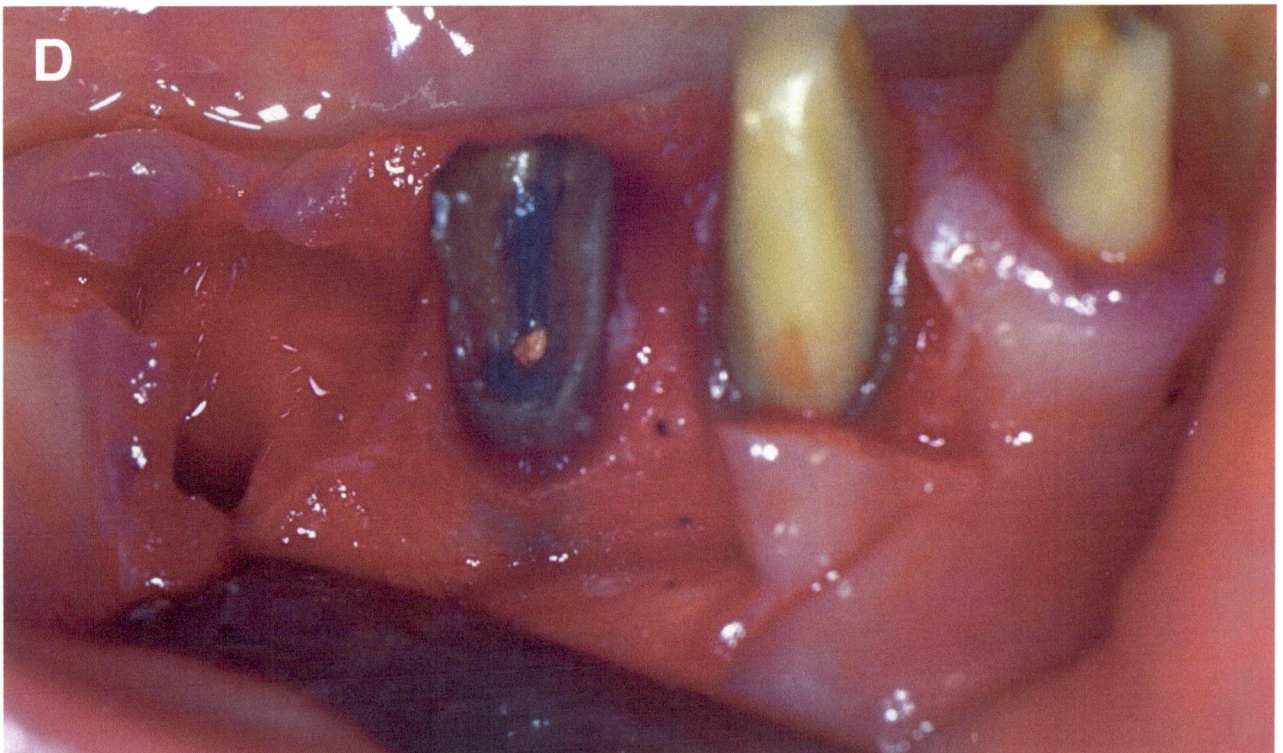

(D, E, F) Periodontal surgery was performed to expose the remaining roots for restoration.

Replacing Failing Prosthetics *(Continued)*

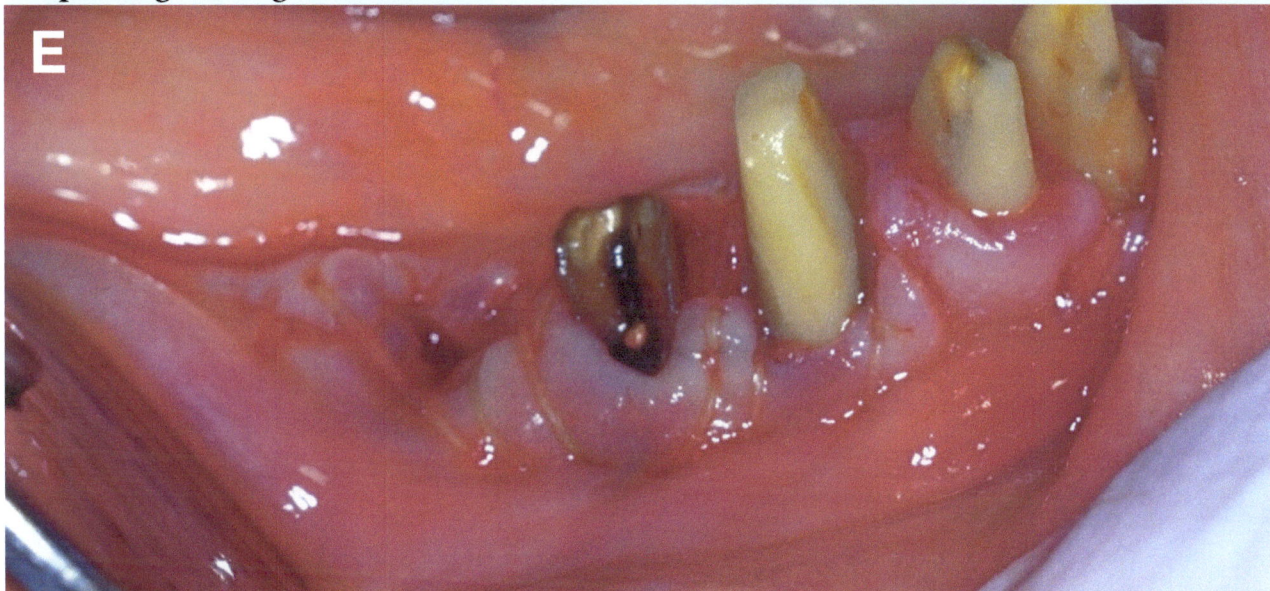

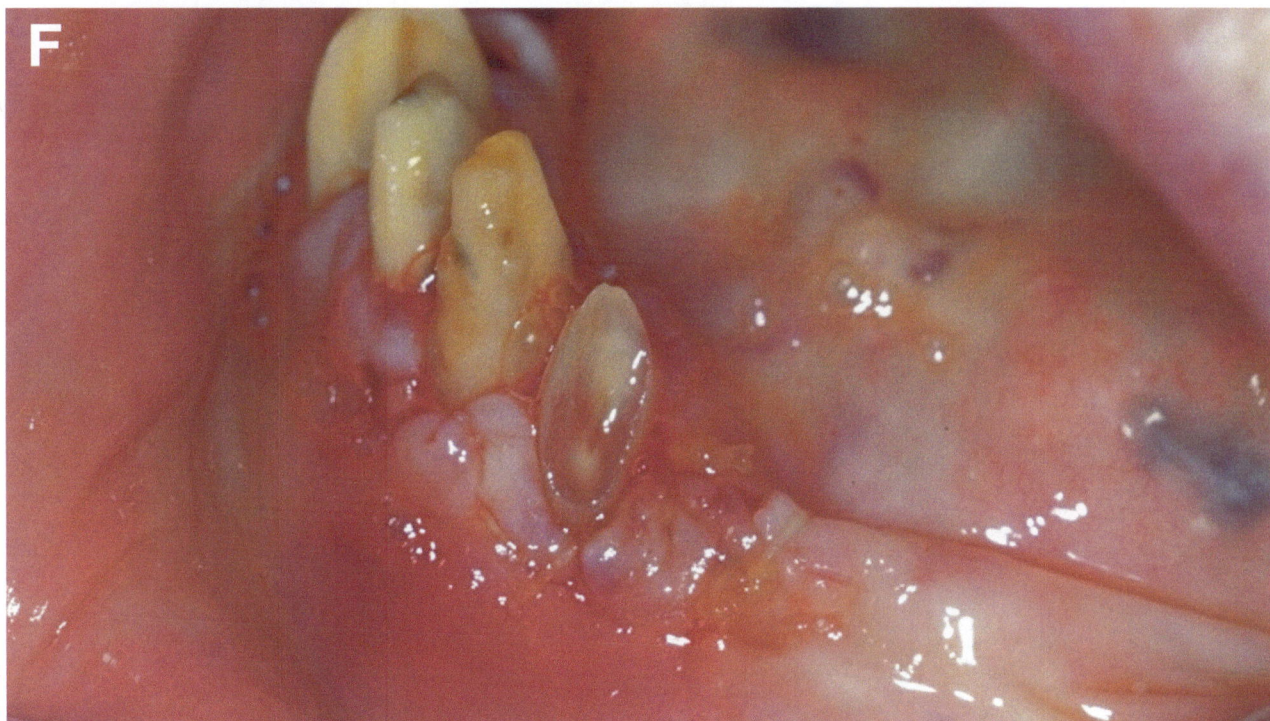

Replacing Failing Prosthetics   (Continued)

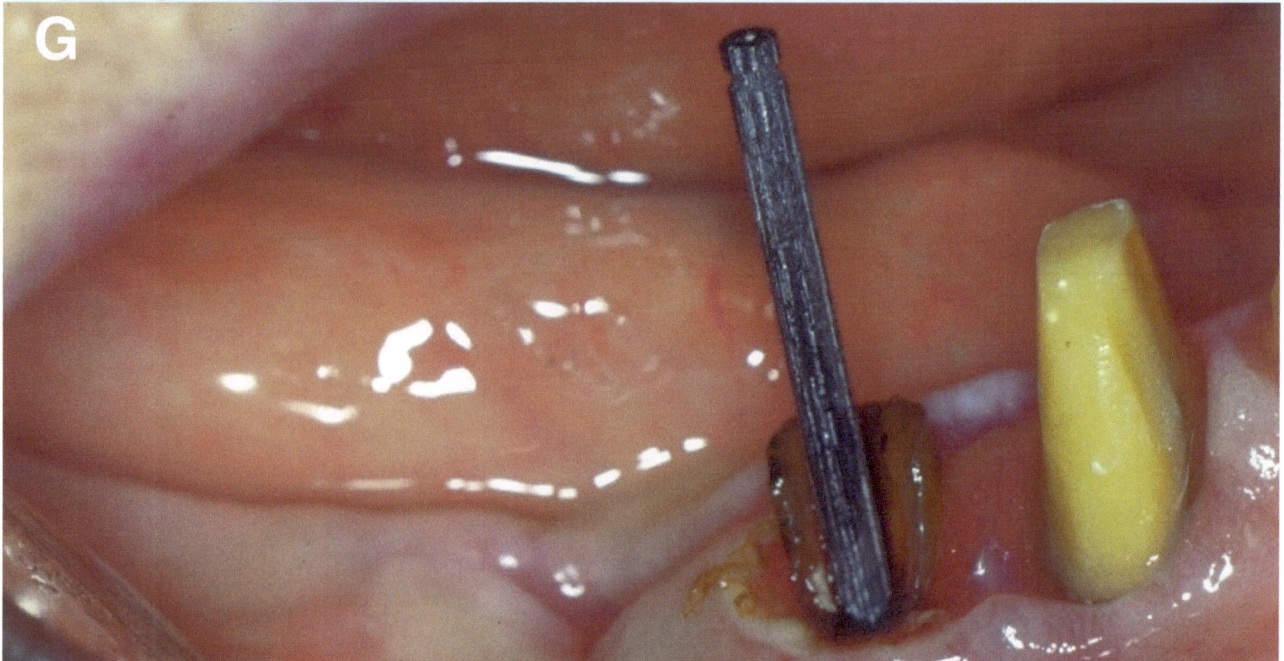

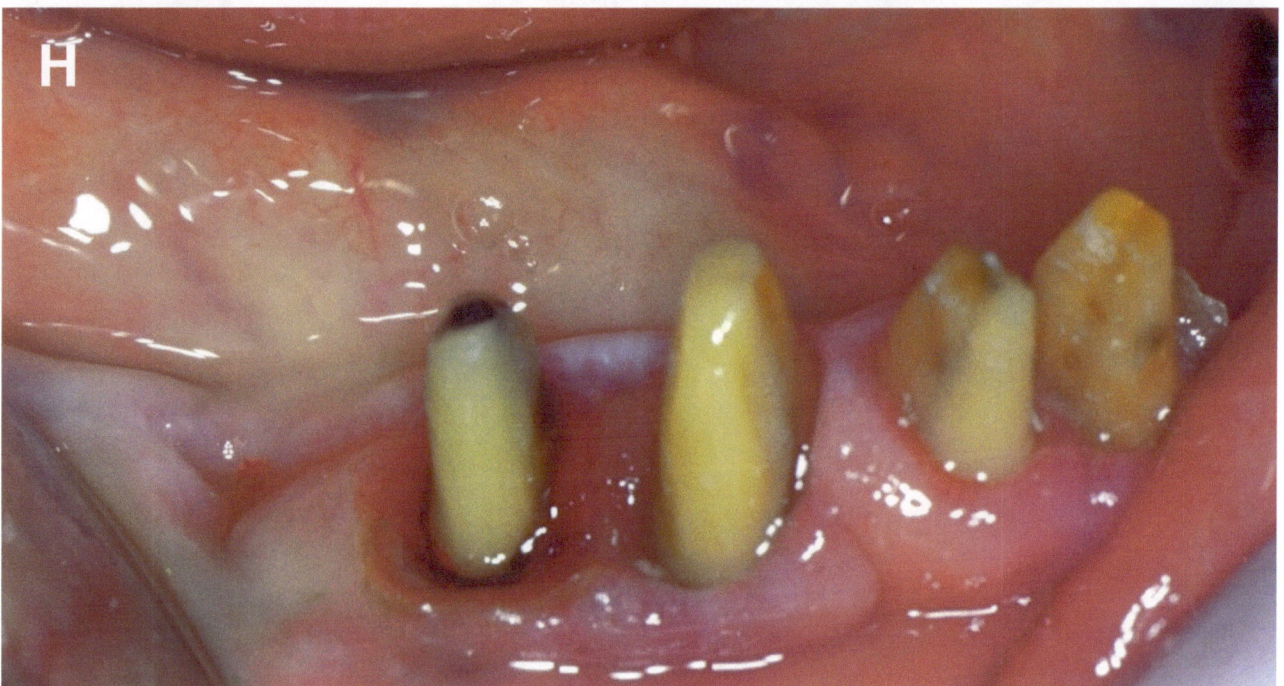

A carbon fiber post and core is bonded to build up the tooth.

Replacing Failing Prosthetics (Continued)

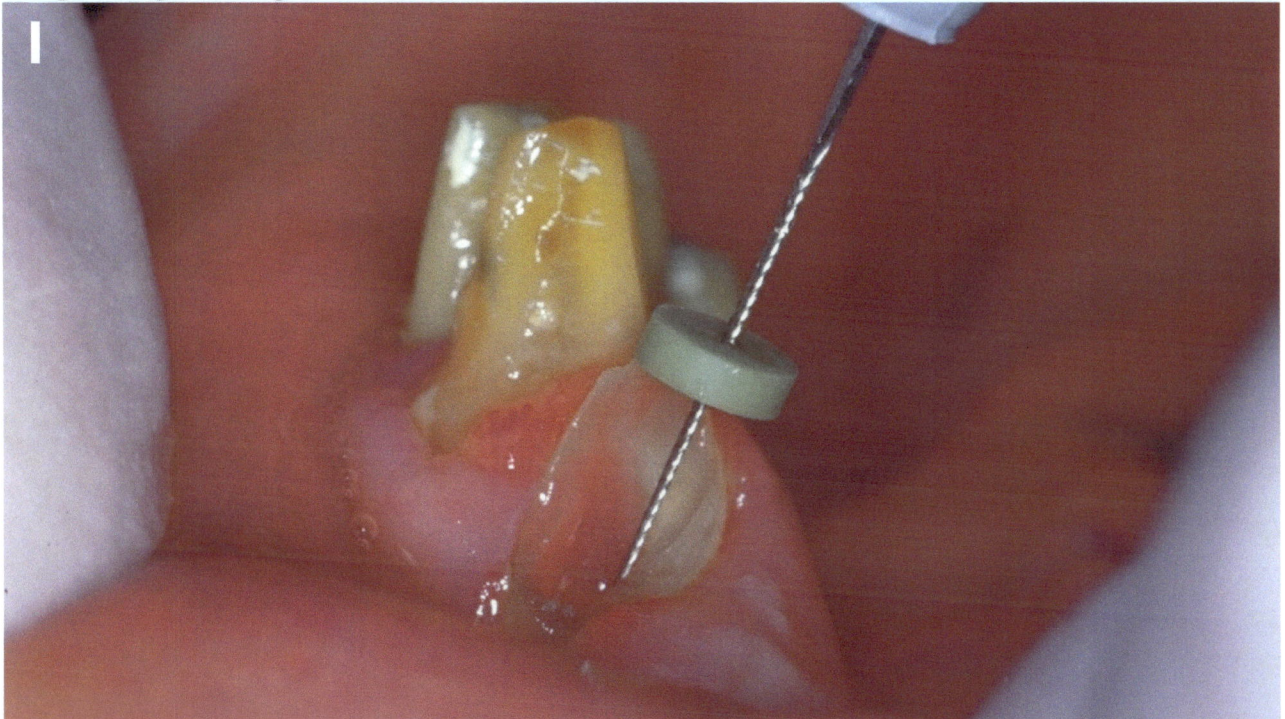

Root canal therapy is performed where necessary.

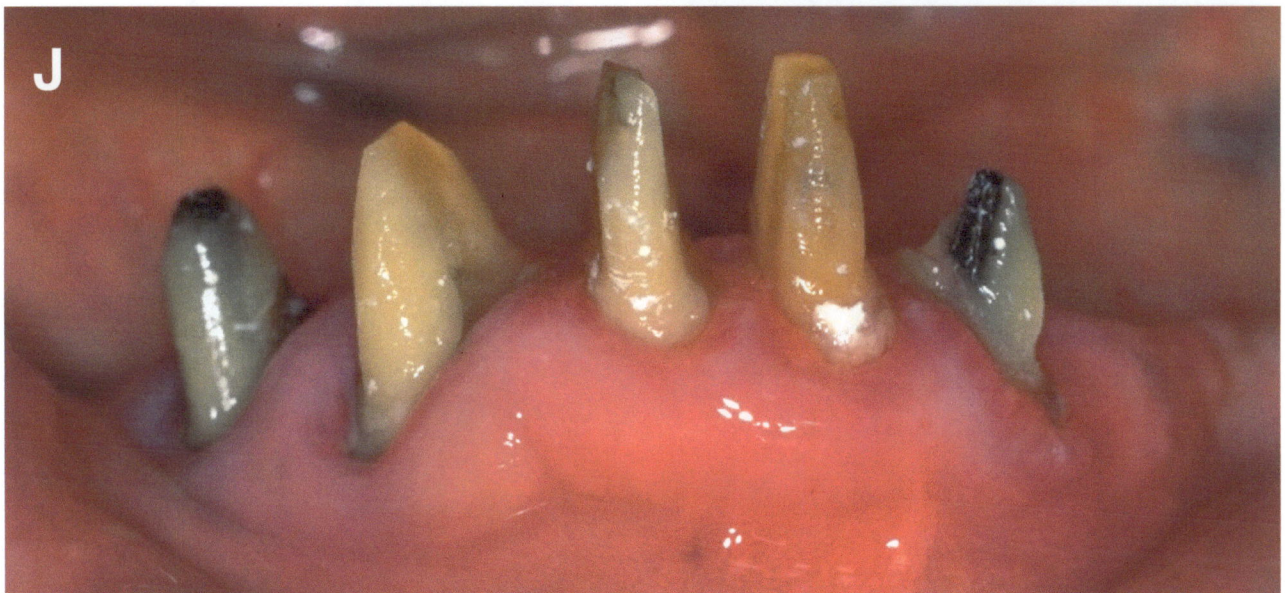

Three months later the tissues are healing and the roots have been built up.

Replacing Failing Prosthetics   (Continued)

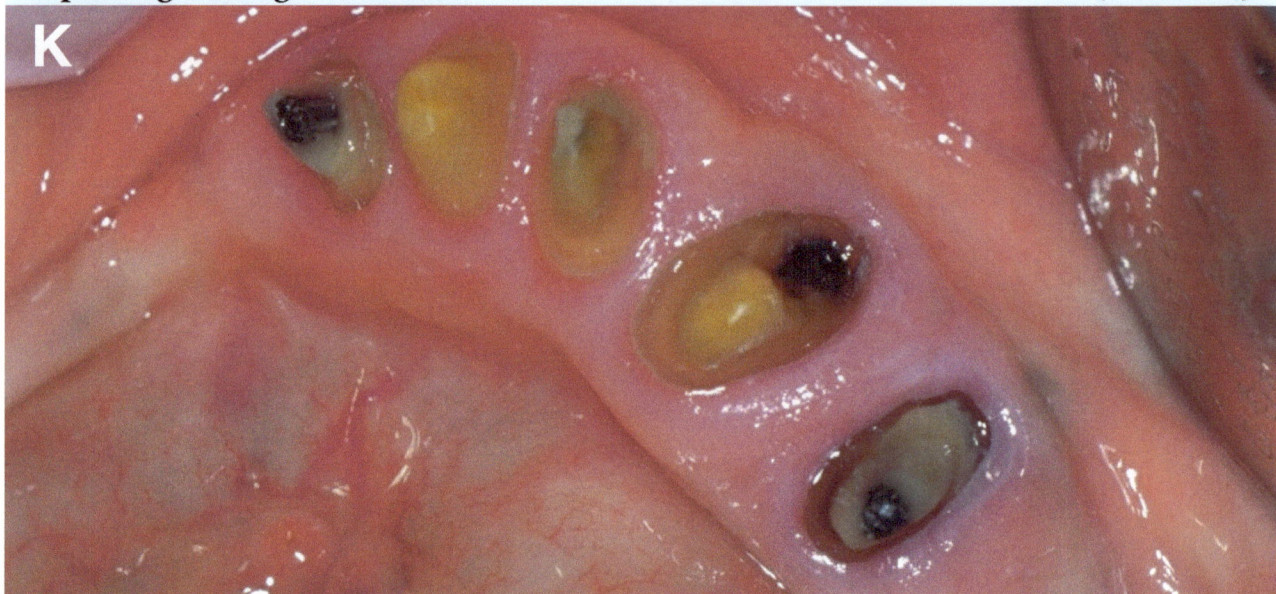

Four months following surgery the tissues appear pink and healthy.

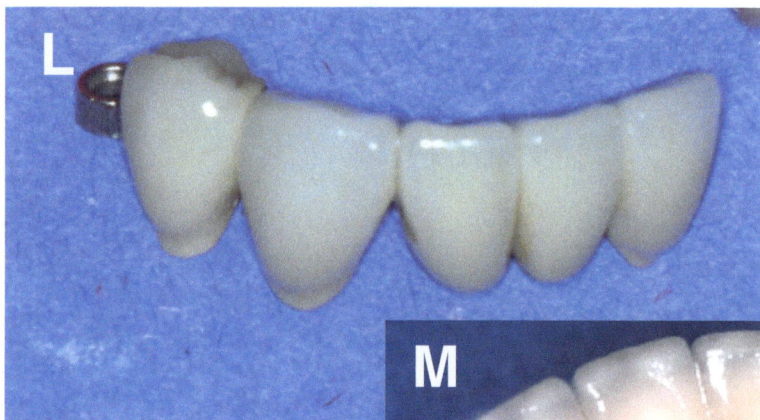

The final splint with attachments. These female attachments will snap on with male attachments on the removable partial denture. This avoids the use of visible clasps.

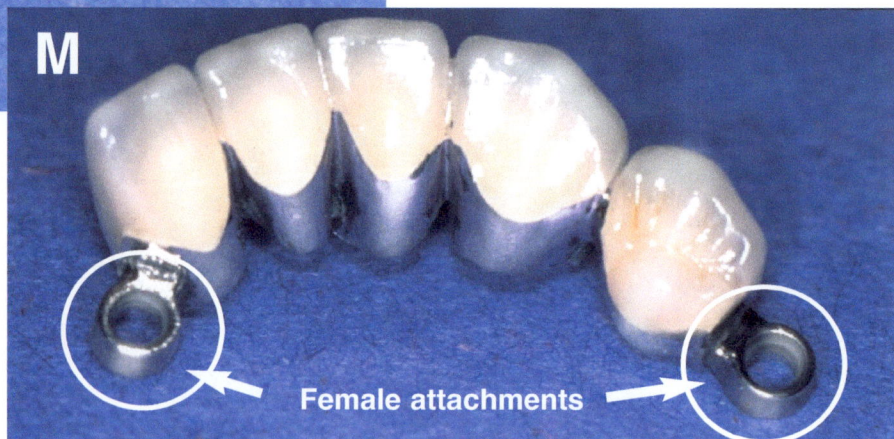

Female attachments

Replacing Failing Prosthetics

(Continued)

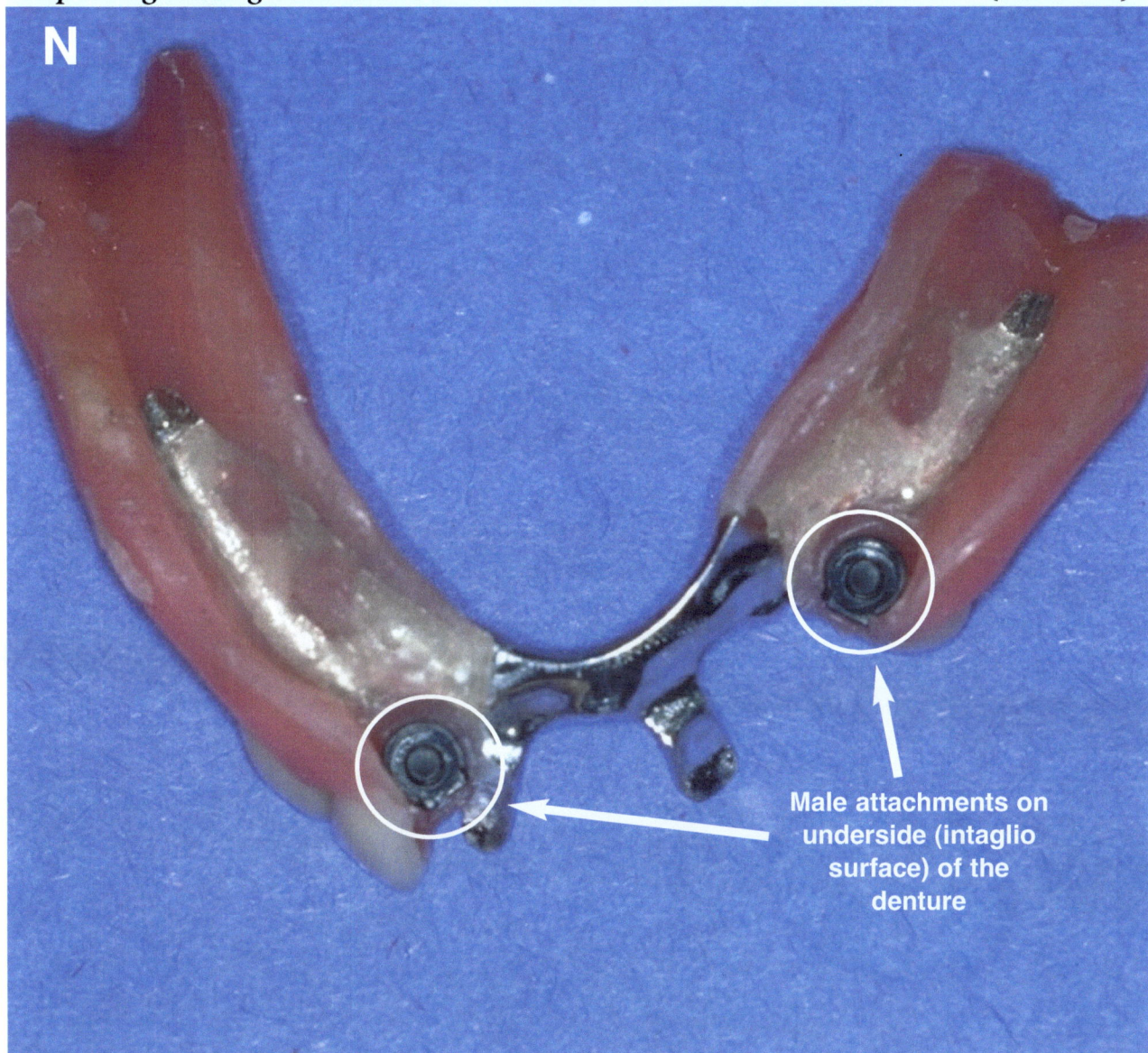

N

Male attachments on underside (intaglio surface) of the denture

Replacing Failing Prosthetics   *(Continued)*

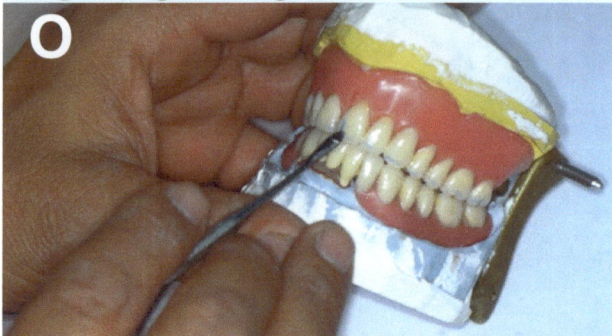

The patient wanted a natural look and this was accomplished through proper shade, tooth mold and tooth arrangement.

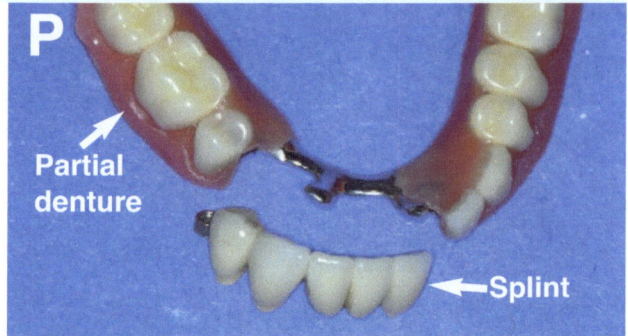

The lower partial denture teeth are placed in wax and tried in the patient's mouth along with the splint to verify fit.

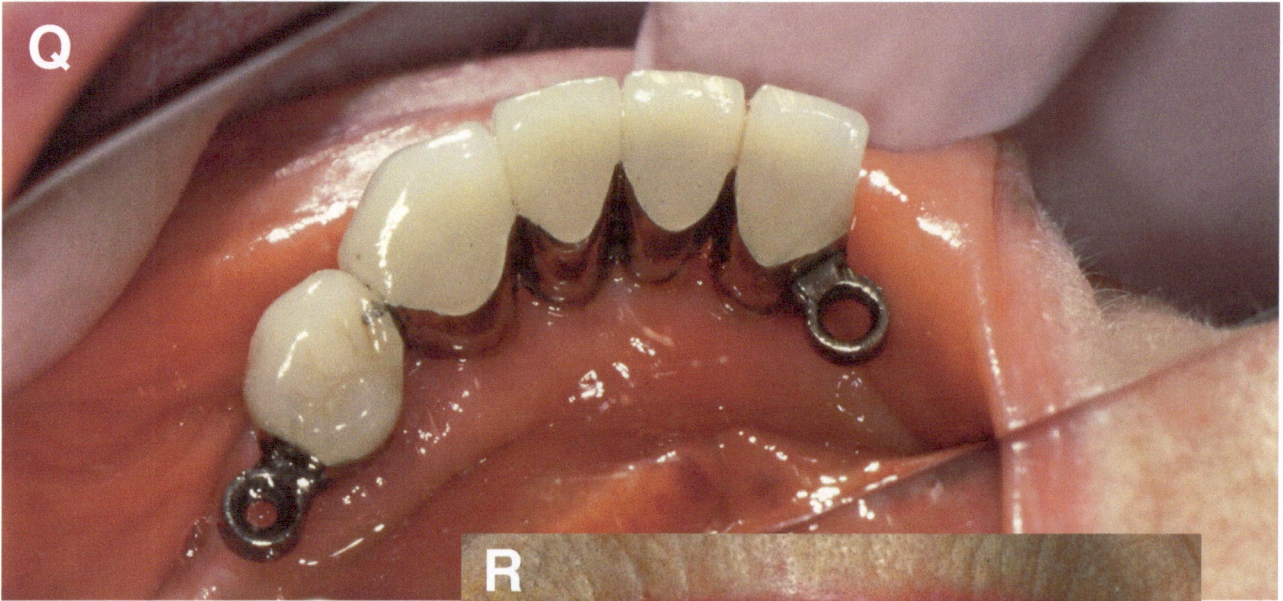

Verification of intra-oral fit of lower splint.

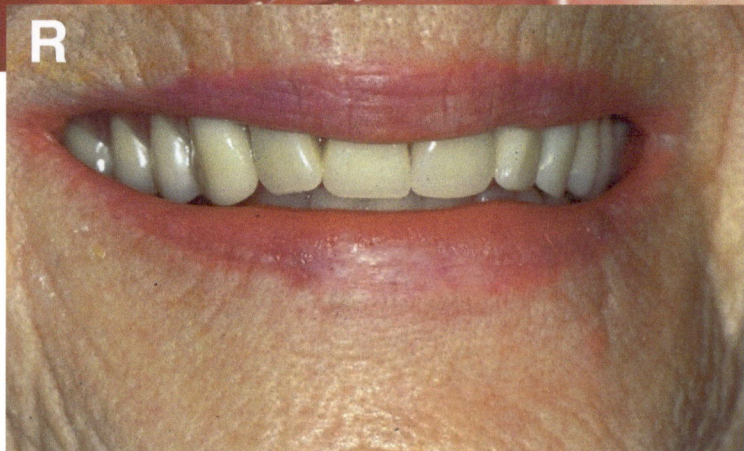

The final dentures appear natural and are functioning well.

FINANCES

Before you can determine the cost of any procedure, you must know approximately what is involved and necessary. According to a recent Reader's Digest article[30] about the diverse treatment recommendations and fees presented to a "test" patient who was sent to various dental offices around the country, an unethical motive is suspected. Rather than address the issues the article presents, many dentists took offense to it (no doubt due to the accusatory slant of the author). I certainly understand a diversity of professional fees (based on variables such as treatment alternatives, geographic dental office location, the dentist's degree of experience, and the value the dentist determines for his or her service) however, this wide range of treatment requirements is somewhat unusual. It would certainly be enlightening to gather all the information together with a panel of experts to explore this further.

In dental school, we were taught to perform proper diagnosis and treatment. Yes, there were differences in opinion however, as facts were revealed and analyzed, most students agreed to a relative degree. The financial pressures of the real world of the dental business unfortunately tend to corrupt the sensibilities of some well-trained professionals. So, a patient should understand these realities, and before accepting a particular treatment (especially if the treatment involves extensive and costly procedures), obtain a second or third opinion. Request written clarification of precisely what needs to be done, why it must be done, and what possible alternatives exist. Then take a good look at the dentist involved (refer to the next chapter on the Best Dentists) and make an intelligent choice.

As to the business side of a dental practice, profit as a result of other people's problems has always bothered me. Fortunately, most patients appreciate the effort that goes into providing quality dental care and legitimate advice on health issues. For my part, I still get euphorically mesmerized when involved in certain intricate and difficult dental procedures. My effort is rewarded not only financially but also with a certain union or partnership that develops between a patient and health care professional.

Everyone Loves Fun – But Do We Really Need a Third Party?

Twenty-nine years ago, I don't remember dealing with dental insurance. Initially, its popularity seemed to be based on a few legitimate "claims." Patients were encouraged to use their benefits to obtain proper health care, dentists experienced increased business and received relatively fair reimbursements, and the insurance companies made a profit. Today, for the most part, the situation has deteriorated. Patients are now encouraged to visit specific dentists (or "providers," as they are now

---

30. "How Honest are Dentists?" by William Ecenbarger. Reader's Digest, February 1997. 50-56.

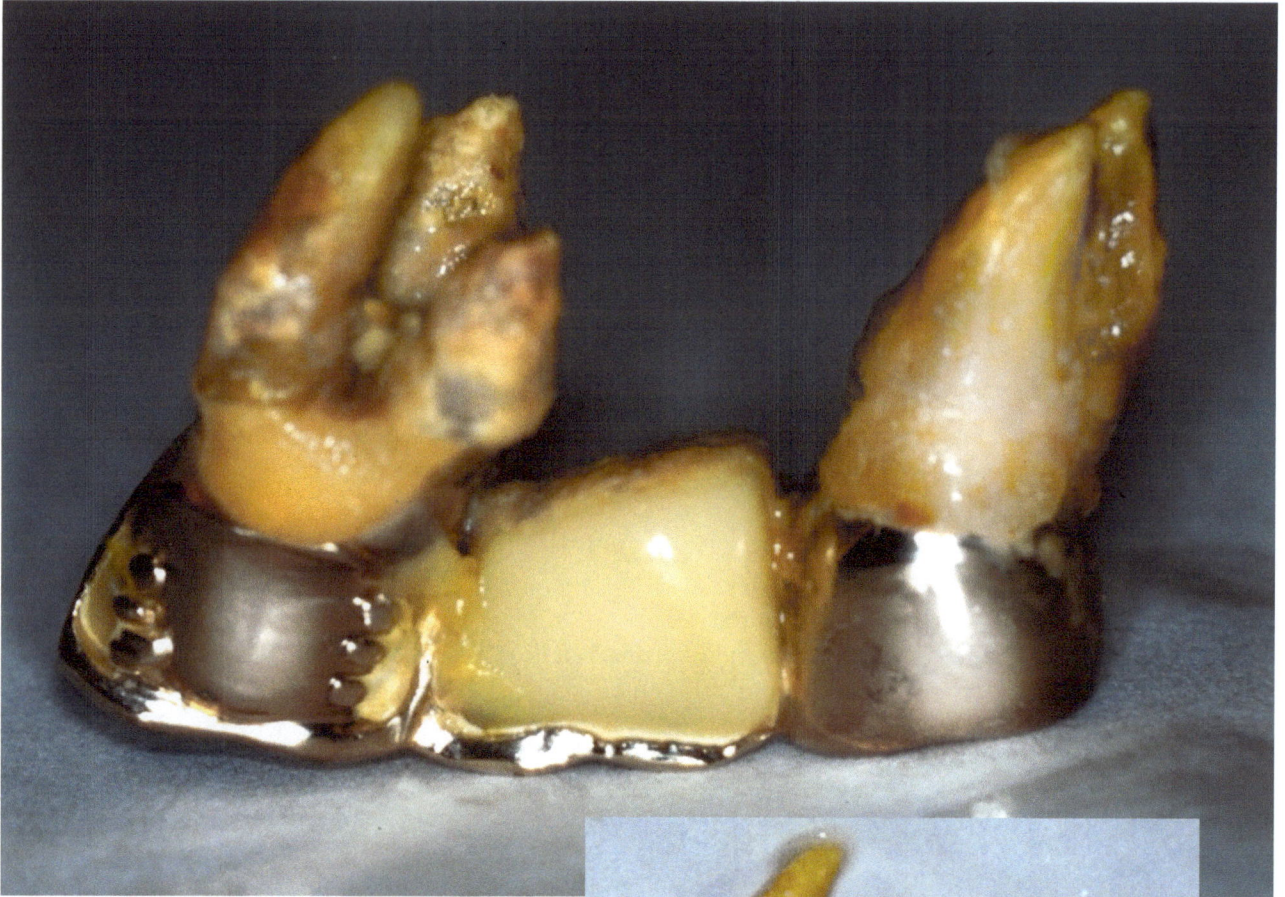

A "successful" long-lasting bridge covering teeth with terminal periodontal disease. This man presented to my office with this condition. He had been receiving his later "dental care" in an HMO environment.

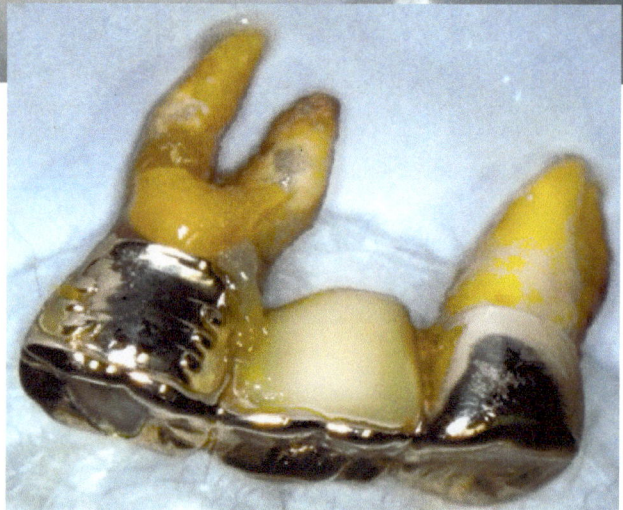

called) who deliver services at a discounted fee in order to receive an increased volume of "heads" from the insurance company. The approval process for many dental procedures has become extremely cumbersome, and the ability of the dentist to provide quality care has suffered. Based on this type of deteriorating arrangement, this "middleman" is a hindrance and should be eliminated.

A wise patient should choose a dentist who will address legitimate dental needs, formulate a written treatment plan, and if possible, arrange financing the patient can afford—regardless of insurance coverage. It's strange, but it seems that if patients don't need a lot of dental care other than a few cleaning appointments and periodic exams, they don't need to be paying insurance premiums—and if they do need extensive dental care, most policies have severe limitations that usually significantly interfere with successful treatment.

Priorities

Several years back, I initiated a $35,000, full-mouth reconstruction case. This case involved periodontal surgery and prosthetic rehabilitation. It was quite complex and time consuming. A few years after completion, the very nice, middle-aged patient passed away. I was aware of her chronic medical problems—diabetes and fluctuations in obesity and blood pressure—but she was regularly visiting her physicians and apparently being treated. I wonder, however, if she had spent as much time and money with her physicians as she had with her dentist—could they have paid more attention to her and possibly intercepted her fatal episode? Please remember that dentistry does not deal with life and death situations. Some people have even called dentistry "elective therapy." *You should prioritize your personal health needs and treat yourself according to what makes sense.*

THE BEST DENTISTS

The perfect dentist knows everything, treats you like royalty, is painless, does not let personal problems hinder his concentration, is asexual, has employees exactly like himself, schedules appointments any time you want and supplies services free of charge. What a great deal!

In reality, the best dentists (as is the case with all professionals) are those who put aside distractions and concentrate on your particular needs in a compassionate manner. The best dentist is knowledgeable in the field and keeps current with improvements. All this costs money, and in order for the best dentists to provide this level of service, the patient must be willing to commit the time and money required. Problems develop usually as a result of differences in opinion regarding the value of the service being performed. Some degree of sacrifice is necessary on everyone's part.

Since most dental procedures are intricate, exacting, and time consuming, a good dentist will not rush. The adage "Haste makes waste" applies here, especially if the results are expected to endure. Good dentists will not compromise quality, and they know the real costs of proper care.

In order to identify the best dentist for your needs, it is important for you to interview him or her. Contact a few dental offices, speak with the receptionist, explain that you are seeking an excellent dentist, and ask if it is possible to arrange an appointment for a consultation. Get as much information as possible from the receptionist, or if possible, ask to speak with the dentist. Prepare a written list of your concerns.

In my office, I often receive telephone inquiries asking what I charge for certain procedures (without an examination). These inquiries raise the concern that the patient is comparison-shopping and basing a decision on fees alone—not a good way to obtain the best value.

When I graduated from the Baltimore College of Dental Surgery in 1972, the last thing I wanted was to open my own practice. I headed for Boston, Massachusetts, where I heard there were plenty of young women, lots of partying, and a beautiful New England setting. Over the years I experienced life, the fun, the disappointments, the exuberance of youth, the tempering of spirits, and finally, the development of a more mature perspective. From more experienced dentists, I learned what I could, not only their "dental lessons," but how they managed and survived in a difficult environment. I saw drug abuse, divorce, premature death, malpractice, but also resiliency among those dentists who seemed able to function well and be happy. Dentists, like all other human beings, are subject to life's pressures.

Your selection of a good dentist should be based on your judgment when evaluating character, no matter what "stage" of life the dentist is experiencing.

THE CONTROVERSIES

The Mercury Issue

A silver filling (also known as an amalgam restoration) is actually an alloy—a combination of metals including mercury. Over the past 20 years, a number of dentists have indicated that this type of restorative material is poison. They say the mercury leaches into the body and causes everything from depression to Multiple Sclerosis. I don't doubt that people differ in their sensitivities to various materials; my experience, however, indicates that amalgam restorations are quite safe and extremely durable. It's interesting, though, to observe the overwhelming emergence of alternative "filling" materials. Composite and porcelain restorations bonded to the teeth not only look great in comparison to amalgam, but also seem to bring the "poison" issue to rest.[31] Initially these replacement materials weren't as durable as amalgam, but as their popularity increased, sales revenues supplied the funds necessary to conduct research and improve the physical properties of these materials. I routinely use these newer materials, but never without a thorough consultation with my patients and an explanation of the pros and cons of the treatment.

Lasers

Lasers always seem to evoke a sense of a "state-of-the-art" means of treatment. I've seen dental offices advertise that lasers are used in their practices for various procedures. This seems at this point to be more of a marketing device rather than a "breakthrough" in superior treatment. However, as with the incorporation and improvement of composite fillings in lieu of the "poisonous" amalgams, laser technology will, I believe, become a more useful technology as improvements continue to occur.

Implants

There is a lot of money to be made in providing implant dentistry, most of it by the manufacturers. I remember when I once brought a patient to an oral surgeon for a consultation. My patient had no back teeth in his lower jaw and had stable, healthy teeth in the front. I was surprised when the surgeon suggested that besides providing implants in the back area of the jaw, the patient's healthy front teeth should be extracted and replaced with implants. In my opinion, this suggestion constituted malpractice.

Implants, which can be simply defined as artificial roots placed in the bone to support teeth, are great when a patient can afford the oftentimes complex treatment and maintenance visits. However, the abusive use of these devices (and by many unqualified dentists) is malpractice. Sadly, this occurs relatively frequently.

31. Unless they also discover "poison" elements in these materials!

Poor Treatment Planning Resulting In Implant Failure   *(Photos A – F)*

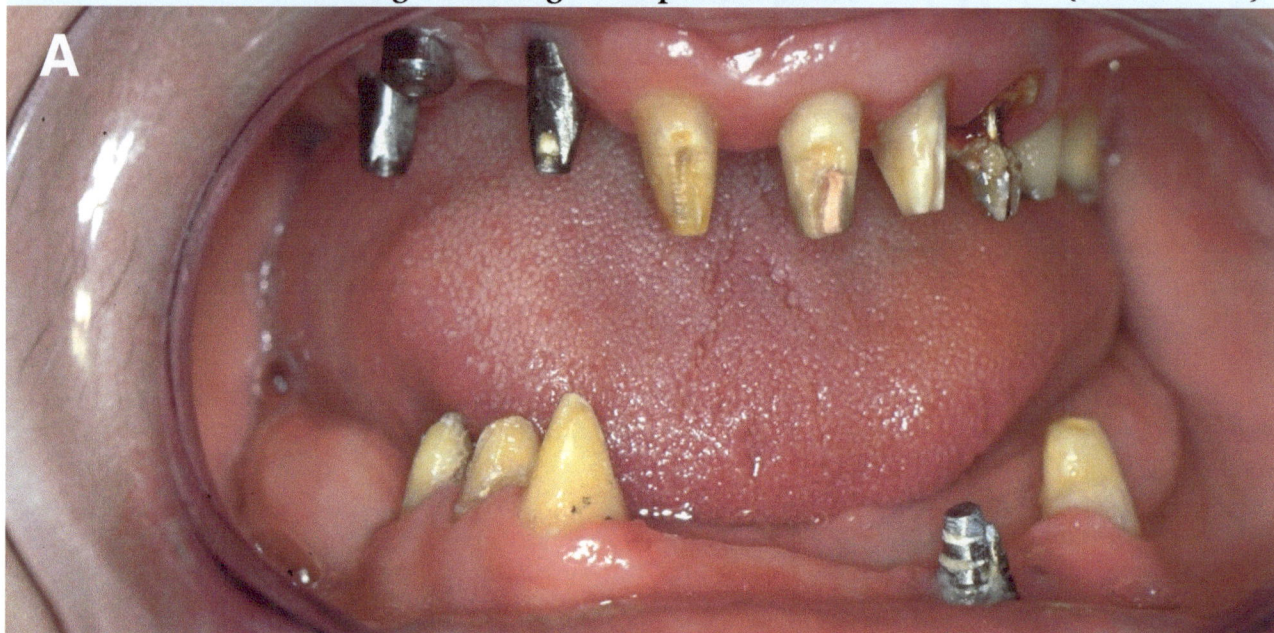

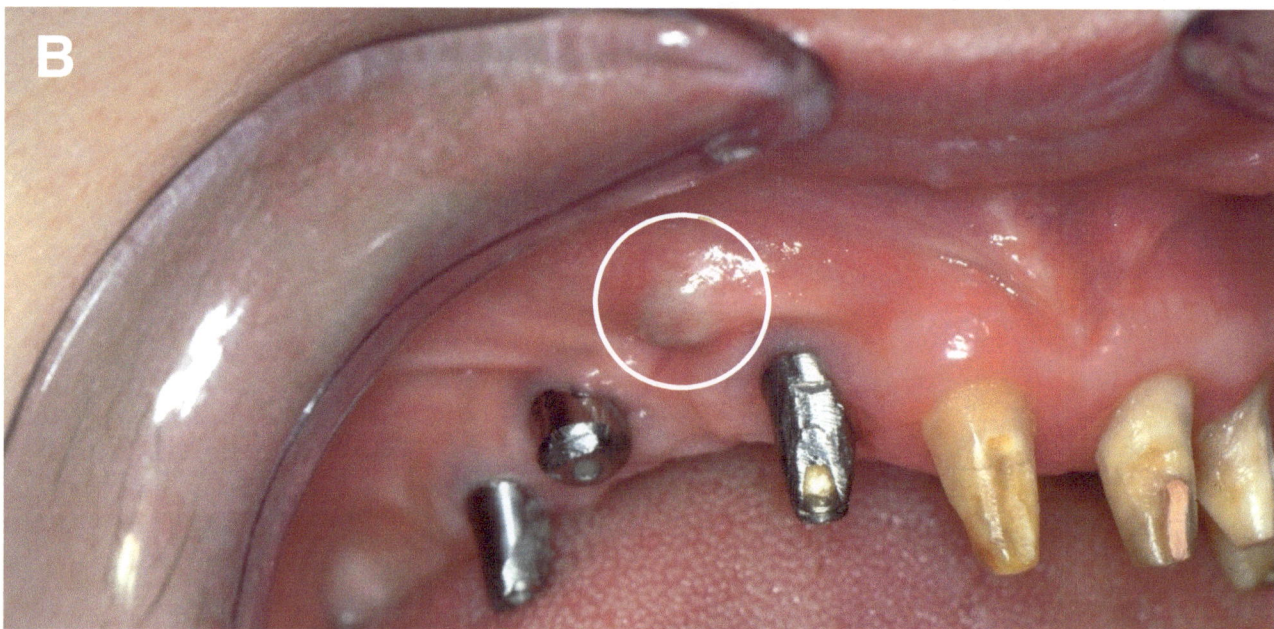

An improperly placed implant is "hidden" beneath the tissue.

Poor Treatment Planning Resulting In Implant Failure   (Continued)

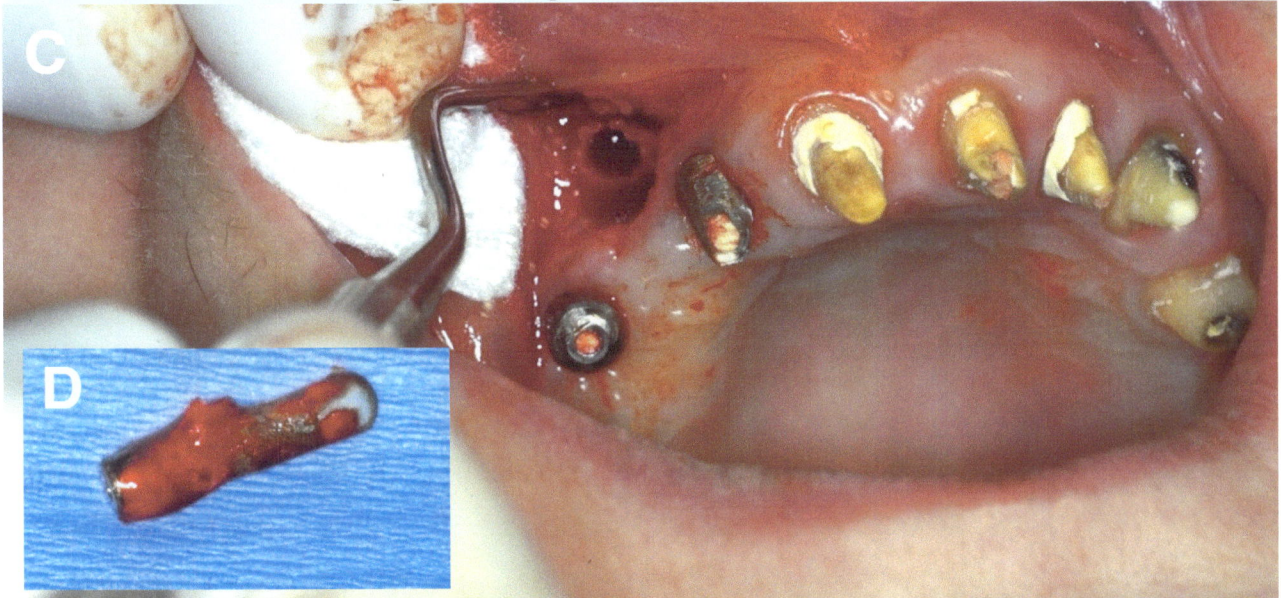

The implant is surgically removed. <u>Proper</u> planning and case study might have prevented this type of failure.

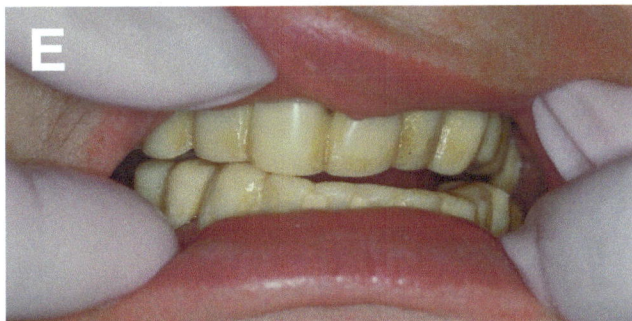

The improperly fabricated temporary splints as seen at this patient's initial visit to my office.

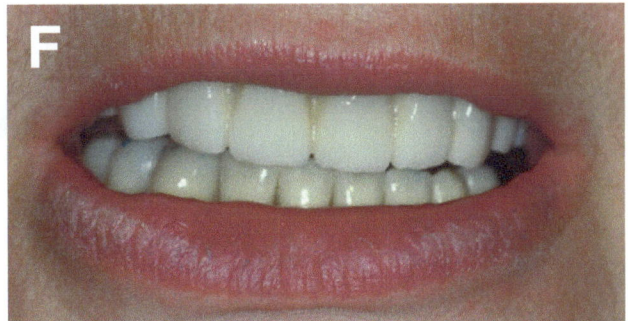

Properly fabricated splints were inserted.

Iatrogenics and Malpractice

Iatrogenics is dentist-induced problems—whether it is a poor quality filling, a badly constructed crown, or a blatant misdiagnosis that leads to the wrong treatment—it is malpractice. In dental school, professors review and grade the quality of work the student produces. In the real world, this safeguard doesn't exist. The reasons for iatrogenics however, are numerous, but it is all malpractice. When third party plans and insurance companies encourage discount dentistry, iatrogenics is often the end result. Independent quality control is necessary, and standards must be established if we are to end this "routine care" that is really only a facade for malpractice.

The Result Of Iatrogenics   (Photos A – H)

A

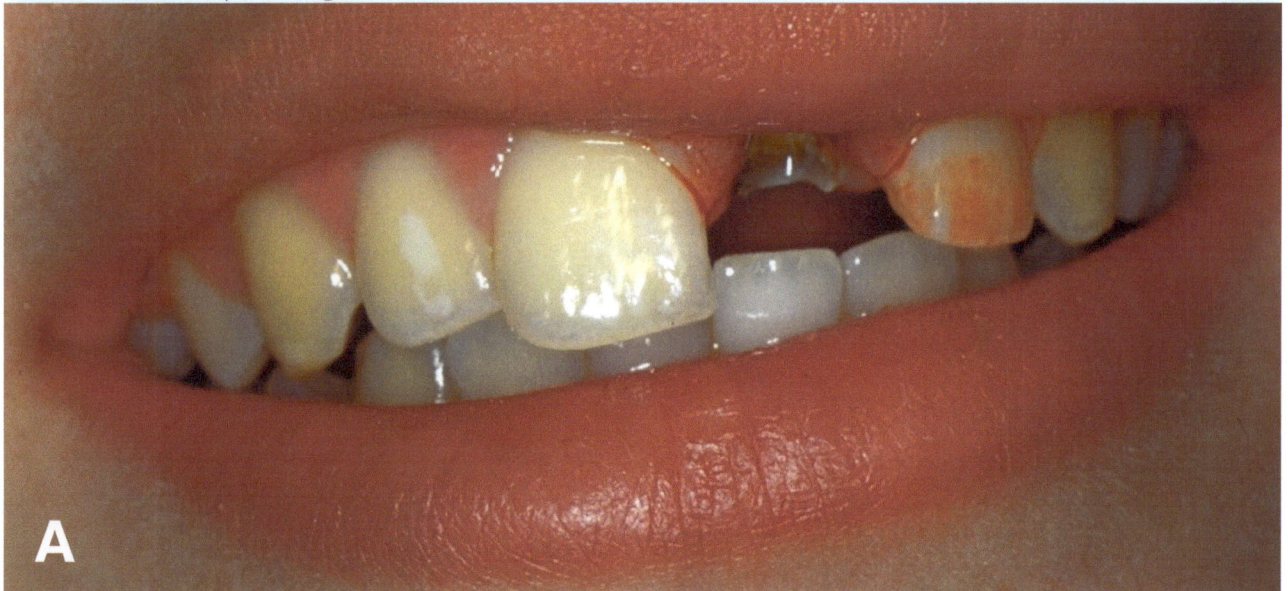

A young girl presented to my office as an emergency patient. This defective restoration was doomed to fail due to the inadequate screw post and poor quality crown.

If this restoration had originally been fabricated properly, the patient (and her mom and dad) would not have had to interrupt their Miami Beach vacation and be subject to emergency dental fees.

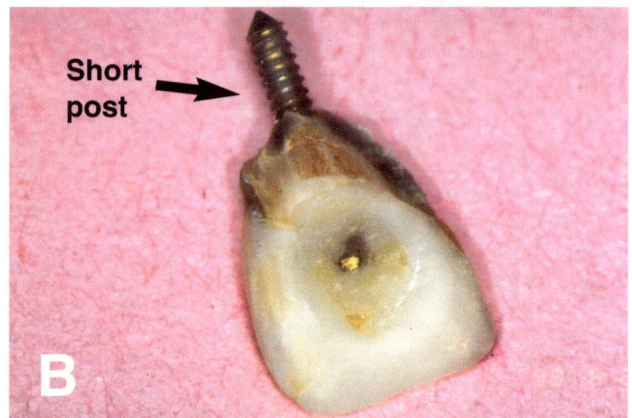

Short post

B

Restoring The Damaged Root   *(Continued)*

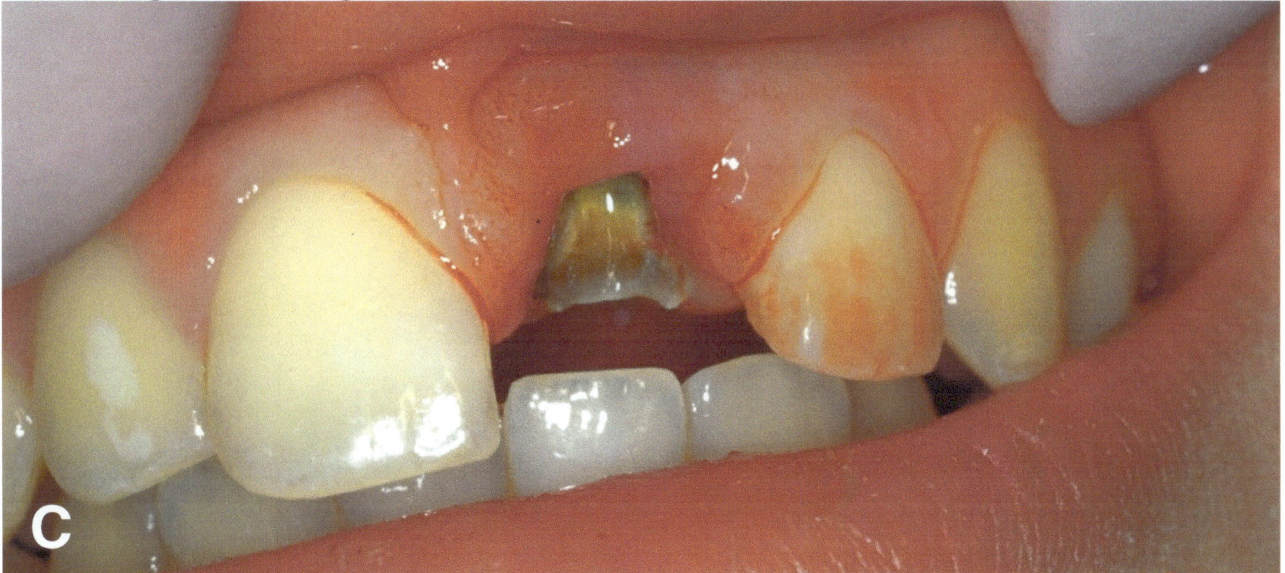

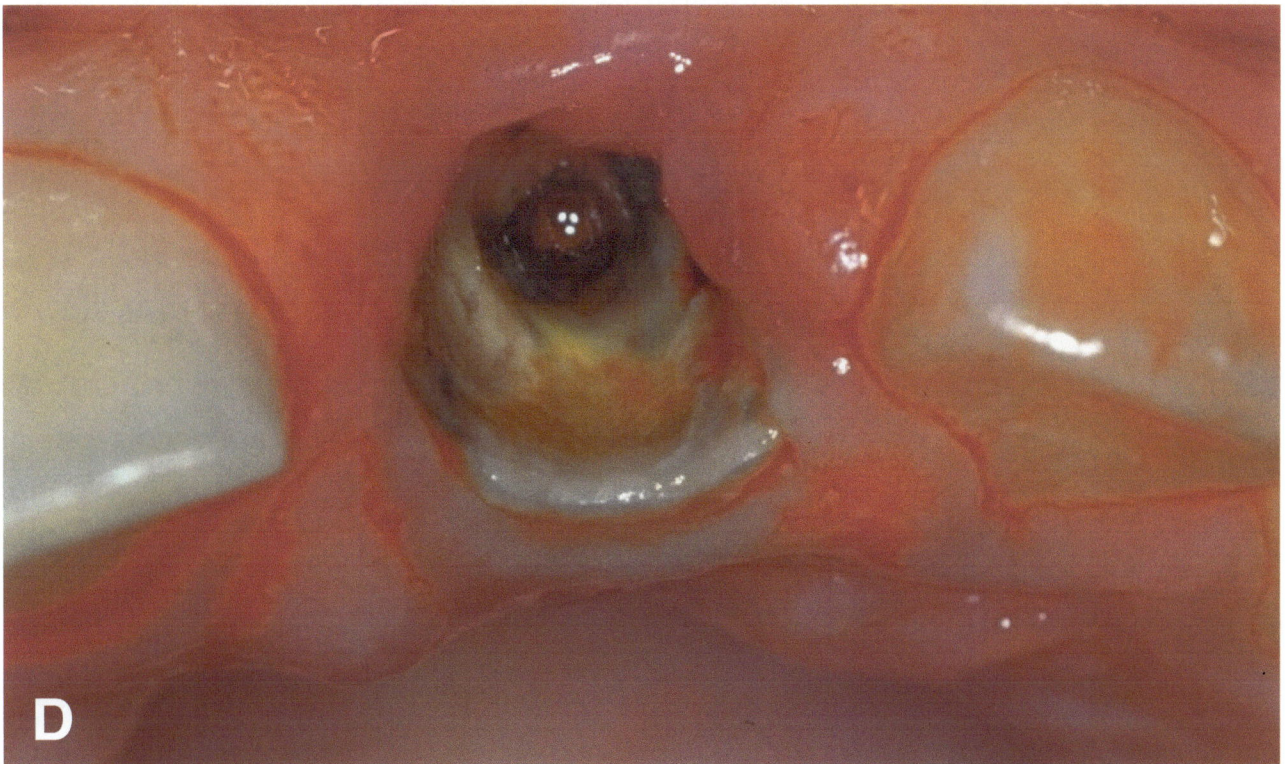

The remaining root was barely salvageable. After discussing treatment options with her parents it was decided to attempt to restore the root.

Restoring The Damaged Root   *(Continued)*

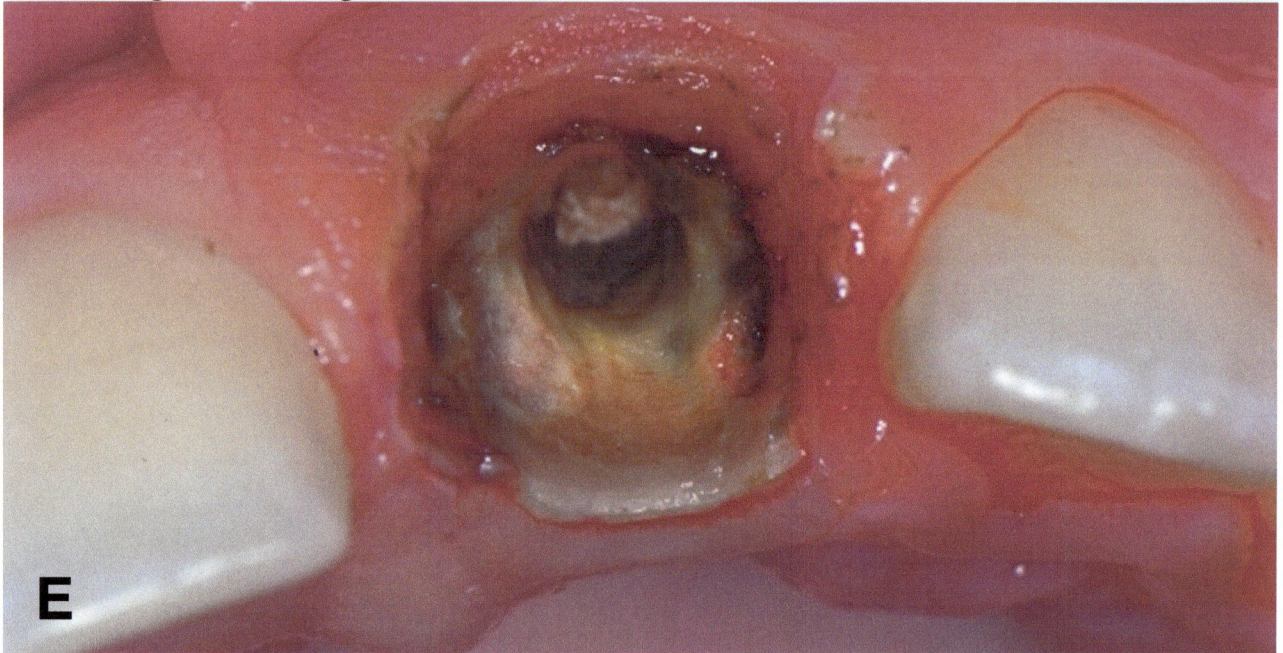

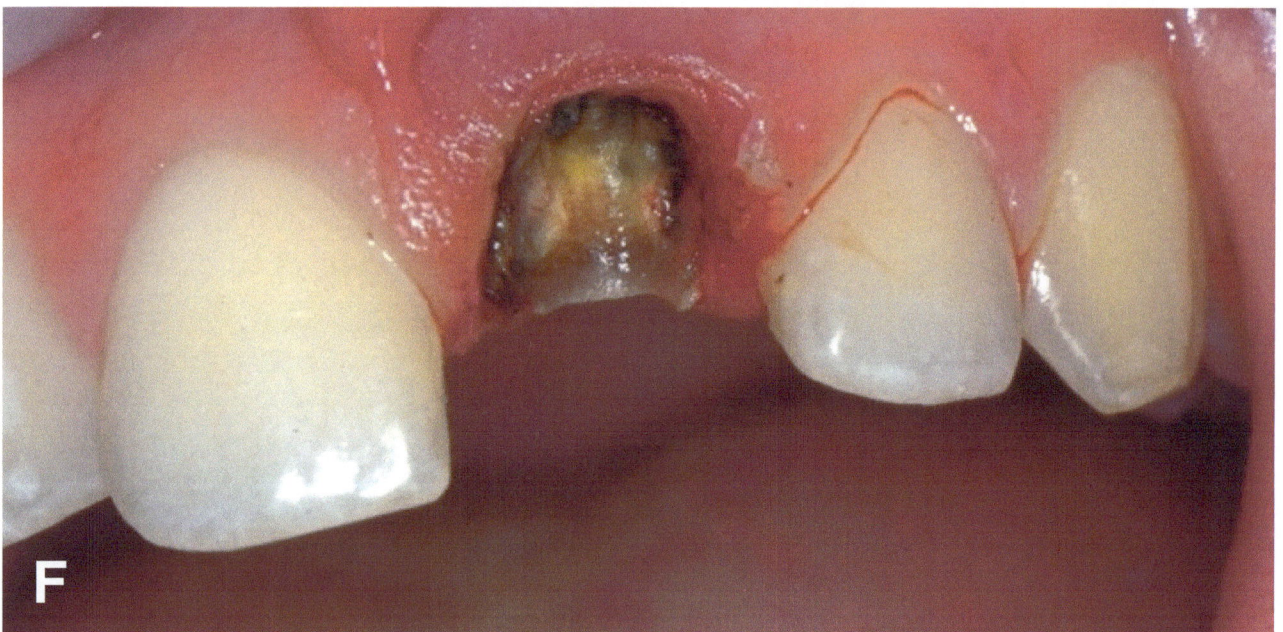

Electrosurgery was performed in order to gain access to the root (definitive periodontal surgery or orthodontic extrusion of this root may be beneficial in the future).

Restoring The Damaged Root   *(Continued)*

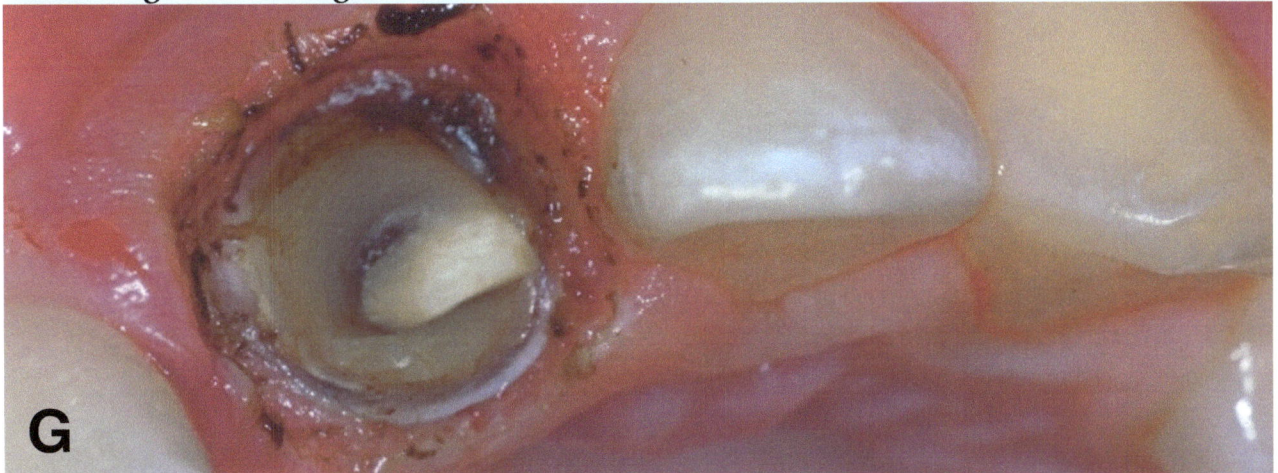

A carbon fiber post is bonded into the canal. A core material will be bonded to this post and remaining root structure.

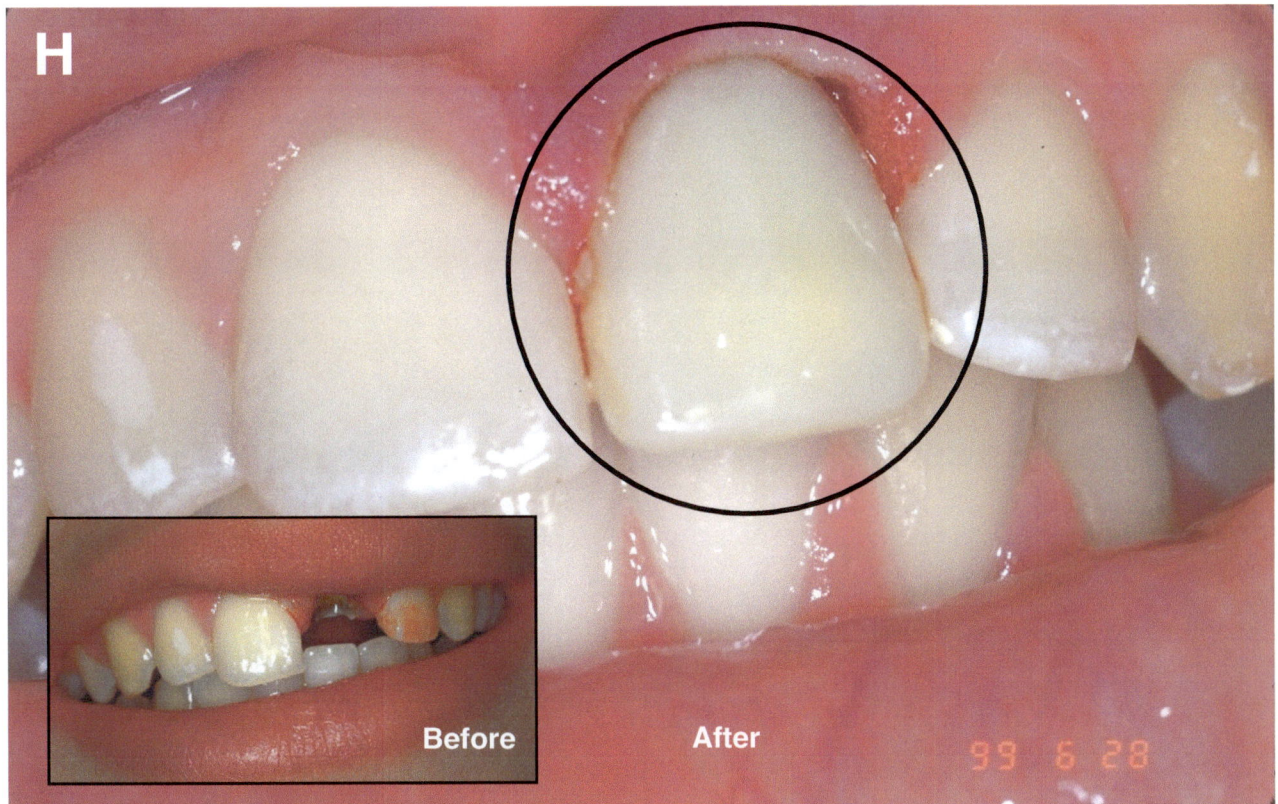

A temporary crown was fabricated and cemented onto the post and core.

A Failed Bridge

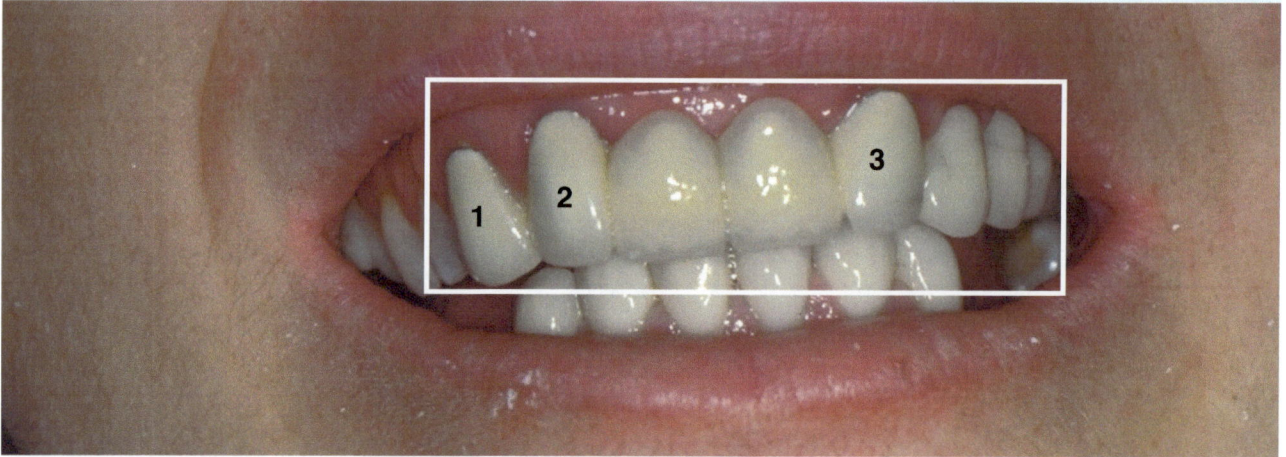

Poor aesthetics and improper fabrication. This defective bridge had open margins that allowed bacteria and debris to collect under the crowns. This resulted in recurrent decay, wash-out of the cement and dislodgment of the bridge.

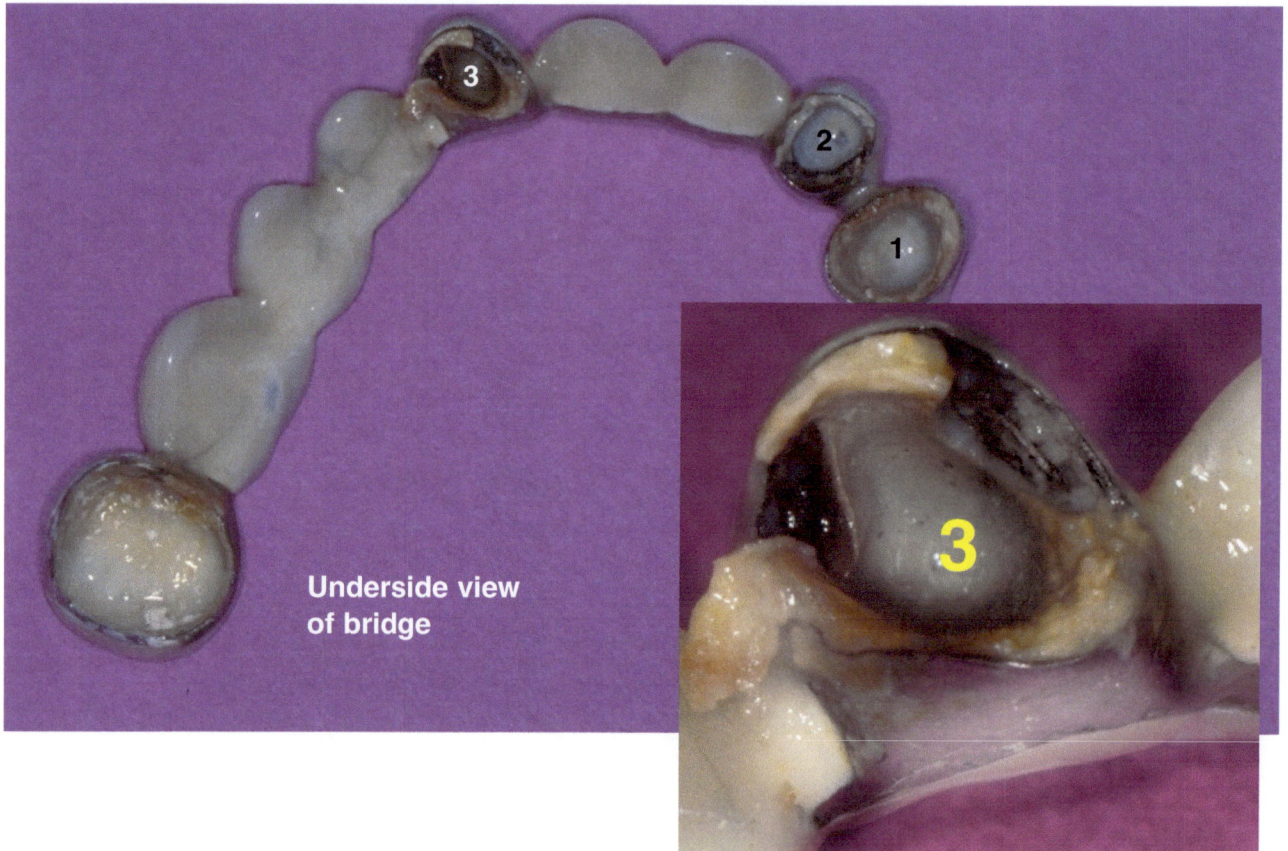

Underside view of bridge

Poorly Fabricated Crown Restoration

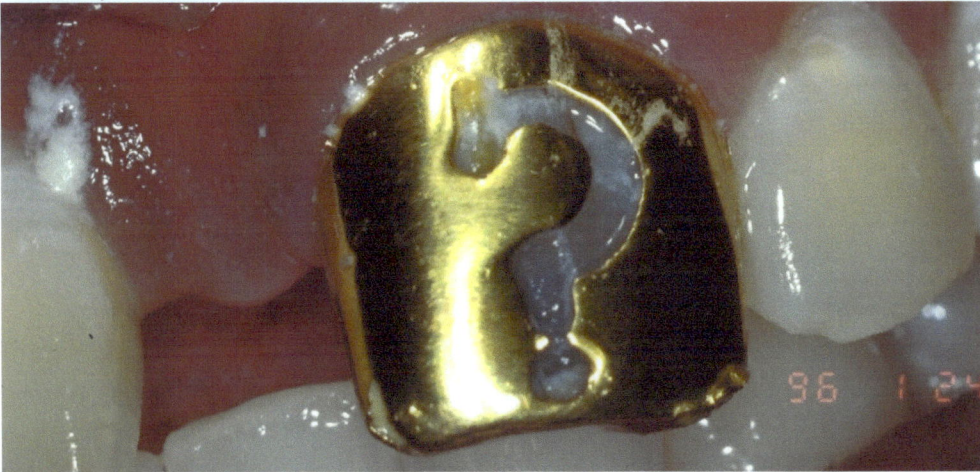

Though creative designs can be incorporated within a good crown, this is a blatant example of iatrogenics. A poorly fabricated crown restoration will cause damage to the tooth and gums, it is unacceptable and it is malpractice.

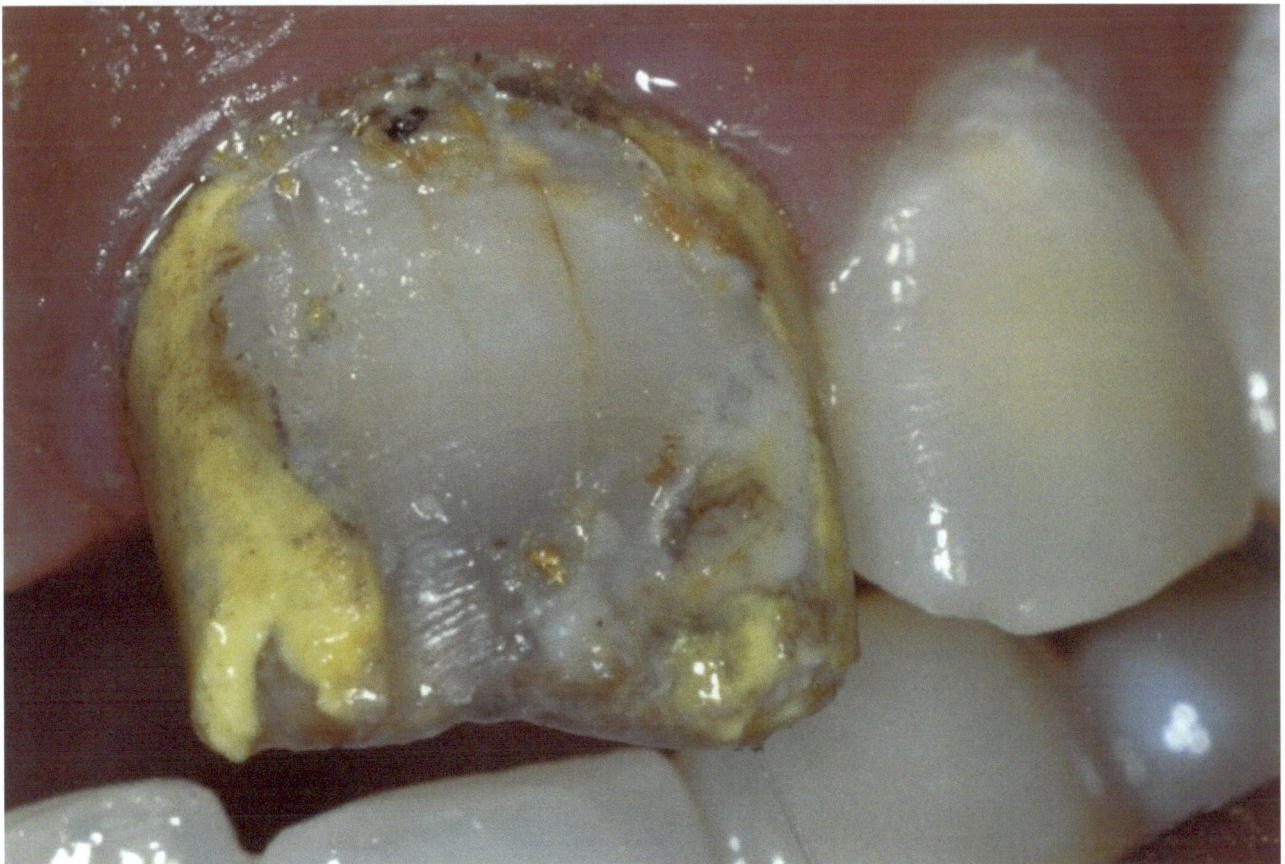

Upon removal of the crown a rotting tooth and inflamed gum tissue is apparent.

Poor vs Good Gold Crown

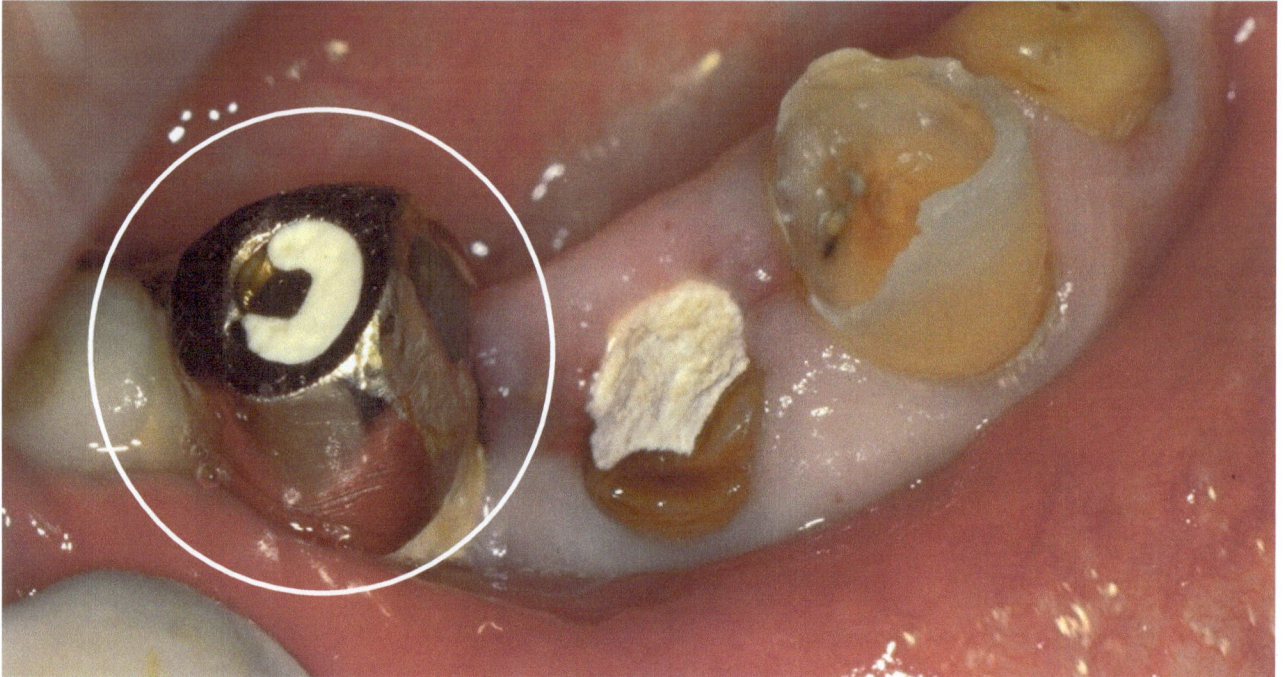

A deteriorating mouth with poor dental work. This crown lacks anatomy, has open margins and an occlusal (top portion of the crown) defect that has been patched with cement.

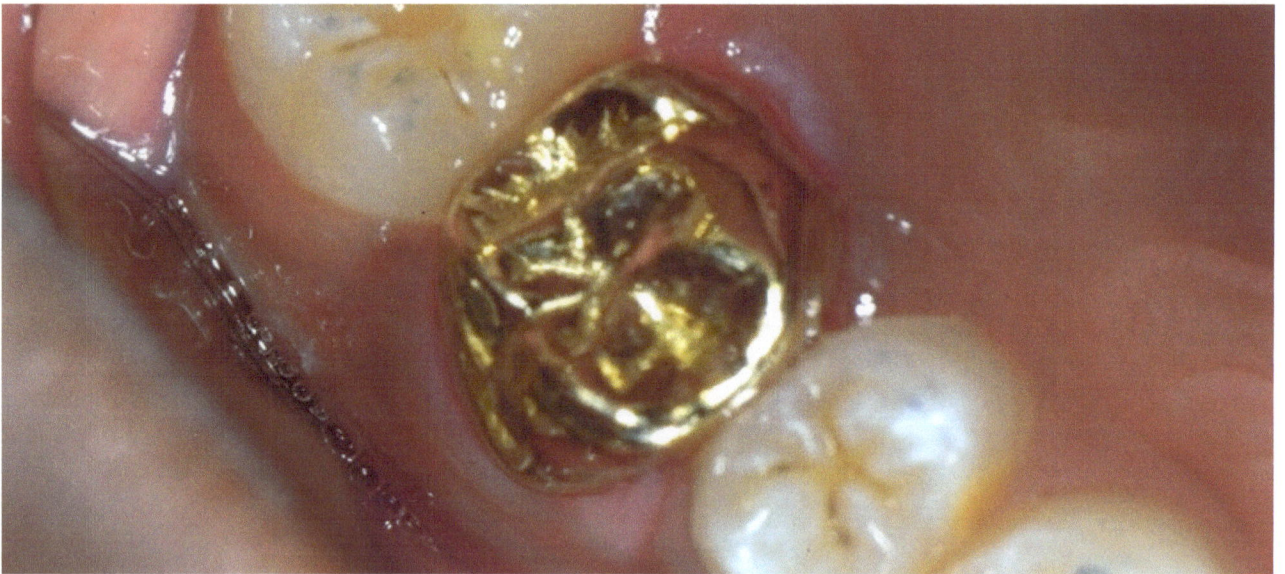

A good quality all gold crown that satisfies all requirements regarding form and function.

Root Canal Failure

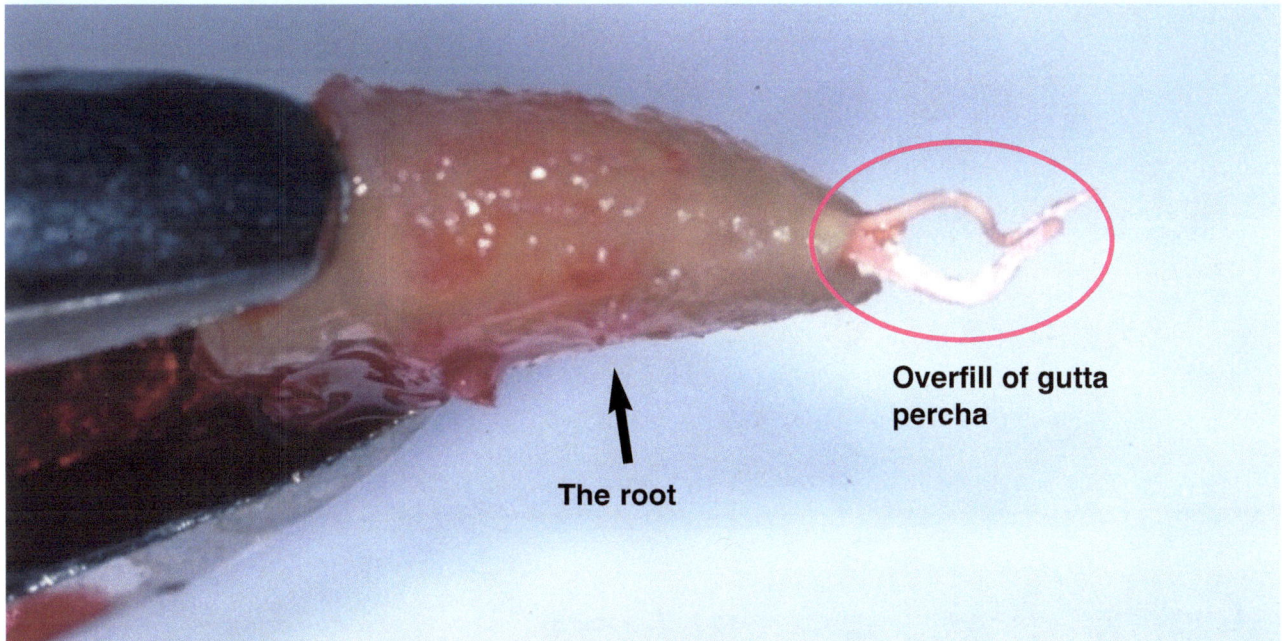

Overfill of gutta percha

The root

A failed root canal due to a poor seal at the end of the root (apex) and overfill of gutta percha.

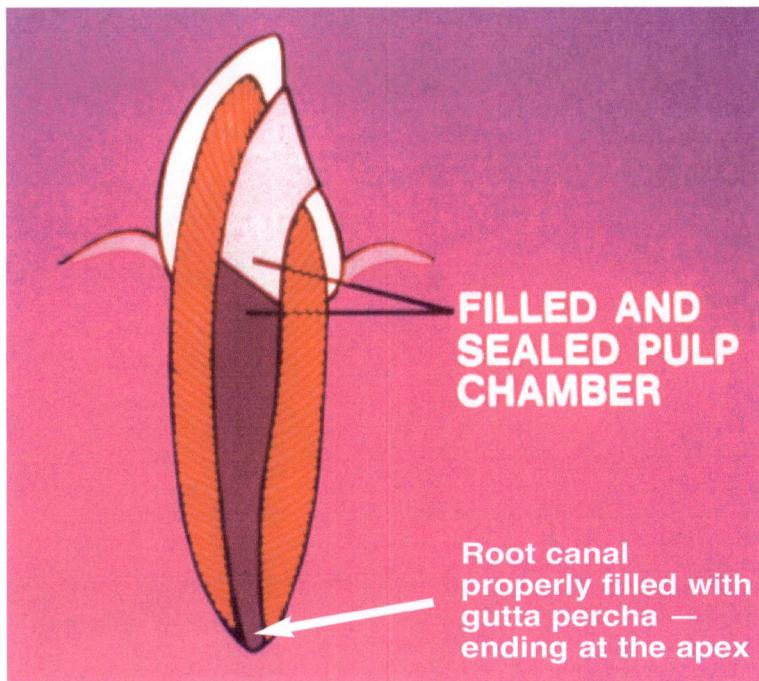

FILLED AND SEALED PULP CHAMBER

Root canal properly filled with gutta percha — ending at the apex

A Failed Bridge

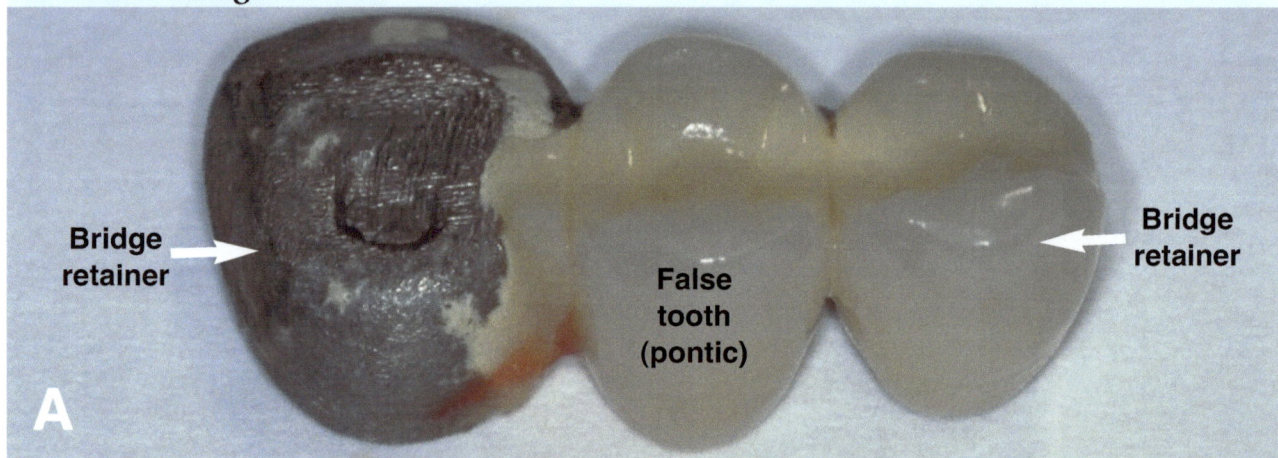

A dilemma regarding a porcelain fracture on a bridge. Strict attention to fabrication methods, utilization of better materials and proper bite adjustment could limit these types of situations. Patients also need to be careful when biting on very hard substances such as ice or bones.

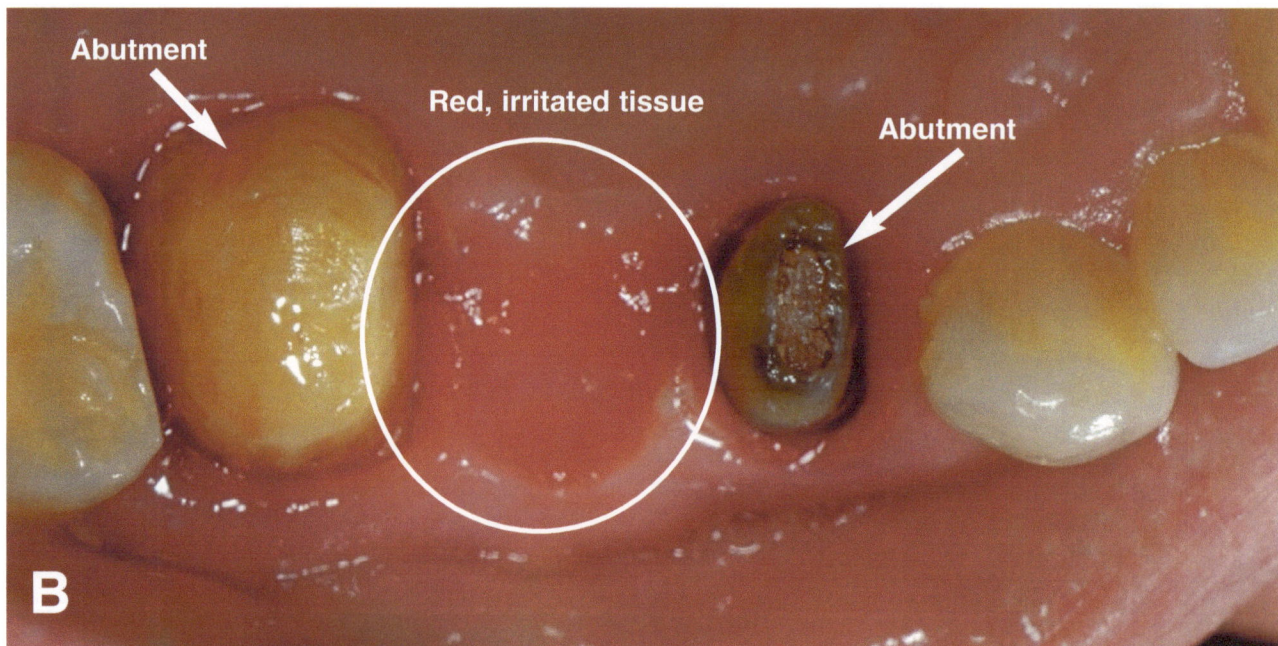

Obvious inflammation is present where the false tooth was sitting. Proper bridge design would have avoided this situation.

Patient's Responsibility — It is incumbent upon a patient to avoid habits that will damage prosthetic appliances. Even if properly constructed, damage can occur due to grinding habits or chewing on ice or other very hard materials.

Design Flaw In A Bridge Compromising Patient's Hygiene

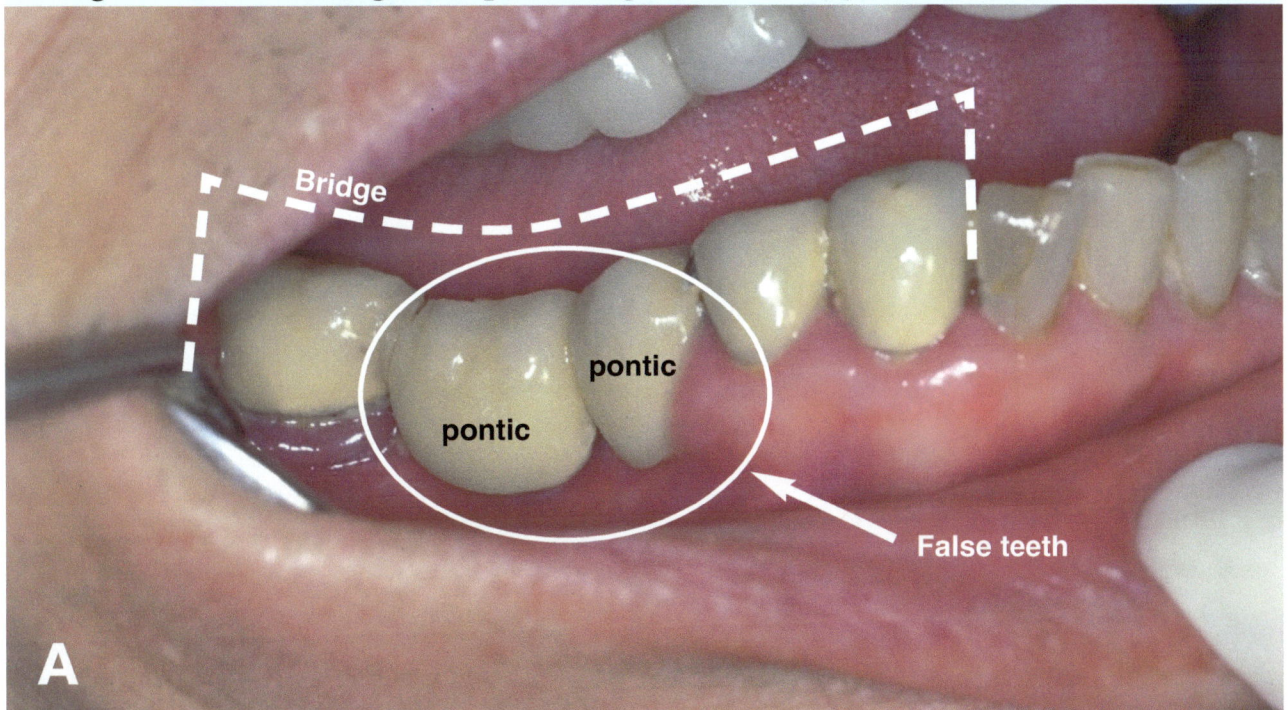

Another defective bridge. The false teeth are positioned in such a way that proper hygiene procedures are impossible to perform.

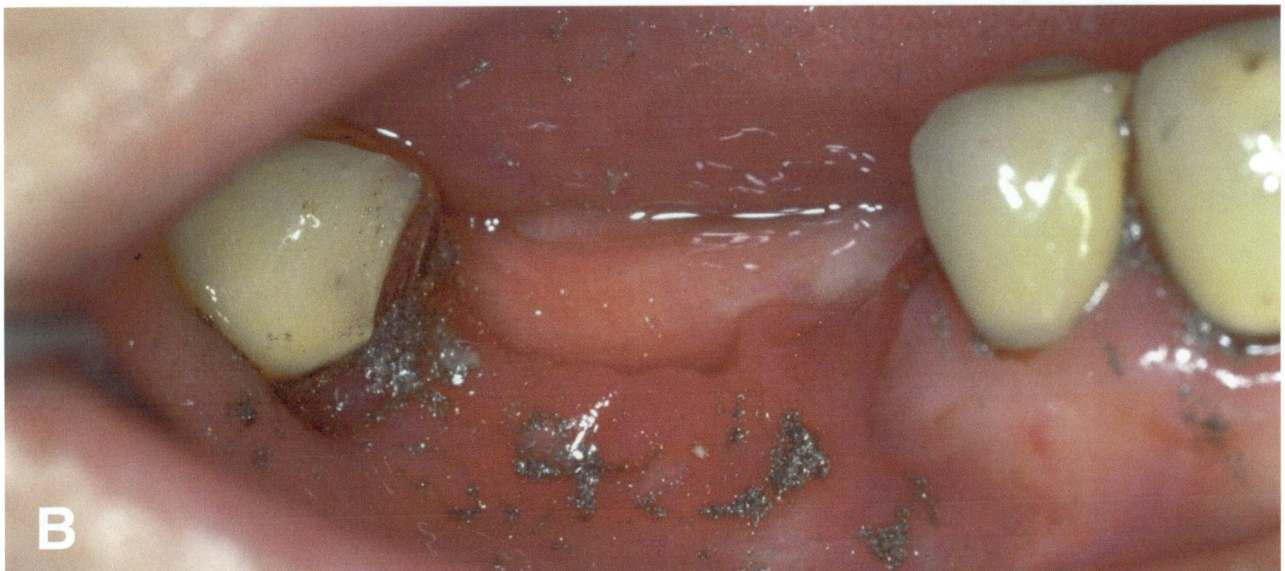

Following removal of the false teeth (pontics) from the bridge, soft tissue inflammation and damage is obvious.

Poor Crowns And Periodontal Disease

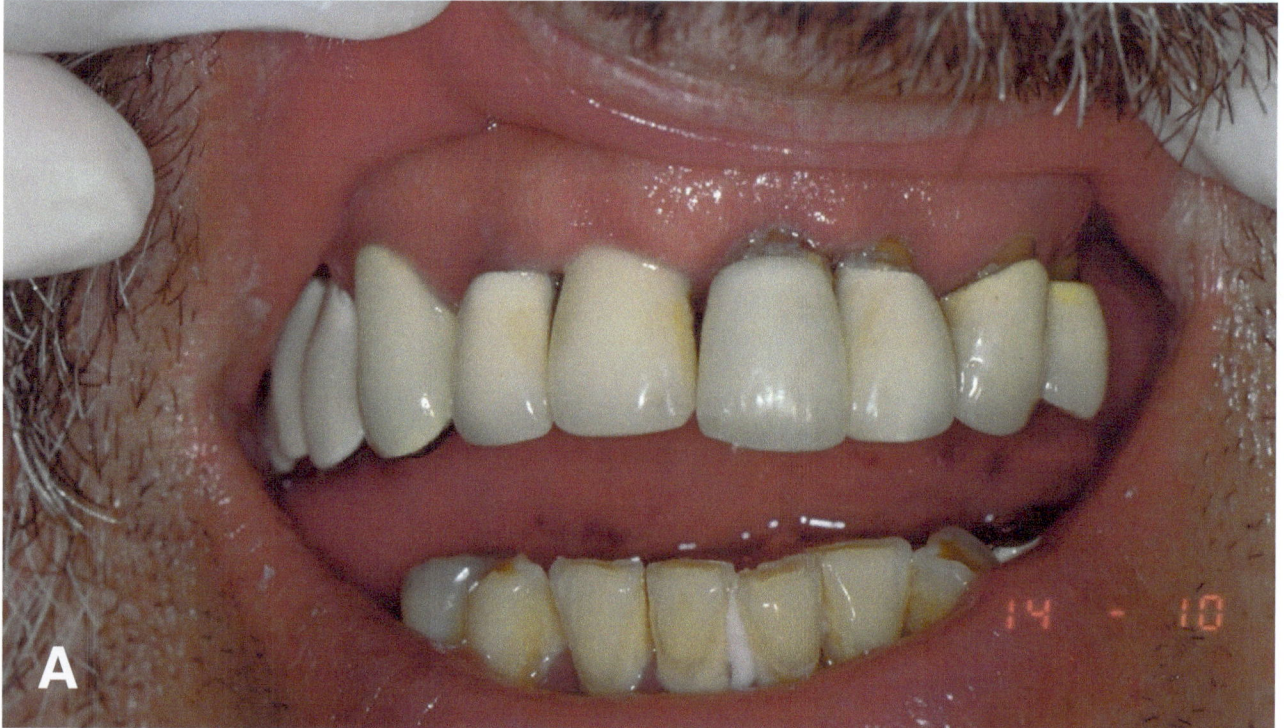

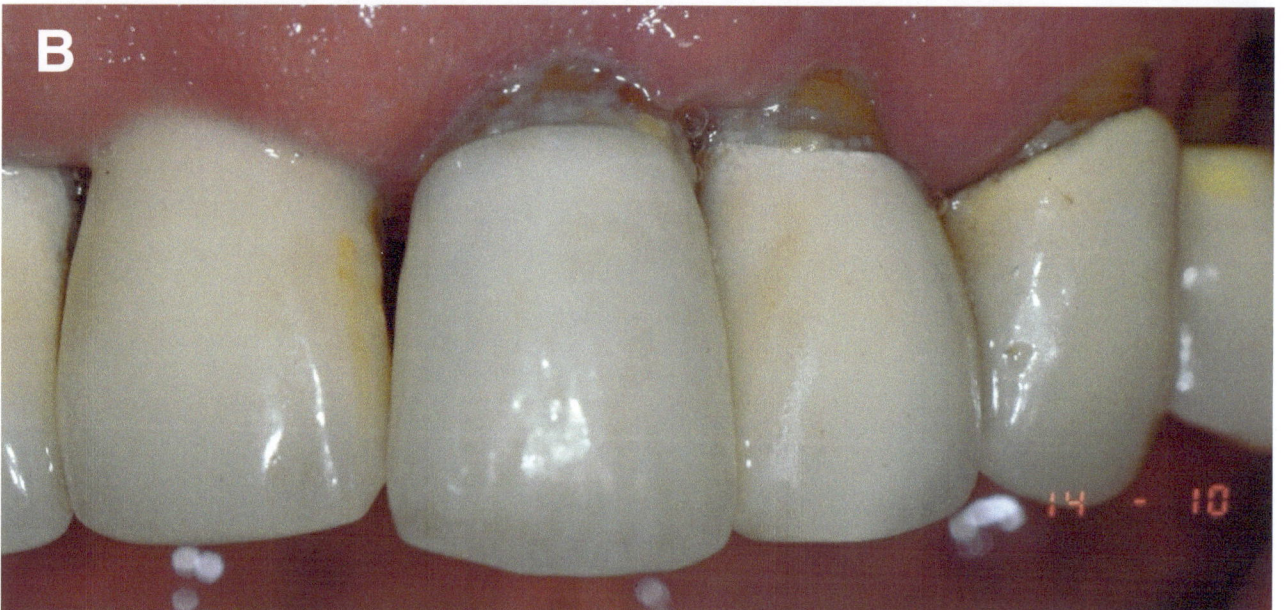

Poor quality crowns along with advanced periodontal deterioration. Healthy gum tissues are incompatible with bad restorative work.

Improper Shade Selection

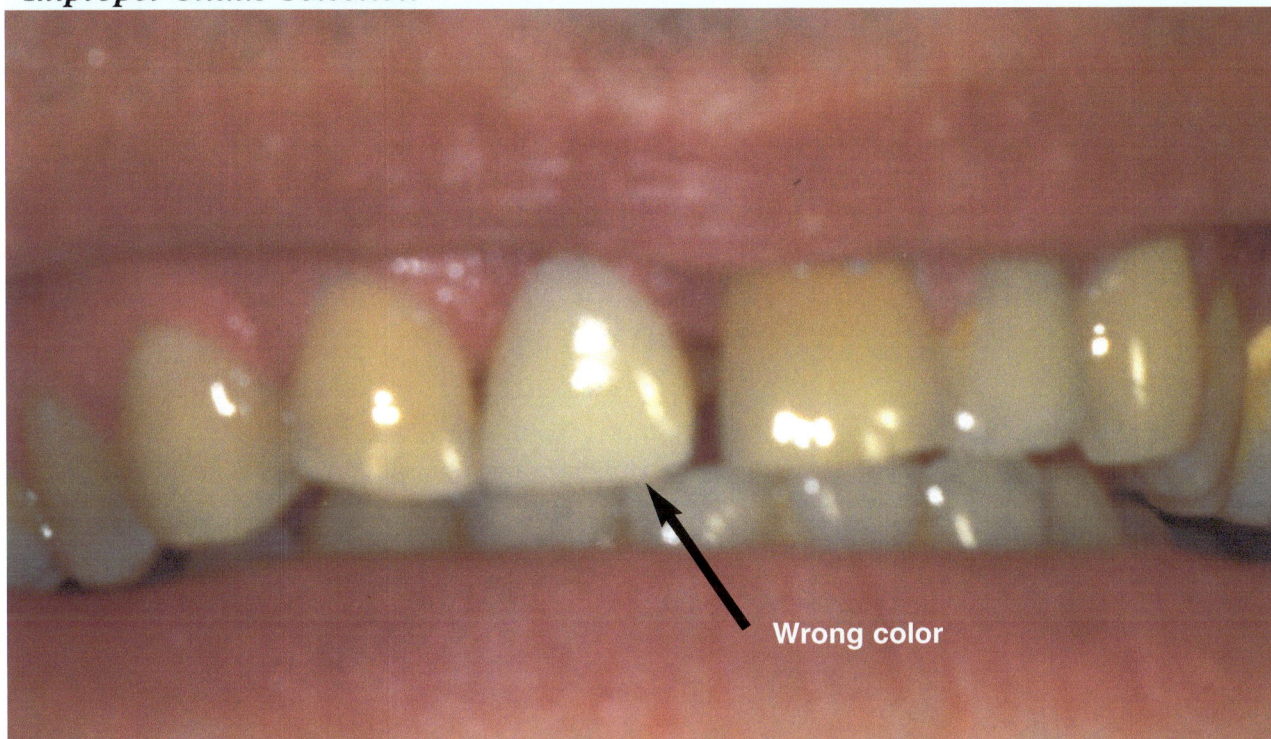

A one-tooth removable partial denture (flipper) with improper shade match.

Antibiotics

When I attended dental school in the early 70s, information about the subject of antibiotics was very limited. I believe this was due to the lack of specific clinical data on a per case basis. While I don't profess to be an expert in the area of pharmacology, I question the proper scientific clinical use of antibiotics. Antibiotics have been advocated in so many different ways and varying dosages that I suspect guesswork and perhaps, financial motives are an integral component of their use. With advances in computerized medical technology, combined with more specific blood or saliva tests, possibly a more rational understanding of the interplay between infection, the host immune system, and antibiotics will result.

The prophylactic use of antibiotics to prevent infection in certain patients is an important issue. Patients with a history of rheumatic fever, certain heart valve disfunctions, or having had some susceptible surgical procedures might benefit from administration of antibiotics prior to certain dental procedures. With the increased utilization of coronary stents, dentists and patients need to be informed regarding proper precautions. There is some evidence that prophylactic antibiotic administration would be beneficial to these patients within three months of stent implantation.

From the book "Coronary Stenting: Current Perspective" by Michael J. B. Kutryk, Patrick W. Serruys. Publisher: Martin Dunitz, Ltd. ©1999, London.

Vitamins and Minerals

The use of vitamins and minerals is an area of "therapeutics" that remains elusive in terms of specific clinical scientific per-case data. Again, my dental school curriculum (and I attended a first-rate dental school — University of Maryland, Baltimore College of Dental Surgery — the *first* dental school of the world) was practically non-existent in this area. There is so much money involved in selling vitamins and minerals that experts can be bought, brainwashed, and used forever. I have made diligent efforts to research this field and I am convinced that, unless specific dosages and requirements are established for individuals and specific results are monitored, the "success" of vitamin and mineral therapy will remain elusive.

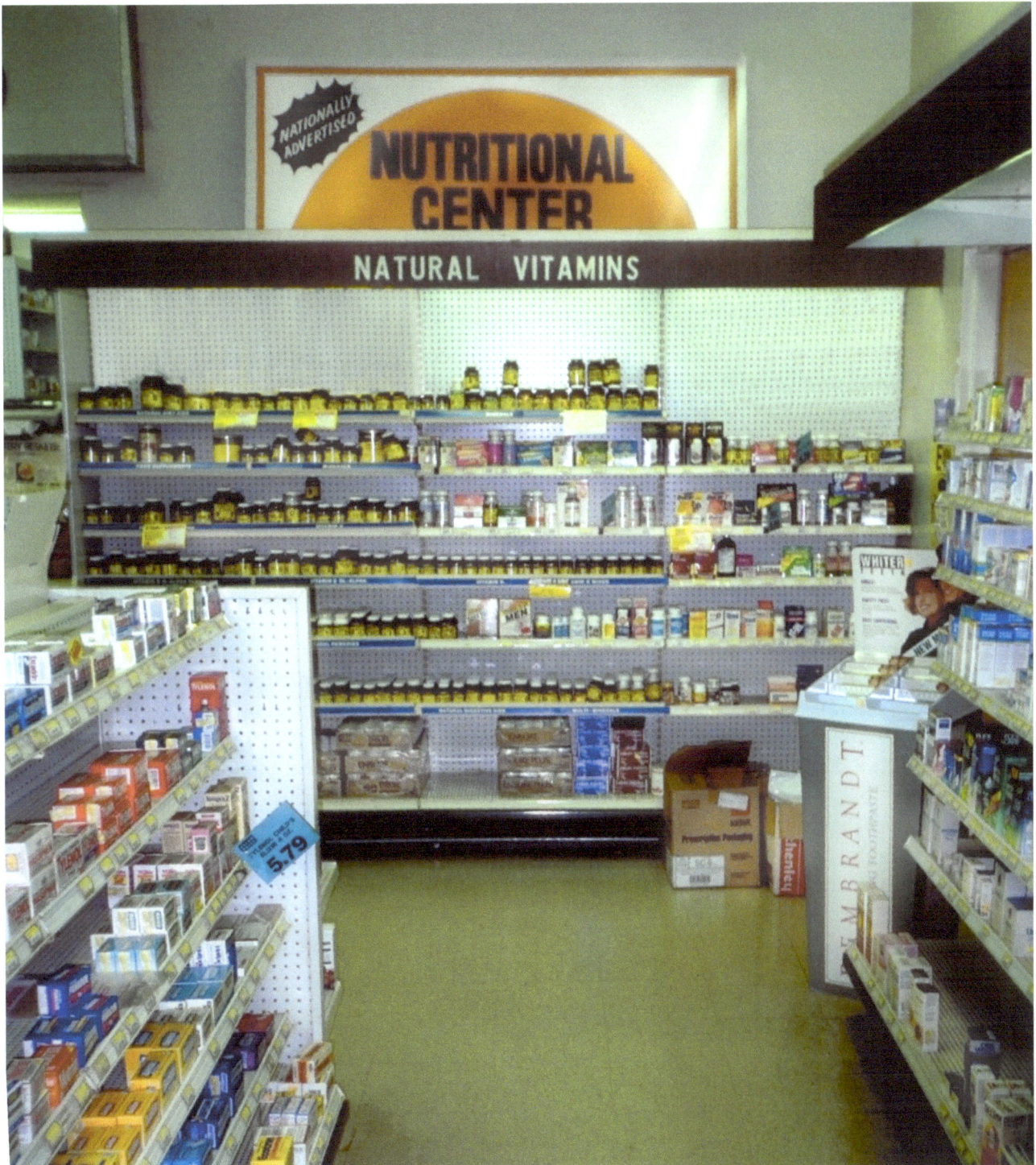

THE FUTURE

Having years of experience and a rather analytical mind, I can make some basic assumptions concerning the future of dentistry.[32]

Dental restorative materials will continue to improve in the near future; research in genetic engineering, however, will provide more natural replacements. Dentistry will become more integrated with medicine in terms of the understanding of the nature of disease and its relationship to a person's physiology and environmental influences.

In terms of prevention, a system will be designed so patients can gain a realistic appraisal of their future medical/dental profile from an early age. The objective is to evaluate needs early on so that prevention and conservative therapy will be much more effective.

Eliminating substandard dental treatment (that seems to exist to a great extent due to financial duress among some "desperate" practitioners and insurance providers) will be difficult without an educational program that explains the difference between poor, average, and legitimately superior treatment. Even then, who will pay for superior treatment? For the time being, the unchanged constant is that most people still dislike visiting the dentist—myself included.

Gene therapy — here's the key to the future! As we age, systems deteriorate, and essential chemicals necessary for normal physiology decrease and may stop being produced. Since the total system is dependent on proper dosages of millions of intricate chemical reactions, an overall diminishing capacity eventually cascades into death. The twentieth century has seen explosive progress in our understanding of the human body. Computer technology has incorporated this understanding into a vast complex data base that, if properly programmed, will help organize a better understanding of the interrelationships that constitute exactly how the body functions and ages.

Genes are the blueprints by which proteins and all vital chemical mediators are produced. Analysis of the aging process and subsequent chemical deficiencies will lead to specific gene therapy replacement.

The question is, how will we adapt to this possible "cure" for aging? I was taught in college that scientific advancements precede social acclamation by about forty years,[33] so there is a lot of time for people to adjust their thinking.

The ability to enjoy life may be somewhat enhanced by the optimistic predictions of an advanced society. However, basic needs and desires can't wait for a rosy future. Most of the information in this book is presented to educate, and therefore, hopefully make people aware of their dental health. In reality, however, trips to the dentist are inconvenient and many times costly. I have always thought it would be nice if convenient and inexpensive therapies were available that would allow for extended longevity in a totally healthy state. What is the benefit if sophisticated treatment meth-

32. Although I wish I had a crystal ball. That way, when I go to the races on Saturday, I'd always have winners! (How boring.)
33. I'm not sure where I read this or if this is the exact wording, and the meaning is broad in scope; however, the general idea seems valid.

ods exist or will exist if the price paid both in time and expense is prohibitive and very stressful in itself? Hopefully, future therapies will address themselves to this practical dilemma, but in the interim some sacrifice is necessary to achieve superior results.

Questions about happiness and the adaptability of humans to an increased life span intrigue me. If, in the Jewish religion, a boy reaches manhood in his 13th year (a Bar Mitzvah) in a time where life spans may increase tremendously, should some sort of adjustment be made so the enjoyment of a longer childhood can be sustained? How will teenagers adapt to the realization that the future may allow them to be around for a very long time?[34] Will college years be increased, and how will people plan their futures and pace themselves? If the ultimate goal of good medicine is to provide physical health and the elimination of death, then is the ultimate goal of emotional health predicated on finding Utopia? Now there's a great question. It is probably the basic idea behind alco-

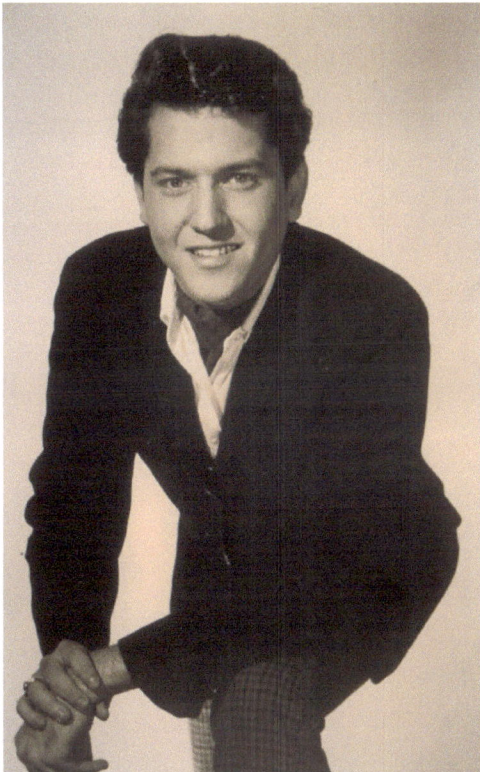

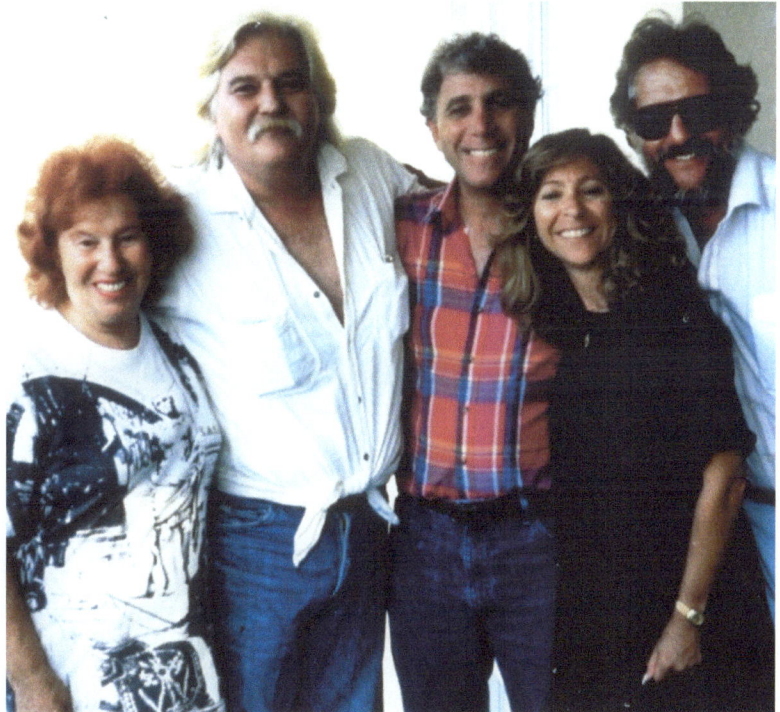

Jimmy Miller surrounded by our family. Left to right: Mom, Jimmy, me, my sister Jodie and her husband Jerry.

My rock producer cousin Jimmy Miller. An early photo of Jimmy during his beginning years in show business as a singer/performer. He eventually moved to England where he became an integral part of the 70's and 80's music scene. Considered one of the greatest groove producers ever, his credits include the sole album by Blind Faith, the single "Gimme some lovin'", albums for the Rolling Stones from 1968 –1973, and much more. Jimmy died prematurely at age 52 – a Rock and Roll lifestyle.

---

34. It most likely won't make too much difference because, as most children can't comprehend death in their future, most teenagers are more interested in fun and adventure in the present.

hol or drug abuse—after all, achieving a euphoric state is easy under the influence of some drugs, but Utopia—a carefree, eternal existence—is somewhat more complex! Of course, the euphoric high of drugs is temporary and paid for with emotional and physical damage, if not death, but all pleasures and happiness are obviously not contingent on drugs. There's love, appreciation of natural beauty, watching children play and grow, and the satisfaction of doing good deeds and helping other people. If medicine can keep us healthy for a longer time, then perhaps we would all be able to perform more good deeds. Or maybe this optimistic outlook is flawed due to the inexact nature of human beings. I just don't know. After all, I'm only a dentist. As a fellow human being, I have natural flaws and a limited vision. It's more comfortable to live with what we know and understand than to contemplate an unknown future.

At the beginning of this book, I wrote that its success would hopefully bring me more money, which I imagine will make my future more enjoyable. The benefits you receive from this book, whether as a patient or student of the health sciences, will hopefully enhance your future too, and maybe this idea of mutual success is the key to happiness. The puzzle of living may never really be solved, but the endless challenges make the journey worthwhile, and extending the game is a natural consequence of our knowledge.

*****

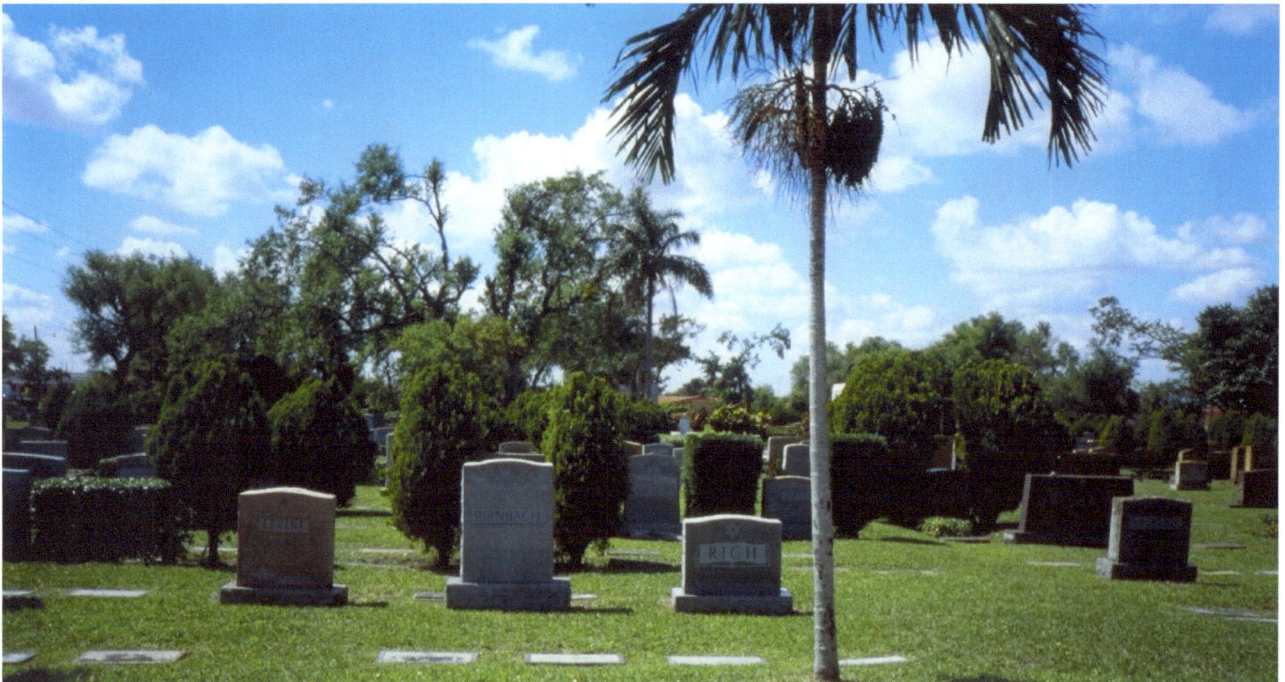

The End... as we know it today.

Postscript

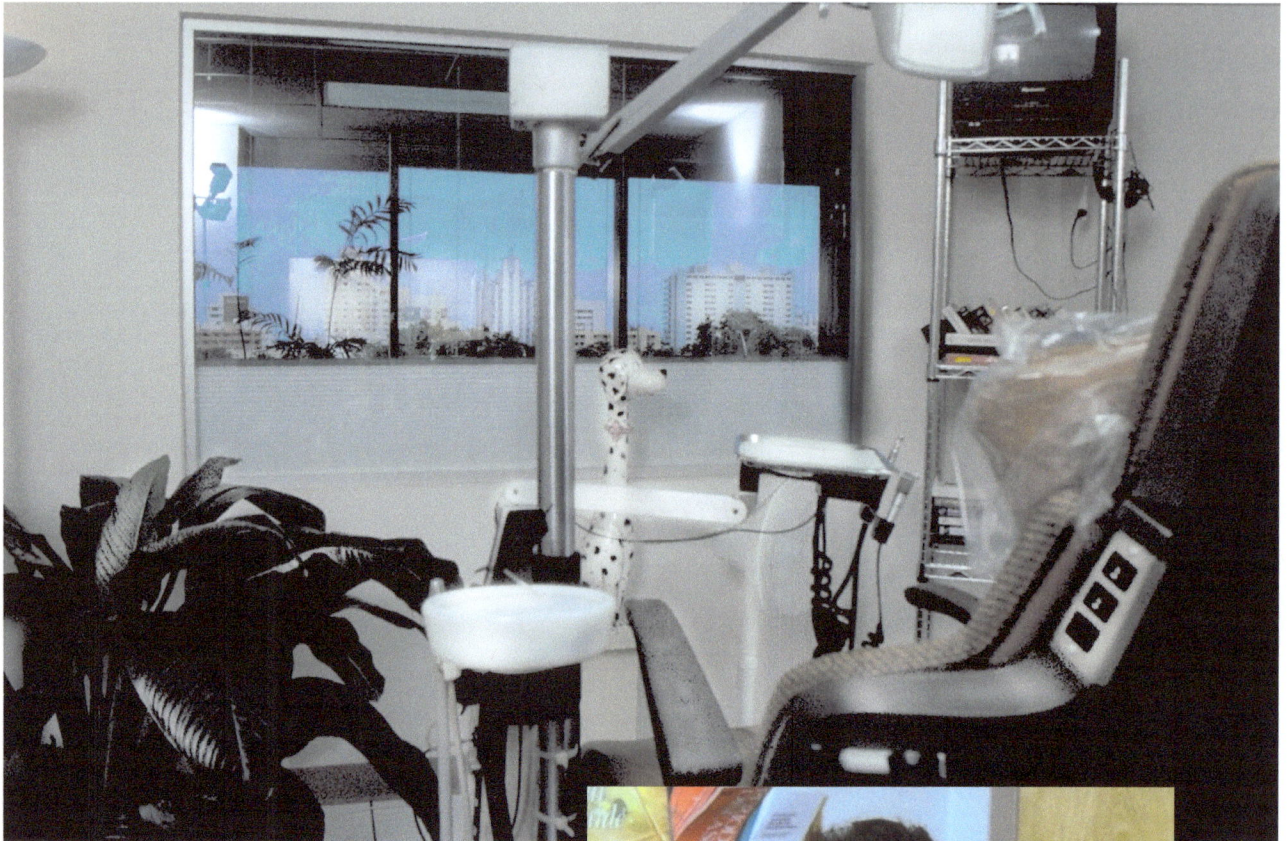

Room with a view — my office.

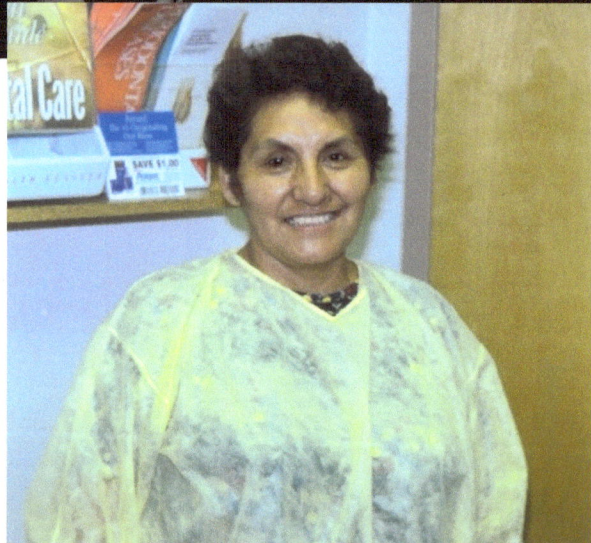

My indispensable dental assistant/office manager Nerida Di Pietro

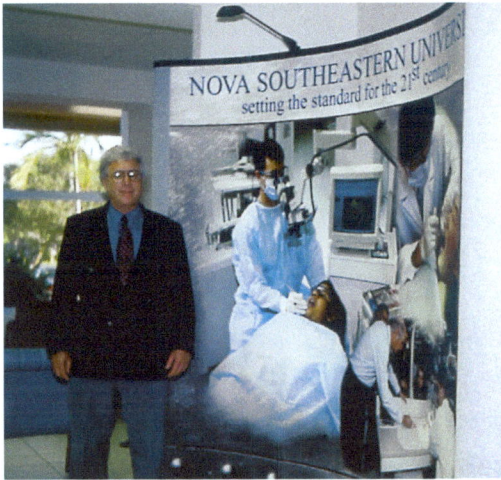

My visit to Nova Southeastern College of Dental Medicine was exciting. This new dental facility exemplifies the advanced state of dental education.

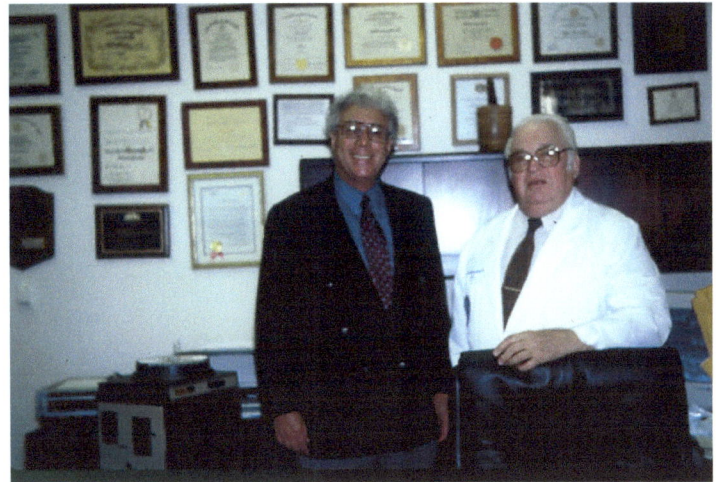

Dr. Seymour Oliet (right), a professor emeritus and former dean of the University of Pennsylvania's School of Dental Medicine. Dr. Oliet is the dean of Nova Southeastern College of Dental Medicine.

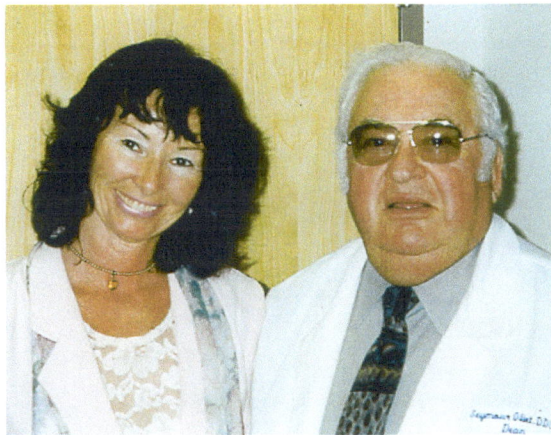

Ann Page, assistant to the dean.

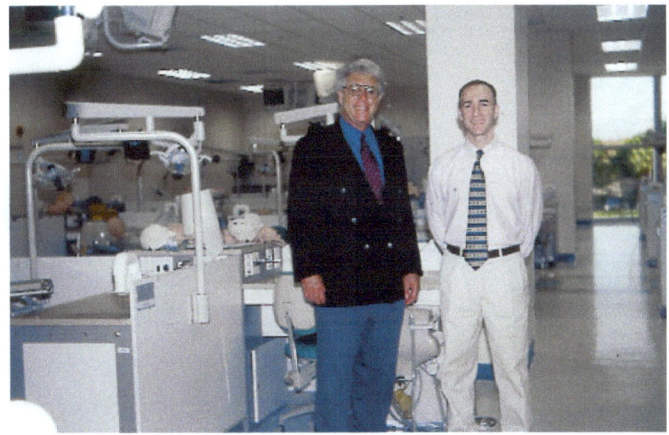

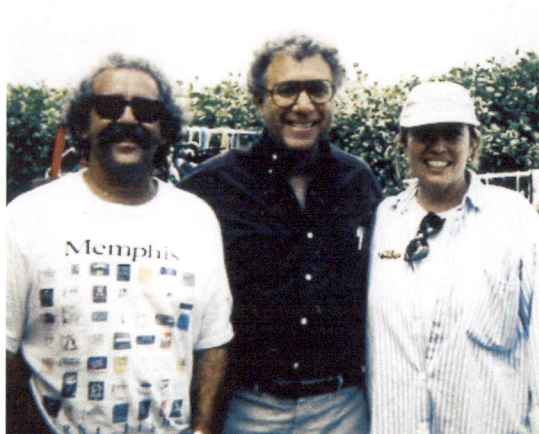

Good friends June and Danny Vargas have provided needed encouragement and lots of laughs over the years. (Me in the middle).

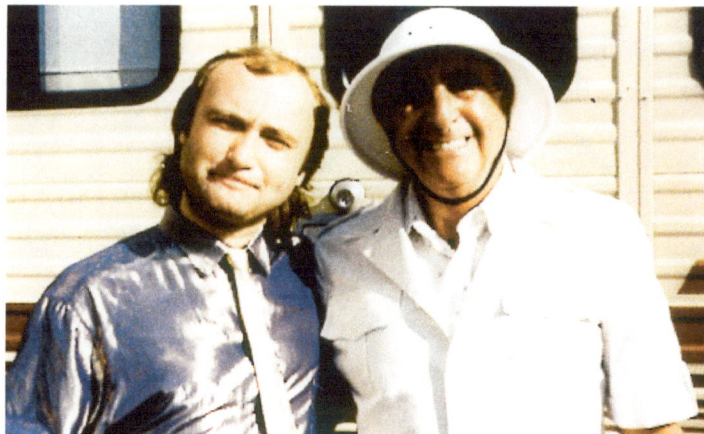

My actor father Abbey Vine (r) next to Phil Collins on the set of a production in South Florida. My dad's outstanding role was in the movie "The Bodyguard" where he played the owner of the Fontainebleau Hilton Hotel in a scene with Whitney Houston and Kevin Costner.

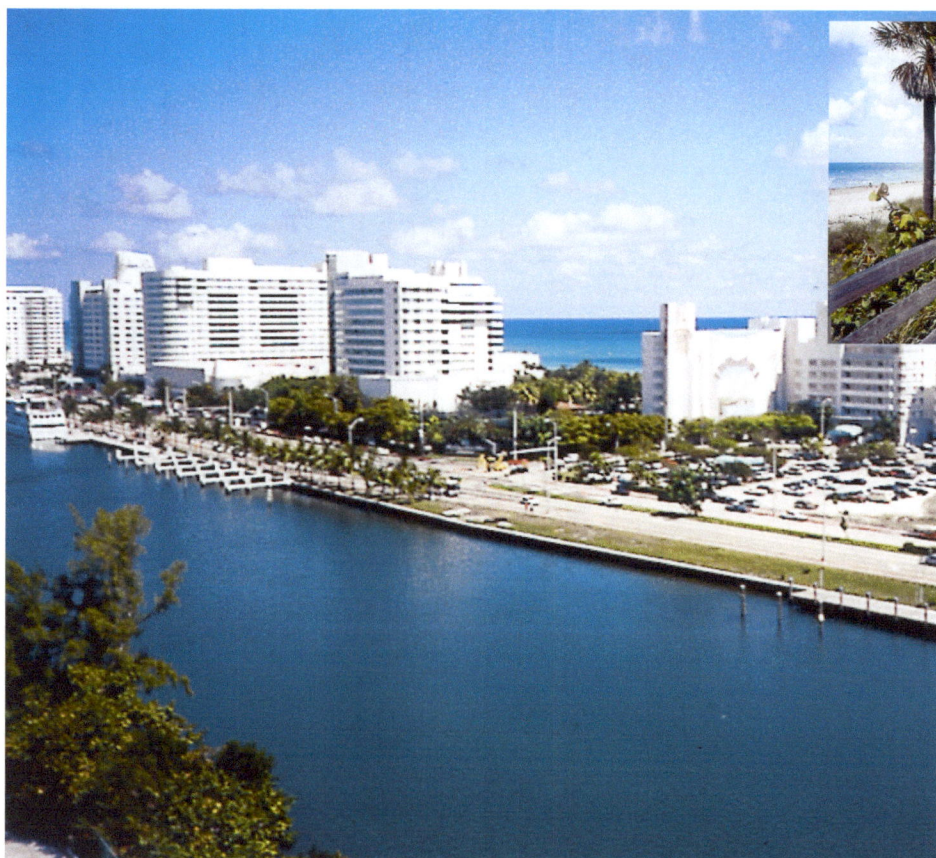

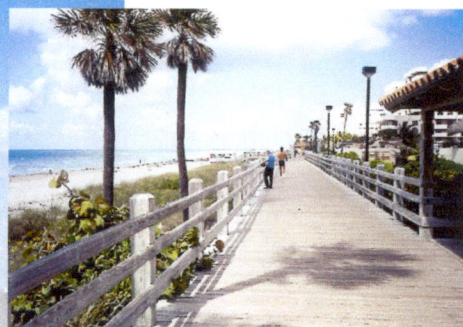

My exercise pathway adjacent to the beautiful blue waters of the Atlantic.

View from my balcony overlooking the Fontainebleau Hilton.

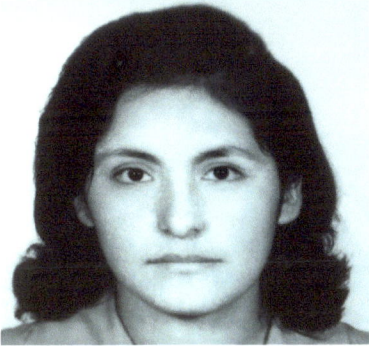

Nerida Di Pietro

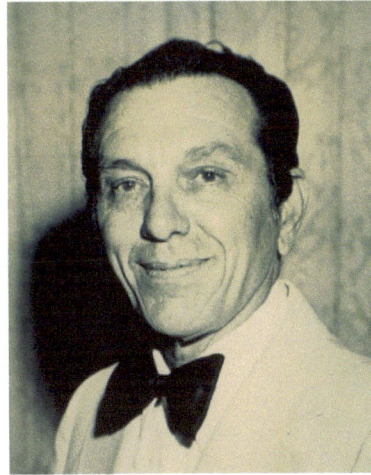

Gino (Louis) Di Pietro — Nerida's very talented husband. Not only did he manage some of the most exclusive night spots in New York, the Bahamas and Miami, but wrote the most romantic ballads I've ever heard.

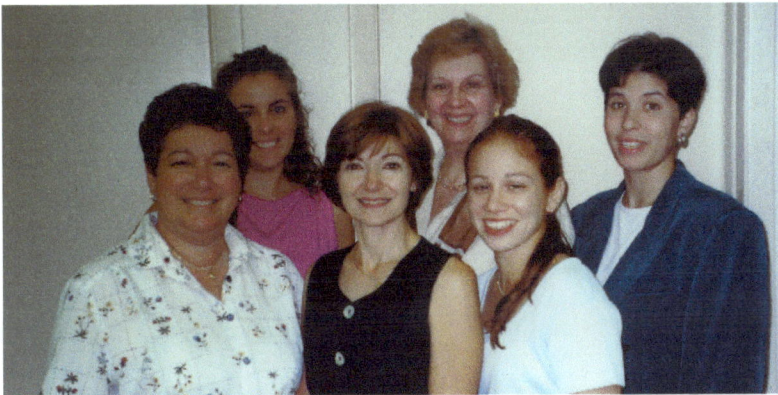

Coral Gables Secretarial Services – First row, left to right: Marcia Brod, Maria Ingelmo, Amanda Barba
Second row, left to right: Ellen Roden, Nancy Morgan (president), Vickie Sfalanga.

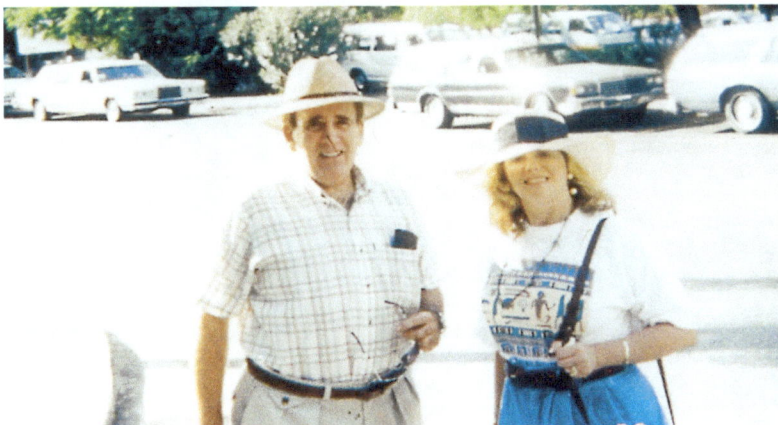

Michele Applebaum with brother Dr. Donald Applebaum, Miami Beach cardiologist.

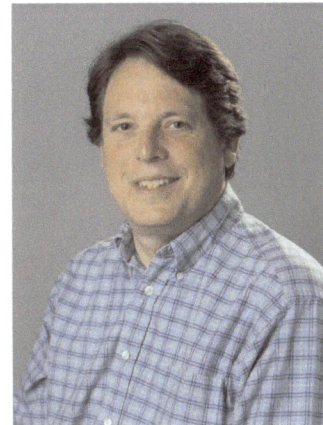

Leonardo Borsten, president of PrePress Consolidated Color, Inc., Miami, Florida. His persistence, talent and desire for excellence in graphic design helped make this book a reality.

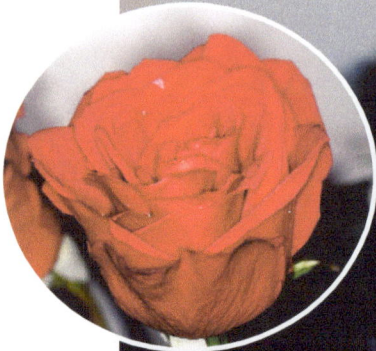

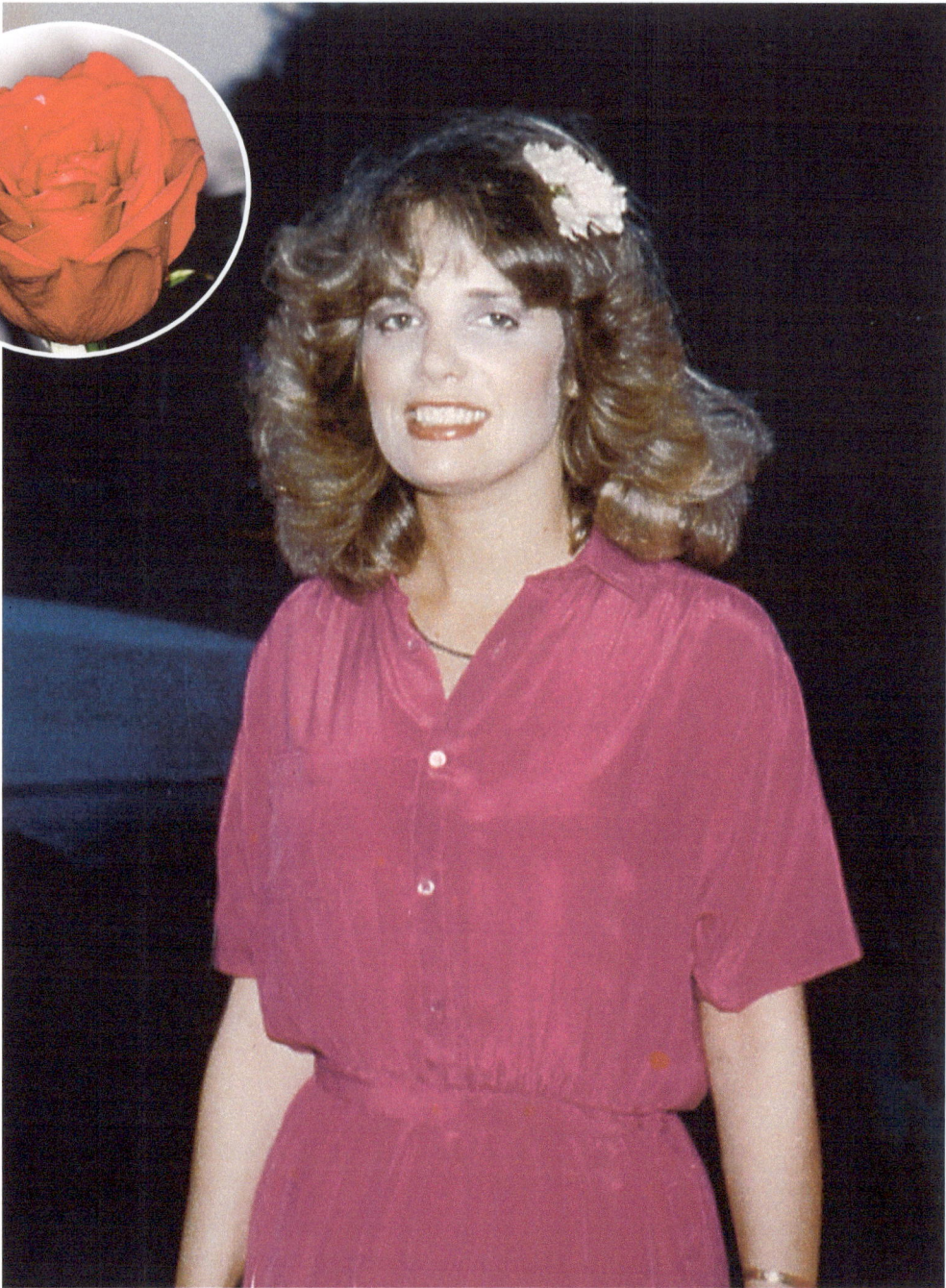

Michele Beth Applebaum

INDEX

You can order this book as a gift for people you care about.

Share the knowledge with students, friends and relatives.

Single copies are $49.00. Discounts are available for bulk orders by Educational Institutions, writing and publishing organizations and industry publications.

Call 1-800-328-5119
or
Fax to 305-538-1129
or
e-mail to dvine@davidvinedentist.com

Give name, address, telephone number,
major credit card number with expiration date
or
send check or money order made out to Dr. David Vine, mail to:

David Vine, D.D.S.
400 Arthur Godfrey Road
Suite 403
Miami Beach, FL 33140

Most U.S.A. orders will be delivered within 7 days.